The pH Balance Health & Diet Guide for GERD, IBS & IBD

Practical Solutions, Diet Management + 175 Recipes

Dr. Fraser Smith, BA, ND
Susan Hannah, BA, BScH
Dr. Daniel Richardson, BS, MSc, PhD

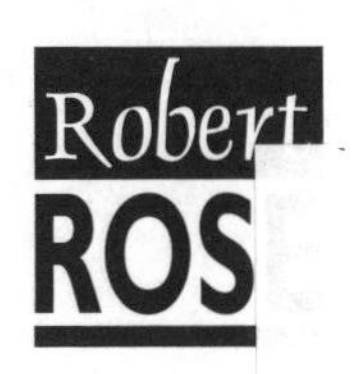

For complete cataloguing information, see page 398.

Disclaimer
This book is a general guide only and should never be a substitute for the skill, knowledge and experience of a qualified medical professional dealing with the facts, circumstances and symptoms of a particular case.

The nutritional, medical and health information presented in this book is based on the research, training and professional experience of the authors, and is true and complete to the best of their knowledge. However, this book is intended only as an informative guide for those wishing to know more about health, nutrition and medicine; it is not intended to replace or countermand the advice given by the reader's personal physician. Because each person and situation is unique, the authors and the publisher urge the reader to check with a qualified health-care professional before using any procedure where there is a question as to its appropriateness. A physician should be consulted before beginning any exercise program. The authors and the publisher are not responsible for any adverse effects or consequences resulting from the use of the information in this book. It is the responsibility of the reader to consult a physician or other qualified health-care professional regarding his or her personal care.

This book contains references to products that may not be available everywhere. The intent of the information provided is to be helpful; however, there is no guarantee of results associated with the information provided. Use of brand names is for educational purposes only and does not imply endorsement.

The recipes in this book have been carefully tested by our kitchen and our tasters. To the best of our knowledge, they are safe and nutritious for ordinary use and users. For those people with food or other allergies, or who have special food requirements or health issues, please read the suggested contents of each recipe carefully and determine whether or not they may create a problem for you. All recipes are used at the risk of the consumer. We cannot be responsible for any hazards, loss or damage that may occur as a result of any recipe use. For those with special needs, allergies, requirements or health problems, in the event of any doubt, please contact your medical adviser prior to the use of any recipe.

Design and Production: Daniella Zanchetta/PageWave Graphics Inc.
Editors: Bob Hilderley, Senior Editor, Health; and Sue Sumeraj, Recipes
Nutrient analysis: Magda Fahmy
Copy editor: Sheila Wawanash
Proofreader: Kelly Jones
Indexer: Gillian Watts
Illustrations: Kveta/threeinabox.com
Periodic Table (p. 22) © iStockphoto.com/Peter Hermes Furian

The publisher gratefully acknowledges the financial support of our publishing program by the Government of Canada through the Canada Book Fund.

Published by Robert Rose Inc.
120 Eglinton Avenue East, Suite 800, Toronto, Ontario, Canada M4P 1E2
Tel: (416) 322-6552 Fax: (416) 322-6936
www.robertrose.ca

Printed and bound in Canada

1 2 3 4 5 6 7 8 9 FP 22 21 20 19 18 17 16 15 14

This book is dedicated to:

FS: My wife, Debra, who has been so supportive of all my writing projects and endeavors, and has encouraged me to keep going, rain or shine.

SH: Those who suffer from gastrointestinal conditions, with the hope that the information provided here will improve your health and quality of life. I also thank my dear friend Sue Price for supporting all of my creative efforts, but especially my writing. And Dr. Shehab El-Hashemy, MBChB, ND, an integrative naturopathic physician and medical doctor at the Canadian College of Naturopathic Medicine, for permission to adapt material from *Family Medicine & Integrative Primary Care: Standards & Guidelines* (2011), pages 133–35.

DR: My great friend and colleague, Professor Joyce Whitehead. Joyce is the Director of the Learning Resource Center at National University of Health Sciences and as such has tirelessly and enthusiastically supported all of my work and the scholarly activity of the entire faculty at our university. Thank you, Joyce, for your many years of friendship and support.

Contents

Part 4: Meal Plans for the pH Balance Diet Program

Part 5: Recipes for the pH Balance Diet Program

Introduction

The World Health Organization (WHO) has defined good health as "a state of complete physical, mental and social well-being and not merely the absence of disease or infirmity." One way of achieving this state of well-being is to adopt a healthy lifestyle, particularly a healthy diet.

At some time in your life, you will likely resolve to go on a diet, typically to lose excess weight but also to improve your health. These healthy diets include gluten-free, lactose-free and allergen-free diets, as well as the DASH (Dietary Approaches to Stop Hypertension) diet, Mediterranean diet, rotation diet, elemental diet, elimination diet and more. The acid–alkaline balanced diet, also known as the pH-balanced diet, is thought to be preventive and therapeutic for a wide spectrum of conditions.

The pH-balanced diet restores the body to a state of homeostasis, or equilibrium, after it has been disrupted or unbalanced by pathogens (bacteria and viruses) and poor lifestyle habits. When we are in a balanced acid–alkaline state, we experience increased vitality, but in an unbalanced state, we experience low energy and fatigue. In this state of ill health, our bodies are more vulnerable to diseases, notably impaired digestion, arthritis, cardiovascular problems and kidney disease.

Fortunately, a pH-balanced diet is not all that difficult to restore and maintain. Despite the somewhat complicated chemistry involved in pH measurements, the diet itself requires only eyeball measurements of servings. For restoring pH balance, aim to eat a ratio of 80% alkalizing to 20% acidifying foods; for maintenance, aim to eat 60% alkalizing to 40% acidifying foods. For some people, this can be quite a leap — the average ratio today is 1 to 10 alkaline to acid. The so-called Western diet, high in red meat and fats, is highly acid–alkaline unbalanced. This imbalanced state is known as acidosis (or alkalosis, which is rare).

The food that we eat every day has some impact on our pH, or acid–alkaline, balance. Eating a diet that is deficient in alkaline-producing fruits and vegetables and high in acid-producing sulfur, processed foods, animal products and sodium can upset the acid–alkaline balance and may lead to serious health problems. Curiously, some foods, such as lemons and grapefruit, are thought to be acidic but actually provide a more alkaline condition in the body, while other foods, such as dairy products, are the opposite and produce an acidifying response even though they are alkaline foods. Of course, other bodily functions and internally produced acids affect the acidity or alkalinity of our system overall, as long as these functions are not overwhelmed. We have systems in place to "buffer" acid levels, which are then removed from the body through our urine or breath. When pH is balanced, our kidneys recover buffering elements and return them to the bloodstream.

Evidence shows that measuring the pH of your urine on a regular basis can provide an estimate of the acid load of your diet. To bypass repeated urine tests, we have provided a list of common foods and their pH level, as well as an extensive list of foods categorized as alkalizing, slightly alkalizing, neutral, slightly acidifying and acidifying. This is adequate for measuring your acid and alkaline load.

A word of caution: Your health-care professional may recommend evidence-based articles and reliable Internet sites for you to explore before beginning a pH-balanced diet. Be cautious of websites that offer products for sale, and beware of sites that are not supported by evidence. See the Resources (page 393) for recommended websites. Books currently in the marketplace focus on different aspects of the pH diet, some educating readers about the health risks caused by the typical Western, or high-acid, diet. Others focus on restoring pH balance through supplements and enzymes. Some describe the foods that are acidifying or alkalizing. Other books are directed to naturopathic care, offering descriptions of supplements and therapies that may rebalance your pH. Finally, some cookbooks offer an array of alkaline recipes to support your efforts to achieve a pH-balanced diet.

A pH-balanced diet is one of the healthiest, most nutritious ways to eat, based on consuming 80% alkalizing whole and fresh foods, lots of vegetables (especially the raw dark green leafy varieties), fruits, roots, legumes and nuts, but also maintaining 20% acidifying foods. We are not asking that you give up all your favorite acid-forming foods — just the processed ones. *The pH Balance Health & Diet Guide* begins with a study of the role a balanced pH plays in achieving general good health and then applies this knowledge to diagnosing and managing selected gastrointestinal disease conditions, namely GERD (gastroesophageal reflux disease), IBS (irritable bowel syndrome) and IBD (inflammatory bowel disease). A pH-balanced dietary program for preventing and treating these conditions includes a 28-day healthy meal plan and 175 recipes. Of special interest is our attention to complementary medical approaches to diagnosing and treating GI conditions and the connections to pH mechanisms as seen from this refreshing medical perspective. We trust that we have provided adequate information and guidelines for you to begin to take control of your health management, including knowing when to turn to health-care professionals for their expertise.

About the Authors

This book has been researched and written by a highly qualified team of health-care professionals with considerable clinical experience.

Dr. Fraser Smith, BA, ND, is the author of the standard textbook *An Introduction to the Principles & Practices of Naturopathic Medicine*, as well as *Keep Your Brain Young: A Health & Diet Program for Your Brain*. He is assistant dean for naturopathic medicine at National University of Health Sciences (NUHS) in Lombard, Illinois. A graduate of the Canadian College of Naturopathic Medicine (CCNM), he became the dean of the naturopathic program before moving to Illinois to work with NUHS in the development and launching of the naturopathic medicine degree program. A contributing editor to the Elsevier Foundations project and textbook, he is regarded as a leading educator, clinical practitioner and author. Dr. Smith lives in the Chicago area with his young family.

Susan Hannah, BA, BScH, is a health writer and former research associate at the Centre for Studies in Primary Care, Department of Family Medicine, at Queen's University. She is the co-author of two previous Robert Rose books: *ASD: The Complete Autism Spectrum Disorder Health & Diet Guide* (2014) and *The Complete Migraine Health, Diet Guide & Cookbook* (2013). Her personal mandate in writing health books is to provide a resource that guides people to attain a state of wellness through lifestyle changes and acts as a bridge between patients and their health-care team whereby patients are able to provide the information that the team needs for optimum decision making and the best outcome possible.

Dr. Daniel Richardson, BS, MSc, DN (Honors), PhD, DAANC, CNC, received his masters degree and PhD in pharmacology and pharmacognosy from the Stritch School of Medicine, at Loyola University. He is a prominent expert in nutrition and botanical medicine, a Diplomate in the American Association of Nutrition Consultants and a certified nutrition consultant. He is a professor in the College of Professional Studies at the National University of Health Sciences in Lombard, Illinois, and assistant dean of the College of Allied Health Sciences. Dr. Richardson has advanced training in phytochemicals and botanical medicine and in sports medicine nutrition.

10 Steps for Implementing the pH Balance Diet Program

Before you begin this diet plan, visit your physician for a physical exam to be sure that other medical conditions are not present.

Testing

1. Test your pH level using a kit from your local drugstore to establish a baseline pH reading.
2. Keep a food journal or diet diary for a few weeks to see the ratio of acid to alkaline foods that you typically include in your diet.

Targeting

3. Establish a pH balance target. If you are suffering from a gastrointestinal (GI) medical condition, an 80% alkaline to 20% acid food ratio may help restore your health. If you are in good health, a 60% alkaline to 40% acid food ratio will help you maintain that state.
4. Follow a meal plan that helps you reach your target alkaline to acid ratio for several weeks. The meal plans in this book have been prepared by a registered dietitian and meet the standards established in Canada's Food Guide and the United States Department of Agriculture (USDA) MyPlate guidelines.

Preparing

5. Based on the meal plans plus the alkaline and acid food lists offered in this book, prepare your shopping list.
6. To reduce acidity, consider your cooking methods. For example, do you cook foods at a high temperature on a regular basis? Steaming, sautéing, roasting and gently cooking all foods will help reduce your acid levels.

Improving Your Quality of Life

7. Reduce the stress in your life by working with experts in massage, yoga, tai chi or other meditative practices. Visit a therapist for cognitive counseling if you are struggling with issues.

8. Exercise regularly (30 minutes a day to get your heart rate elevated). Gentle exercise is recommended for some people with GI conditions. Discuss any new exercise program with your health-care professional.

Looking for Support

9. Be attentive to the people who mean the most to you. Having a support network of family, friends, workplace colleagues and caregivers can improve your quality of life and help you to overcome medical conditions.

10. Check back with your physician or dietitian periodically to check that nothing has gone wrong — and to confirm your success in balancing your pH levels.

If you follow these steps, you should be able to improve your health and maintain a better state of wellness.

Part 1
pH Basics

Chapter 1

What Is pH?

CASE STUDY

Metabolic Acidosis

Nancy sighed again and leaned her head on her hand, trying to catch her breath. She was dizzy and felt really weak. After a four-day session of diarrhea, she was left with rapid breathing, a pounding headache and a strange taste in her mouth. As she pressed her other hand to her chest, hoping it would relieve the scary pain there, she heard voices in the hallway and looked up, very anxious and hoping her husband had returned to explain where she was and what was going on.

Nancy suffered from Crohn's disease, a form of inflammatory bowel disease (IBD). Her recent flare-up was a source of concern because she'd been exhausted before it began. Her husband, Rory, had decided to take her to emergency when she couldn't remember where she was or what day it was.

The nurse hustled back into the room and set up an ECG monitor, another monitor to assess levels of oxygen and a blood pressure monitor. He expertly inserted a needle into Nancy's arm to begin an IV that would slowly deliver high-alkaline fluids. He had quietly explained to Rory that having such severe diarrhea for such a long time had put her in a state of metabolic acidosis — her body's pH levels were seriously out of balance, along with being dehydrated and having lost a lot of electrolytes, minerals such as potassium and magnesium that are critical to many body functions. Nancy's pH level was much lower than normal, meaning her blood was very acidic, and she had used up the natural buffers (sodium, calcium, potassium and magnesium) that help restore normal acid–alkaline balance. In metabolic acidosis, enzymes do not work properly and many body functions might stop, so immediate care is critical. Now that Nancy was in hospital, she was getting the care she needed; Rory could breathe a sigh of relief ... (*continued on page 32*)

During high school chemistry class, our teachers introduced us to the complicated concept of "potential for hydrogen," or pH, by using litmus strips, the standard test for determining the acidity or alkalinity of chemical compounds. When a litmus strip is dipped in an alkaline liquid, it turns blue; when dipped in an acidic liquid, it turns red.

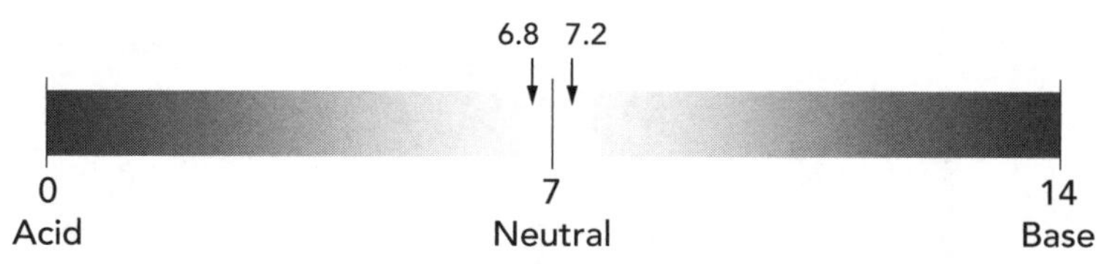

pH Measurement

In chemistry, pH is a universal measure for acidity or alkalinity (also known as basicity) that is stated on a scale of 0 to 14. A pH under 7 is acidic; over 7 is alkaline. For example, the pH of lemon juice (acidic) is around 2.0, and the pH of household ammonia (alkaline) is 11.5. Pure water has a pH very close to 7. A pH level of 7 at 77°F (25°C) is defined as "neutral" because the concentration of H_3O+ (hydronium) equals the concentration of OH– (hydroxide) in pure water.

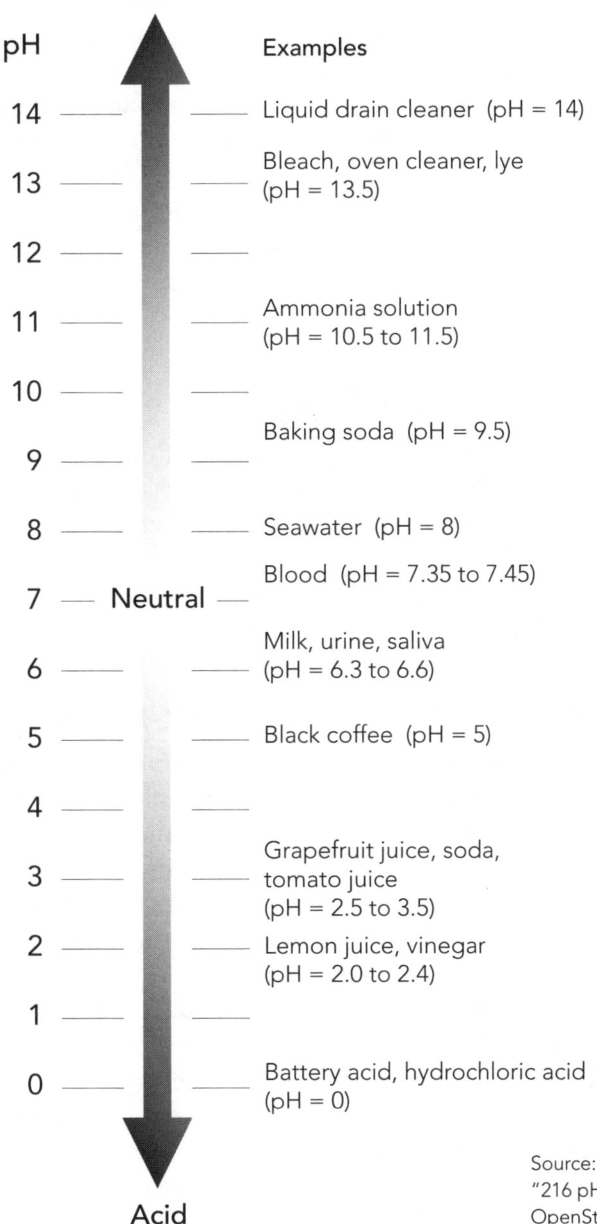

Source: Adapted from OpenStax College. "216 pH Scale-01." *Anatomy & Physiology.* OpenStax-CNX Web site, May 16, 2013. CC by 3.0.

Did You Know?

Range of pH Readings

Our world is full of substances that fall somewhere on the scale between acid and alkaline — ranging from the most acidic (0 on the pH scale) to the most alkaline substance (14). Most of the fluids in our bodies are around pH 6 to 8, except for stomach acid, which is usually around pH 2 because of the presence of hydrochloric acid, used to help digest food. The normal pH for human blood is on average 7.4. If your pH deviates significantly from this range, your health suffers.

Did You Know?

pH Accounting

Our bodies are excellent accountants when it comes to pH. Various mechanisms make every effort to neutralize excess acid and restore homeostasis, and the biochemical processes involved in maintaining homeostasis are necessary for our survival — the homeostasis process helps us survive in environments that could otherwise kill us. These processes operate best within a limited temperature range and at a specific pH of acidity. For example, shivering is a response to cooler weather, because small movements of muscles release heat and warm the cooling body.

Homeostasis

Understanding pH measurements is important not only in the natural sciences but also in the food and health sciences. The makeup of our bodies is 75% fluid, including blood, urine and water. Weighed together on the pH scale, these bodily fluids are slightly more alkaline than acidic, around 7.36 to 7.44. To be healthy, the body needs to maintain this alkaline to acid balance. When this balance or equilibrium is lost, the result can be a serious negative impact on our health.

The proper balance of various factors in our bodies, in this case alkaline to acid, is known as homeostasis. Various other mechanisms, notably body temperature and cellular hydration, work to keep us within the bounds of homeostasis. The homeostatic process occurs not only in the blood but also in other systems of fluids found in the body — in our urine, saliva and stomach acids, for example. Homeostasis also monitors and regulates the oxygen and carbon dioxide levels involved in pH mechanisms. Homeostasis is at work on the molecular level in every cell and even in intestinal bacterial populations.

Feedback Loops

The acid–base (or acid–alkaline) balance of our blood is carefully controlled through a communication feedback loop using the endocrine and nervous systems. Feedback can be negative, when the response reduces the original stimulus, or positive, when the response increases the original stimulus. Feedback also limits or stops processes.

Negative Feedback Mechanisms

When you set the temperature on your home thermostat, you are setting up a negative feedback mechanism. If you have the thermostat at 68°F (20°C), a sensor in the thermostat turns on the furnace whenever the temperature drops below that point. The sensor responds once again to turn off the furnace when the temperature in the room reaches 68°F, thus maintaining the selected temperature.

In our bodies, insulin's management of blood sugar levels is a negative feedback mechanism. Body receptors sense an increase in blood sugar and send a message to the pancreas, where insulin is secreted into the bloodstream and sugar is moved out of the bloodstream into cells. After the blood sugar level is within normal homeostasis range, insulin is no longer produced and released by the pancreas.

Negative Feedback Loop for Regulating Body Temperature

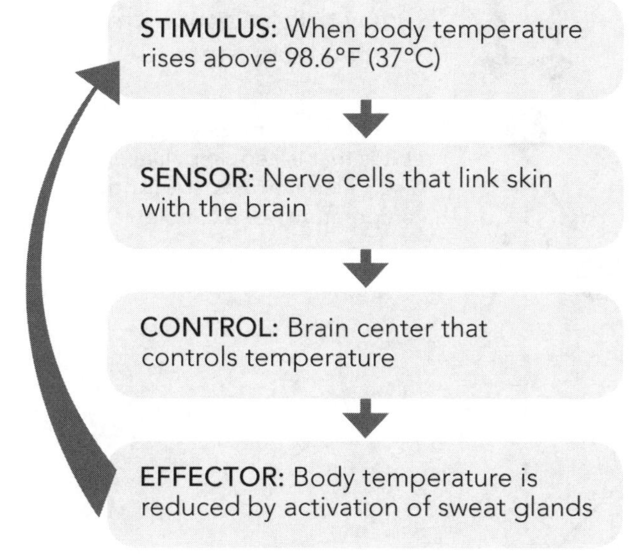

Sensors are triggered when body temperature rises beyond set point

An automatic response is sent from nerves in the skin to the brain

An automatic response to reduce body temperature is sent out

Sweat helps to release heat from the skin

Source: Adapted from OpenStax College. "105 Negative Feedback Loops." *Anatomy & Physiology*. OpenStax-CNX Web site, April 5, 2013. CC by 3.0.

Positive Feedback Mechanisms

The positive feedback mechanism differs from the negative process because it is additive. The molecule involved in the process continues to increase until the goal is reached, at which point it stops being produced. For example, when a blood vessel is damaged, a cascade of events is set off. Platelets are attracted to the injury and, once in place, release more chemicals to continue the cascade. The piling on of platelets continues until a blood clot forms. The goal is reached and the cascade ends.

Nervous System Control

The nervous system manages homeostasis by regulating organs and processes in the body, using set points intended to protect the integrity of hydration, body temperature and pH balance. When any change occurs that is outside the comfort range for this set point, a message is sent to the brain's regulatory centers from sensors in the skin and other organs. A response to return the body to the set point takes place — through sweating, for example, if the body temperature is too high. Once the body temperature has

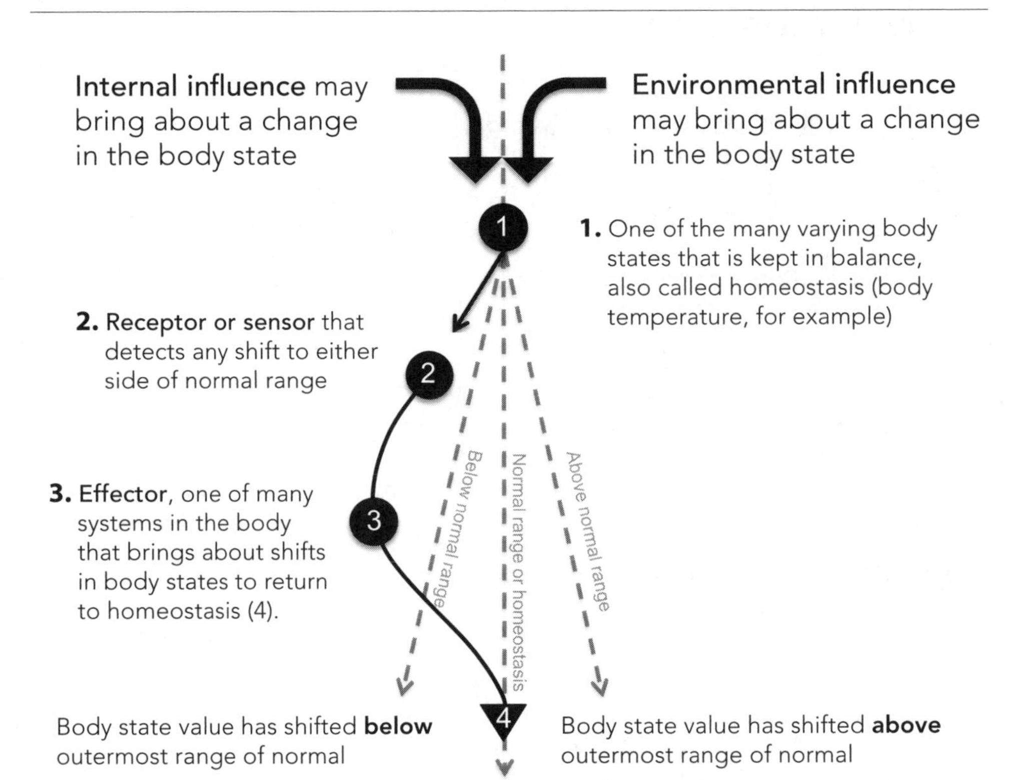

returned to normal, the areas involved in the regulatory process stop the activity, called negative feedback. The nervous system responds quickly to changes in homeostasis.

Did You Know?

Endocrine System

The endocrine system is the collection of glands that help with communication throughout our bodies by secreting different hormones into the bloodstream, where they are carried to the target location to deliver their message. The endocrine system regulates metabolism, sexual development and sexual function. Messages from the endocrine system take longer to reach their target but last longer.

Blood pH

In the blood, the acid level rises due to increased intake of acid-forming foods, reduced excretion of acids and/or increased intake and excretion of alkaline-forming foods. When alkaline substances in the body are reduced through intake, production or increased excretion, acid levels rise.

Tolerance Limits

When we are healthy, our bodies maintain, within limits, adequate concentrations of fluid components, even when the external environment changes. Going beyond these tolerance limits can lead to illness or death.

Acidosis and Alkalosis

Our bodies function properly when our blood is around 7.4 on the pH scale, which is just slightly alkaline. Any time our bodies move away from that value, conditions called acidosis or alkalosis occur, depending on whether the value is lower than 7.35 or higher than 7.45. Here are some examples of dysfunctions as a result of acidosis or alkalosis.

- **Proteins:** Proteins are the basic building blocks for our body tissue. Their three-dimensional structures hold their shape when the body is at pH 7.4, but these shapes may deform if alkalosis (above 7.45) or acidosis (below 7.35) occurs.
- **Enzymes:** Enzymes are specific proteins that are involved in many processes throughout our bodies. They function best at pH 7.4. Normal function will be affected at values outside of 7.35 to 7.45.

> **Did You Know?**
>
> **Enzyme Function**
>
> The countless biochemical reactions that happen inside our bodies are either catabolic (breaking down into smaller units to produce energy) or anabolic (building up by combining smaller units) and are managed by special protein molecules called enzymes. Enzymes are the catalysts that make it possible for metabolism to happen in an efficient way. Biochemical reactions grouped with relevant enzymes achieve physiological goals to form metabolic pathways, and different metabolic pathways link up and react with each other to form bodily systems. A dysfunctional or unfolded enzyme can have a profound impact on many systems in our bodies.

pH Diet

Our Western diet is poorly balanced for pH, overabundant in acidic-forming foods and insufficient in alkaline-forming foods. On the one hand, the typical Western diet contains too much acid-forming processed food preserved and flavored with sulfur and sodium. On the other hand, this diet is often deficient in leafy vegetables and fresh fruits — foods that are highly alkalizing. This imbalance creates excess acid and insufficient alkaline content in the body. The inability to manage excess acid in the body is called metabolic acidosis. Likewise, we can eat an overabundance of alkaline foods, leading to a state of metabolic alkalosis, though this state is less common and less dangerous to our health.

Kinds of Acidosis and Alkalosis

Depending on the cause, acidosis and alkalosis are classified as being metabolic, respiratory or renal.

- **Metabolic:** All the chemical reactions that keep the cells in your body in a living state are collectively referred to as your metabolism and can be classified as catabolic (breaking down molecules for energy) or anabolic (building up molecules from simpler compounds). Metabolism is a balance between these anabolic and catabolic reactions.

Without it, life ends. Our thyroid gland secretes the hormone thyroxine, which sets the pace of metabolism. Nutrients from our diet provide the building blocks for our bodies to metabolize food into heat energy to meet daily requirements. An inability to break down excess acid from the diet — to the point of toxic accumulation — is called *metabolic* acidosis.

- **Respiratory:** Changes in exhaling carbon dioxide from our lungs or breathing problems can also cause acidosis or alkalosis. Carbon dioxide is a slightly acidic product of oxygen metabolism and is produced in every cell, then excreted into the blood and carried to the lungs. Carbon dioxide is exhaled from the lungs as part of the cycle of respiration, and the loss of carbon dioxide increases the amount of oxygen picked up by the lungs. As our bodies work to produce oxygen, carbon dioxide continues to be carried to the bloodstream and the pH of the blood decreases. When higher levels of carbon dioxide are sensed by the brain, the speed and depth of breathing changes to increase the amount exhaled and maintain the levels of carbon dioxide and oxygen. This is *respiratory* acidosis.
- **Renal:** Kidneys affect the acid–alkaline balance of our bodies because acids and bases are also excreted by the kidneys. This process is slower than respiratory excretion. The kidneys reduce acids by providing buffers that are then excreted. When a healthy balance is maintained, the kidneys are able to recapture the buffers and send them back to the bloodstream to capture more acid. Changes in urine excretion from acids to bases typically take a few days rather than seconds. This is *renal* acidosis.

Acidosis Symptoms

High acidity can contribute to illness in most body systems, but especially in the gastrointestinal system, where acids are already active in the digestion of food and absorption of nutrients. Symptoms of acidosis may include:

- **Central nervous system:** Headache, sleepiness, confusion, loss of consciousness, coma
- **Respiratory system:** Shortness of breath, coughing
- **Heart:** Arrhythmia, increased heart rate
- **Muscular system:** Seizures, weakness
- **Digestive system:** Nausea, vomiting, diarrhea

Alkalosis Symptoms

A high level of bicarbonate in the bloodstream is called metabolic alkalosis, or primary bicarbonate excess. Brief periods of alkalosis can occur after the ingestion of excessive bicarbonate, antacids or citrate, often to relieve stomach acid reflux. Alkalosis also occurs as a result of excessive vomiting, excessive use of laxatives or the use of diuretics for high blood pressure. Symptoms include:

- **Central nervous system:** Confusion, lightheadedness, stupor, coma
- **Peripheral nervous system:** Hand tremors, numbness or tingling in the face, hands or feet
- **Muscular system:** Twitching, prolonged spasms
- **Digestive system:** Nausea, vomiting

Common Acidic and Alkaline Elements

You may also remember from chemistry classes the periodic table of elements, which categorizes similar elements into families. Some elements from the metal family are alkaline-forming when dissolved in water. Certain elements, when in compounds, have unfilled outer orbitals and are thus able to donate or accept electrons and serve as buffers against acidosis or alkalosis. These elements may need to be administered as mineral supplements to prevent imbalance. Sodium and potassium are the chief buffers, along with bicarbonate of soda (baking soda).

Did You Know?

Balance and pH Proportion

The term "balance" suggests that two equal components weigh the same on a balance scale. While "balance" is the term commonly used in discussing the respective levels of acid and alkaline chemicals in the body — potassium to sodium, for example — "proportioned" is more accurate. The ideal proportion of alkaline to acid chemicals is 3 to 1, but the proportion in most individuals is closer to 10 to 1 (acid to alkaline). This proportion is dangerous to our long-term health.

Periodic Table

1 H Hydrogen																	2 He Helium
3 Li Lithium	4 Be Beryllium											5 B Boron	6 C Carbon	7 N Nitrogen	8 O Oxygen	9 F Fluorine	10 Ne Neon
11 Na Sodium	12 Mg Magnesium											13 Al Aluminium	14 Si Silicon	15 P Phosphorus	16 S Sulfur	17 Cl Chlorine	18 Ar Argon
19 K Potassium	20 Ca Calcium	21 Sc Scandium	22 Ti Titanium	23 V Vanadium	24 Cr Chromium	25 Mn Manganese	26 Fe Iron	27 Co Cobalt	28 Ni Nickel	29 Cu Copper	30 Zn Zinc	31 Ga Gallium	32 Ge Germanium	33 As Arsenic	34 Se Selenium	35 Br Bromine	36 Kr Krypton
37 Rb Rubidium	38 Sr Strontium	39 Y Yttrium	40 Zr Zirconium	41 Nb Niobium	42 Mo Molybdenum	43 Tc Technetium	44 Ru Ruthenium	45 Rh Rhodium	46 Pd Palladium	47 Ag Silver	48 Cd Cadmium	49 In Indium	50 Sn Tin	51 Sb Antimony	52 Te Tellurium	53 I Iodine	54 Xe Xenon
55 Cs Cesium	56 Ba Barium	57 La* Lanthanum	72 Hf Hafnium	73 Ta Tantalum	74 W Tungsten	75 Re Rhenium	76 Os Osmium	77 Ir Iridium	78 Pt Platinum	79 Au Gold	80 Hg Mercury	81 Tl Thallium	82 Pb Lead	83 Bi Bismuth	84 Po Polonium	85 At Astatine	86 Rn Radon
87 Fr Francium	88 Ra Radium	89 Ac** Actinium	104 Rf Rutherfordium	105 Db Dubnium	106 Sg Seaborgium	107 Bh Bohrium	108 Hs Hassium	109 Mt Meitnerium	110 Ds Darmstadtium	111 Rg Roentgenium	112 Cn Copernicium	113 Uut Ununtrium	114 Uuq Ununquadium	115 Uup Ununpentium	116 Uuh Ununhexium	117 Uus Ununseptium	118 Uuo Ununoctium

*	58 Ce Cerium	59 Pr Praseodymium	60 Nd Neodymium	61 Pm Promethium	62 Sm Samarium	63 Eu Europium	64 Gd Gadolinium	65 Tb Terbium	66 Dy Dysprosium	67 Ho Holmium	68 Er Erbium	69 Tm Thulium	70 Yb Ytterbium	71 Lu Lutetium
**	90 Th Thorium	91 Pa Protactinium	92 U Uranium	93 Np Neptunium	94 Pu Plutonium	95 Am Americium	96 Cm Curium	97 Bk Berkelium	98 Cf Californium	99 Es Einsteinium	100 Fm Fermium	101 Md Mendelevium	102 No Nobelium	103 Lr Lawrencium

Some elements are naturally acidic, others alkaline:

Acidic elements

Phosphorus (P)
Chloride (Cl)
Fluorine (F)
Lead (Pb)

Alkaline elements

Sulfur (S)
Sodium (Na)
Potassium (K)
Calcium (Ca)
Magnesium (Mg)
Zinc (Zn)
Iron (Fe)

Bicarbonate Buffer

Carbon dioxide (CO_2) is metabolic waste carried in the blood to be deposited in the lungs and exhaled. More than 75% of the CO_2 in your body is in the form of bicarbonate (HCO_3-), which is produced by the kidneys. In metabolic acidosis, the bicarbonate buffer fails to remove this acidic metabolic waste, leaving the body with an acid overload. Further, the typical Western diet raises the amount of acid taken in by the body and increases the loss of bicarbonate. One of the functions of the kidneys is to excrete acid and, at the same time, produce bicarbonate. Some acids depend on potassium or sodium to be excreted, which may result in a loss of minerals or electrolytes.

GI Balance

The gastrointestinal (GI) tract manages acid–alkaline balance through the movement of hydrogen and bicarbonate ions through the gut. When normal gut function is somehow disrupted — through disease symptoms or acid–alkaline imbalance, for example — homeostasis can be upset. The area of the GI tract that is affected and the nature of the fluid loss may determine whether metabolic acidosis or alkalosis (rarer) will occur.

Paleo pH

Since the prehistoric era of the hunter-gatherer, the net acid load in the human diet has grown significantly. Simply stated, we are eating more foods containing more acidic chemicals than our Paleolithic ancestors did. The hunter-gatherer diet had a ratio of potassium (K) to sodium (Na) of 10 to 1, for example, while the modern diet, as described by Dr. Abram Hoffer, has a ratio of 3 sodium to 1 potassium. Since the agricultural revolution (about 12,000 years ago) and, more recently, the Industrial Revolution (about 250 years ago), the ratio of potassium to sodium has decreased and the ratio of chloride to bicarbonate has increased in our diet. These molecules all impact cell-to-cell communication in our bodies, and changing the balance has a negative impact on our health.

High-Acid Diet Dangers

Today, many people consume a diet low in magnesium, potassium and fiber but high in acid, saturated fat, simple sugars, sodium and chloride. This diet may induce a mild to severe form of metabolic acidosis in many people, and with aging, there can be a gradual loss of kidney function. A low-carbohydrate, high-protein diet, with its increased acid load, may not cause much change in blood pH but will result in many changes in other bodily systems. Eating high-acid foods may cause:

- Abnormal or low thyroid gland activity (mild hypothyroidism).
- Increased amounts of cortisol circulating in the blood (hypercortisolemia), which affects pain levels and quality of sleep.
- Decreased insulin-like growth factor (IGF1) activity. IGF1, a protein similar to insulin, stimulates growth hormone (GH), is an anti-inflammatory and antioxidant, protects cells and is involved in the breakdown of tissues and cells. Decreased IGF1 activity in an adult may lead to cardiovascular or neurological disease or aging in general.
- Increased GH resistance, which can lead to failure to grow and thrive.
- Hormonal dysfunction, insulin resistance, protein breakdowns and interruption of enzyme activity.

Eating Trends

Today, most people eat an unbalanced diet. Their meals are deficient in alkaline-supportive nutrients, such as magnesium, potassium and fiber (which help to buffer acids in our bodies), but high in saturated fat, simple sugars, sodium and chloride. This diet can induce a mild form of metabolic acidosis. Aging can also lead to a gradual loss of kidney function, followed by an increase in diet-induced metabolic acidosis — based on the modern diet.

In addition, the amount of water in the typical diet is insufficient and may include bottled or filtered water made with processes that remove those important buffering minerals (check labels for minerals). Since our bodies are mostly water, an easy way to improve your diet is to make sure to drink enough water throughout the day, and not just when you feel thirsty. This is especially important during times of greater physical exertion or hot weather. Adding a squeeze of lemon to a glass of filtered water is a great way to kick-start your optimum health regimen.

How to Measure pH Levels

There are several tests commonly used to determine the pH level of fluids in your body and in the foods you eat.

Testing Saliva pH

Although relatively easy to do, testing the pH levels in saliva is not the most accurate procedure. If, on the one hand, the saliva pH is below 6.5, you may be producing a high level of acids, or you may be unable to remove acids from your body through your kidneys and urine. If, on the other hand, the saliva measurement is over 6.8, you are on the alkaline side and may be suffering from excess gas, constipation, yeast, fungus or mold. Because the bloodstream has its own intrinsic buffer system, salivary pH changes do not absolutely tell us about what is going on in the bloodstream.

Testing Urine pH

Using pH strips to test your urine may show whether you are able to excrete acids or take in buffer minerals, such as calcium, sodium, magnesium and potassium. If your urine pH test is below 6.5, the reading suggests that your body's buffering system may be overwhelmed and acid levels may need to be reduced.

Analyzing Ash

To identify acid- and alkaline-forming foods, the foods in question are combusted and the ash that results is analyzed to calculate the amounts of alkaline and acid. This method has shown that food with acidic anions include phosphorus, chloride and sulfates, and foods with alkaline cations include potassium, magnesium, sodium and calcium. Ash analysis is not a perfect measure of pH because the bioavailability of nutrients in foods is not taken into account and the actual acid–alkaline balance of the body after eating the foods does not match the ash analysis. This technique is not recommended.

FAQ

Q. What are cations and anions?

A. If an atom loses one or two electrons to another strongly charged atom, it becomes what is called an ion, and has a positive charge overall, since one or two negatively charged electrons have been lost. This positive ion is called a cation. If an atom gains electrons, it becomes a negatively charged ion called an anion.

Calculating the Net Acid Excretion

This technique measures the acid and ammonium in your urine by taking away the amount of bicarbonate found there to give a net acid excretion (NAE). Rather than measuring the acid or alkaline load of individual foods, this final acid load measurement represents the food taken in over a period of time. The NAE can also be calculated by adding up all urinary acidic anions and then subtracting the bicarbonate in the urine. The final value is the total acid and alkaline load from all foods eaten over a period of time and does not provide the acid count.

Calculating the Potential Renal Acid Load

The potential renal acid load (PRAL) provides a measure of the net acid or alkaline load of your food intake, which will help you calculate the approximate load from the makeup of the food. This technique includes the bioavailability of each micro- and macronutrient, sulfur content and protein to create an index of the acid–alkaline load based on the food eaten.

PRAL Values of Some Common Foods

The foods on this list are categorized alphabetically within groups for quick reference. A negative value means the food has an alkaline-forming (or base-forming) load; a positive value means the food has an acid load. All foods values are per 3½ oz (100 g) of food before cooking. If you eat, for example, 7 oz (200 g) of amaranth, the PRAL value for the amaranth in your meal is 14.6 (7.3 x 2). The PRAL measure for many of the foods on this list indicates the acid and alkaline load of each food, which enables more precise selection for meals.

Food	PRAL
GRAINS	
Amaranth	7.3
Barley	2.5
Buckwheat	3.4
Buckwheat flour, whole-grain	–0.5
Bulgur	3.8
Millet	8.8
Oat bran	16.9
Oats	13.3
Quinoa	–0.2

Food	PRAL
Rice, brown, long-grain	7.5
Rye	12.0
Wheat, hard red spring	9.1
Wheat, hard red winter	5.6
Wheat, sprouted	5.0
FRUITS	
Apricots	–4.3
Apples, with skin	–1.9
Avocados	–8.2
Bananas	–6.9
Blackberries	–2.8
Blueberries	–1.0
Cherries, sweet	–3.8
Dates, Medjool	–13.7
Figs, dried	–14.1
Figs, fresh	–4.9
Grapefruit, pink and red	–2.5
Kiwifruit	–5.6
Lemons, without peel	–2.3
Mangos	–3.0
Melons, cantaloupe	–5.1
Oranges	–3.6
Pears	–2.2
Pineapple, canned in juice, solids and liquids	–2.7
Pomegranates	–4.8
Prunes (dried plums)	–13.4
Raisins, seedless	–12.0
Raspberries	–2.4
Strawberries	–2.5
Tangerines (mandarin oranges)	–3.1
Watermelon	–2.0
LEGUMES	
Adzuki beans	–6.7
Chickpeas (garbanzo beans)	0.3
Great Northern beans	–9.1
Kidney beans, all types	–8.4
Lentils, green and brown	5.4
Lentils, red	8.6

Food	PRAL
Lima beans	–18.3
Mung beans	–7.5
Navy beans	–5.3
Peanuts, all types	6.2
Pinto beans	–9.6
Soybeans	–4.7
Tofu, regular, prepared with calcium sulfate	–0.3
White beans	–23.2
NUTS AND SEEDS	
Almonds	2.3
Brazil nuts	8.1
Cashews	8.9
Flax seeds	2.1
Hazelnuts (filberts)	–1.9
Macadamia nuts	–1.4
Pecans	2.1
Pistachios	2.2
Sunflower seeds	12.1
Walnuts, English	5.6
VEGETABLES	
Alfalfa sprouts	1.8
Asparagus	–1.9
Beet greens	–16.7
Beets	–5.4
Bok choy	–5.0
Broccoli	–4.0
Broccoli raab (rapini)	–1.8
Carrots	–5.7
Cauliflower	–4.4
Collard greens	–4.1
Cucumber, with peel	–2.4
Dandelion greens	–7.9
Eggplant	–3.9
Kale	–8.3
Leaf lettuce, green	–3.1
Leeks, white and light green parts	–3.2
Mung bean sprouts	–0.4
Onions	–2.1

Food	PRAL
Purslane	–10.7
Radishes	–4.4
Red bell peppers	–3.4
Spinach	–11.8
Squash, summer and zucchini, with skin	–4.1
Sweet potatoes	–5.6
Swiss chard	–8.1
Tomatoes, red, ripe, year-round average	–4.1
Turnip greens	–7.2
Turnips	–3.2
Source: Adapted from data at the USDA National Nutrient Database for Standard Reference, Release 18 (SR18).	

Short Course in the Atomic Structure of pH

To understand pH, we need to review how positive and negative particles can move within substances to change their acidity.

Everything in the universe is made from atoms, which in turn are composed of protons, which have a positive charge (+); electrons, which have a negative charge (–); and neutrons, which have a neutral charge (+/–). Atoms are the basic building blocks that make up matter, the basis for everyday objects, and become the building blocks for molecules — the components in compounds. Most atoms are balanced so no overall charge is present, but if an atom is out of balance, it will take on a positive or negative charge. The ability of atoms to move from a neutral to positive to negative state allows electrons to move from one atom to another, which causes electricity to flow. The signals sent by our brains are powered by this kind of instantaneous electricity.

Signaling

Electrical and chemical signaling are the two forms of power that keep our bodies working. To use hydrogen as an example, combining two hydrogen atoms with one atom of oxygen forms a molecule of water (called a compound). Physically, these building blocks consist of electrons revolving around a nucleus that contains the protons and neutrons. The periodic table tells you how many protons are included in one atom for each element. For water, the atomic number is 10 (1 + 1 + 8 = 10) because each of the 2 hydrogen molecules has 1 electron and 1 proton and each oxygen molecule has 8 electrons and 8 protons, which all combine in a stable molecule of water, or H_2O. When the number of electrons and protons is equal, the atom is considered electrically neutral.

continued...

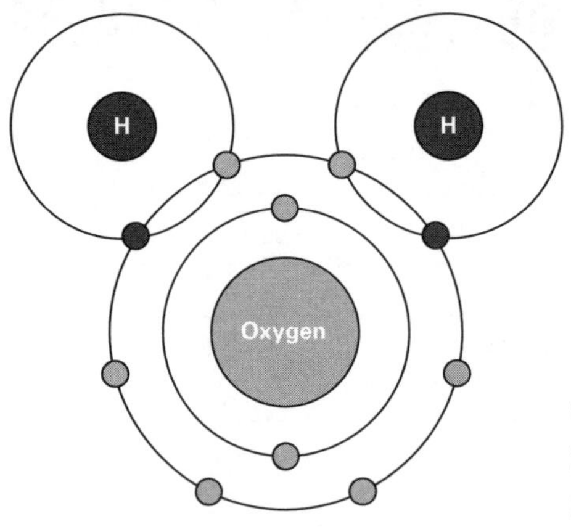

Water molecule (H_20) showing shells around nucleus and covalent bonding through sharing electrons

Source: Adapted from OpenStax College. *Atoms, Isotopes, Ions and Molecules: The Building Blocks*. OpenStax-CNX Web site, February 20, 2014. CC by 3.0.

Bonding

When free-floating atoms come near each other, they may stick together through a few different kinds of bonds to form a molecule. A covalent bond happens when two atoms share electrons that are in the outer ring.

The electrons are shown in rings (called shells) around the nucleus. Each shell holds a set number of electrons: the first (K shell) has 2, the second (L shell) has 8, the third (M shell) has 18, the fourth (N shell) 32, the fifth (O shell) 50 and the sixth (P shell) has 72. Most of the time, the electrons will fill the lower-energy shells first and move outward until all electrons have been placed. An atom is at its most stable when the outer shell that contains any electrons is full and the two outermost shells are able to interact with other atoms when the outer shell is not completely filled.

An atom might gain or even lose an electron to be able to reach the electrically neutral status of having a full outer shell. In the element table, atoms that have full outer shells are not reactive (called "inert") because they are very stable.

For hydrogen, since there is only 1 shell and it has only 1 electron, the atom is not fully stable and is able to lose or donate an electron to another atom. If a hydrogen atom donates an electron, the electric charge changes to a positively charged ion (shown by a + symbol). When an atom gains an electron, it becomes a negatively charged ion (shown by a – symbol).

With a water molecule, two of the electrons from the outer shell of the oxygen have been shared with the hydrogen atoms to achieve a stable form and build a covalent bond between the atoms.

Sometimes water molecules split apart (this does not happen to all water molecules at the same time) and both hydrogen ions and hydroxide ions result. The hydrogen ion, with a positive charge, is then able to combine with any atoms or elements with a negative charge, and an acid may be the result. An acid is any molecule that is able to release hydrogen ions when it splits apart after being added to water. A base, on the other hand, is able to release a hydroxide ion, which may combine with any other hydroxide ions to form a water molecule.

The reactions of acids and bases in water is how the pH scale is measured. Essentially, the pH (potential hydrogen) scale is a measure of the hydrogen ions in a fluid (concentration). The hydrogen ion becomes positive in the water (at which point the ion is called a cation) because the electron (with a negative charge and thus called an anion) is still attached to the molecule. The water-based fluid that the acid has been mixed into will have a higher positive charge.

If a base or alkaline is mixed into the same water-based fluid, it will attract the hydrogen ions and the fluid will become more negative.

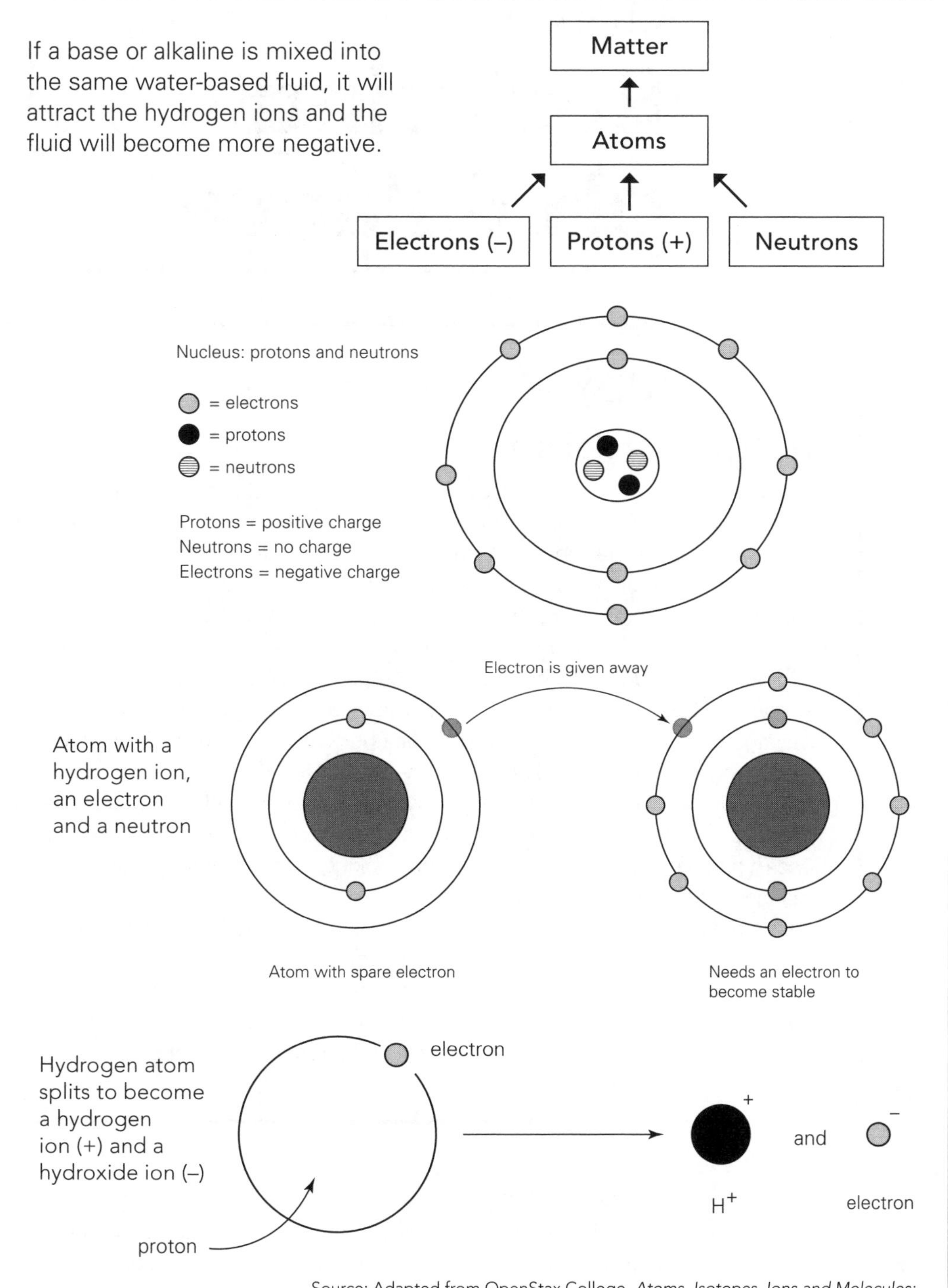

Source: Adapted from OpenStax College. *Atoms, Isotopes, Ions and Molecules: The Building Blocks*. OpenStax-CNX Web site, February 20, 2014. CC by 3.0.

The pH scale, with acid at the negative end (value of 0 to less than 7) and alkaline at the positive end (value of more than 7 to 14), is used to test the acidity or alkalinity of a substance. And since each of these numbers indicates a value 100 times stronger than the previous value, very small changes on the pH scale indicate a large number of H+ ions increasing or decreasing.

Chapter 2

Restoring pH Balance

CASE STUDY *(continued from page 14)*

Metabolic Acidosis

Nancy suffered from a chronic low-level metabolic acidosis because of her Crohn's disease. Because she had many flare-ups with diarrhea, she was often dehydrated. Her body's ability to maintain a state of homeostasis (the point where all her body systems could function) was compromised, and as a result, she was often anemic, with slightly high blood acid levels. In Nancy's case, monitoring her diet, IBD symptoms and stress levels had helped to reduce the number of flare-ups but not to get rid of them altogether. She was signed up to try some yoga breathing classes to manage her stress and help her to reduce her weight gradually. She was also trying a pH-balanced diet where she ate 80% alkaline foods compared to 20% acidic. The diet was pretty easy; you just eyeballed amounts of the food types. Changing patterns of cooking helped too — no more frying, occasional barbecue only, using gentler cooking methods instead, such as roasting, steaming or slow cooking.

In 3 days, Nancy was ready to go home. The hospital had been able to provide meals high in green leafy vegetables, small servings of protein and as much fruit as she wanted, with advice to keep going with her diary practice, since it was a great help for her physician to see possible relationships between foods, symptoms and stressful situations.

Once lost, pH balance can be restored by supplementing buffering agents, increasing the intake of alkaline water, maintaining electrolyte levels and following a diet rich in alkaline-forming foods. These strategies are the basic components of a pH-balanced diet.

Acid Buffers

To govern the effect of pH fluctuation, the body has buffer systems that act almost instantaneously to restore homeostasis:

- Bicarbonate buffer
- Ammonia buffer
- Protein buffer
- Phosphate buffer

Bicarbonate and ammonia are two external buffering agents that bind and unbind hydrogen ions, while internal buffers include protein and phosphate. These buffer systems function to shift strong acids or alkalines to weaker ones, moving them up or down the pH scale and making them more negative or positive by offering ions that balance the molecule. Internal buffers are found in bodily fluids. They work very quickly, in fractions of a second, to prevent large changes in acidity or alkalinity. Buffering agents, along with the renal and respiratory systems, keep arterial blood at a healthy pH between 7.35 and 7.45.

Did You Know?

Bicarbonate Buffer

The bicarbonate buffer reaches every cell in our bodies, acts continuously and is responsible for removing approximately 50% of the acids from our bodies.

The Isohydric Principle

Hydrogen ion activity in a solution occurs because multiple buffers pass hydrogen ions from one to another (called the isohydric principle). A buffering agent, a weak acid or base, maintains the pH close to a specific value even after other acids or bases are added. The buffers donate a hydrogen ion or claim a hydrogen ion, depending on the direction of any shift, to maintain the same pH level (homeostasis).

Alkaline Water

The average amount of water in our bodies differs according to gender, age and fitness level. You begin to feel thirsty when 2% to 3% of your bodily water is lost, but even if you are only 1% dehydrated, your mental abilities and physical coordination are reduced.

The kind of water you drink may also affect the acidity of your body. Choosing distilled, reverse osmosis, bottled or deionized water may increase acidity, while adding minerals to your water can increase alkalinity.

Did You Know?

Rebalancing with Sea Salt

Adding mineral supplements or unrefined sea salt to your diet is one option for balancing out the pH level of the water you drink. Sea salt has more than 80 trace minerals and elements. It offers a mineral balance, with its elements in close proportions to our internal world. Sea salt may help to rebalance excess acidity, restore good digestion, relieve allergies and skin disease, and increase resistance to infection.

Electrolytes

Electrolytes manage energy production, storage and use. They also regulate body fluid levels. Regulation of body fluids is managed by the kidneys, the adrenal glands and the brain. Two-thirds of the water in our bodies is in the intracellular fluid, and the rest is in fluids outside of cells. The water held in tissues — collections of cells that have functions — is involved in chemical and biochemical distributions inside and between tissues and cells, which affects function; the distribution of nutrients, hormones and heat around the tissues; the carriage of oxygen throughout the body; and the management of carbon dioxide levels in the bloodstream. Water in tissues is also responsible for carrying wastes through the liver, kidneys and bladder that are finally excreted through the urethra.

FAQ

Q. Does the pH imbalance of our water, soil and food affect our health?

A. We know that the water we drink has an increasing level of acid minerals, and our soil has a decreasing level of alkaline minerals. The resulting lower pH of our soil may be affecting the levels of minerals in the foods we eat. Reduced levels of calcium and magnesium in the soil may have reduced the availability of iron, manganese, copper and zinc. These factors influence our bodies and our food sources, leading to problems with our diet overall. In general, our water, soil and food are poor in magnesium and potassium and lower in fiber than is healthy, and most people eat too much saturated fat, salt and processed sugars and flours. This diet may lead to a mild form of metabolic acidosis, which can also be a result of aging for many people. Although our blood acid levels may not show much of a change in acid levels from this diet, risks of chronic disease may increase.

pH Balance Diet Principles

The pH Balance Diet Plan is based on complex pH chemistry but operates more simply, almost as common sense.

1. The aim is to increase the intake of alkaline-forming foods and reduce acid-forming foods. In brief, eat more alkaline-forming foods and less acid-forming foods.
2. The target is to eat 4 alkaline-forming foods to 1 acid-forming food to restore good health, and 3 to 1 to maintain good health.
3. Acid–alkaline balance can be restored by focusing on eating foods with balanced pH levels.
4. Reducing the proportion of acidic food we eat may help prevent current and chronic illness. A pH-balanced diet may also be therapeutic in treating other health conditions.
5. Eating a higher percentage of alkaline-forming foods will reduce the need for buffers against acid, which reduces the body's store of these minerals. To protect us from acidosis or alkalosis, our bodies need these buffers.

Once you have confirmed that your pH level is overly acidic, you can start to correct that imbalance by selecting alkalizing foods and avoiding acidifying foods. To satisfy your desire for favorite acidic foods, substitute another alkaline food from the same food group. For variety, try combining any number of alkaline foods. As your health improves and as your diet habits change, your desire for acidic foods may begin to wane.

Did You Know?

Positive Side Effects

By reducing mild to moderate levels of metabolic acidosis, the pH diet may also reduce the risk of hypertension and strokes and improve cardiovascular health, cognition and memory overall. Reducing acidity through a more alkaline diet may also remove built-up toxic waste and improve your body's ability to remove acid as it develops. Restoring pH balance may reduce GI tract symptoms, such as reflux, diarrhea or constipation, pain or bloating. If hormones are again balanced as a result of the pH diet, any issues related to disordered menstruation (cramps, diarrhea) will be reduced as well.

Food Groups

For most diets, the majority of calories come from carbohydrates or fats. To break down these foods, oxygen and insulin must be present, and the byproducts are carbon dioxide (CO_2) and water (H_2O). When the lungs are working properly, the CO_2 is excreted in the breath, with no final impact on the body's acid–base balance.

Breaking down amino acids from proteins can produce acids or, more rarely, alkali, depending on the amino acids. The acids produced are quickly taken up by buffers, and CO_2 is produced. The byproduct from digestion of protein is excreted through the kidneys rather than the lungs. Typically, most fruits and vegetable digestion results in alkali, and the digestion of processed foods, grains, meat or dairy products leads to acids.

Essential Nutrients

Food consists of macronutrients (carbohydrates, fatty acids and proteins) and micronutrients (minerals, vitamins, amino acids and essential fatty acids), and some of these nutrients are considered essential. Essential nutrients are the chemicals necessary for the constant building, maintenance and repair of tissues. Although normal metabolism provides some of the essential nutrients needed for optimum health, not every essential nutrient can be synthesized by our bodies, so some essential fatty acids, amino acids, vitamins and most of the minerals need to be acquired from our food as part of a healthy diet. Each person's requirements for essential nutrients to maintain good health are unique.

RESEARCH SPOTLIGHT

Gut Disruption

The GI tract manages acid–alkaline balance with the movement of hydrogen ions and bicarbonate ions through the gut. When normal gut function is somehow disrupted through GERD, IBS or IBD symptoms, for example, acid–alkaline homeostasis can be upset. The area of the GI tract that is affected and the nature of the fluid loss may determine if a mild form of metabolic acidosis or alkalosis (rarer) will occur. Metabolic acidosis may result in hormonal changes, insulin resistance, protein breakdown and interruption of enzyme activity. Balancing your pH through diet may have some general effects and some effects that are specific to any medical conditions you have — we are each individuals when it comes to the impact of the foods we eat.

Benefits of an Alkaline–Acid Balanced Diet

- Increased consumption of fruits and vegetables improves the potassium to sodium ratio, preventing metabolic acidosis and promoting general good health.
- High concentrations of calcium in your urine help reduce acids. Although theories have posited that calcium loss may affect bone mass, recent research suggests that other factors appear to protect bone calcium levels in the presence of high acid levels.
- High concentrations of nitrogen in your urine from a high-protein diet allow glutamine to bind with acidic hydrogen ions to form ammonium, which, like calcium, is lost to the urine (in the form of amino acids) to reduce acid. Skeletal muscle has the largest stores of glutamine, so muscle breakdown may be a consequence of a high-acid diet. A pH-balanced diet may help preserve the integrity of your muscles.
- Increased growth hormone (GH) production as a result of alkaline supplementation is known to improve outcomes in health conditions such as cardiovascular disease and gastrointestinal conditions (GERD, IBS and IBD). It also improves mental health (memory and cognition).
- Increased intracellular magnesium activates vitamin D, supporting the maintenance of many systems in the body and preventing disease states.
- Reports of the use of alkaline diets for GI conditions attest to improvements of symptoms to the point of being able to reduce medication for some people.

Did You Know?

The Effect of Exercise on pH

Exercise is known to improve health and physical stamina. It also affects homeostasis. When we exercise, our metabolism speeds up and more CO_2 and hydrogen ions are produced in our muscles. We breathe more deeply and quickly to increase the amount of oxygen that is needed to power the sped-up metabolism. If strenuous exercise continues, the needs from the sped-up metabolism exceed the oxygen supply, so other biochemical processes that don't need oxygen are put into action. As a result, lactic acid is produced and enters our bloodstream, increasing overall acid levels.

To Reduce Acid in Your Diet

- Eat plenty of vegetables, fruits, seeds and nuts.
- Avoid excess fats, sugars, refined foods, salt, alcohol, tobacco, coffee and tea.
- Reduce acidic meat and dairy foods to 20% or less of your daily diet.

Part 2

GI Basics and Therapies

Chapter 3

What Are GI Conditions?

CASE STUDY ✍

GERD

Robert is a 56-year-old contractor with a thriving business, a new house he built in the past year and a cottage that he and his two sons, along with other family members, have been working on, hoping to get it built for the summer. He has always liked food, and his wife is a great cook, but lately, dinner has become something he'd rather avoid. A few bites into one of his favorite dishes and he would find himself gasping for air, feeling like he couldn't breathe as a balloon of pain caught him in the lower chest. He would wrap his arms around his large stomach and bend over, trying to catch his breath. Walking a few steps would lighten the pain.

It was always a surprise to him to discover which foods would bring on the pain. Some days, Robert has even passed on his morning coffee, knowing that the terrible burning sensation would follow him through his day. He was finding that he was making errors on job quotes due to his distraction either from the pain or the fear that the pain would start up again. Without breathing a word to his wife, Robert finally made an appointment to see his family physician. His doctor diagnosed him as having gastroesophageal reflux disease, a fairly common diagnosis.

Of all our bodily systems, our gastrointestinal (GI) system is the largest, extending the full length of our torso — from head to tail, so to speak. The GI system protects us from outside attack by bacteria, viruses and other pathogens, and feeds us the nutrients we need to thrive. When the GI system fails, we are subject to illness and disease, ranging in severity from common heartburn to colorectal cancer. Clearly, maintaining GI health should be a priority in our lives. One way of doing so is to eat a nutrient-rich, pH-balanced diet.

The GI Tract

The gastrointestinal system can be seen as a long pipe, or tract, that begins at the mouth and ends at the anus, with separate sections throughout that each have a particular function. Also known as the alimentary canal, this tract allows us to take in many different forms of foods and break them down to capture molecules that can be used by our bodies to build or repair tissue, or as a source of energy to support our bodily movements. Any material that is unable to be digested is expelled.

GI Functional Anatomy

The GI tract has several related anatomical features and functions, some related to pH levels that may require "balancing" to prevent related illness or to treat related illness.

pH Connection: Some people with GI disorders have an increased risk of metabolic acidosis, or high acid levels, because of the loss of bicarbonate from chronic diarrhea — one of the most important buffers for balancing pH in the body. Typically, only a small amount of buffer is lost with the stool every day, but when normal GI function is disrupted, acid–alkaline balance can be overwhelmed, and either metabolic acidosis or alkalosis may be the result. Bicarbonate supplementation, delivered in a hospital setting or under the direction of a health-care professional, is the usual therapy. Side effects of high doses of bicarbonate can be harmful, even fatal.

Mouth

Located below your nose, the mouth takes in food, which is chewed by the teeth, lubricated by saliva and swallowed into the esophagus.

pH Connection: Metabolic acidosis as a result of disrupted gastrointestinal function may affect the alkalinity of the salivary glands in the mouth, which likely has some role in protecting the mouth, throat and esophagus against acids. Possible impacts include cavities, inflammation of the gums, ulcers in the mouth, herpes and cracked corners of the mouth. Increasing fluid and electrolyte intake may help to rebalance pH in the GI system.

GI Tract Anatomy

The gastrointestinal system can be seen as a long pipe, or tract, that begins at the mouth and ends at the anus, with separate sections throughout that each have a particular function.

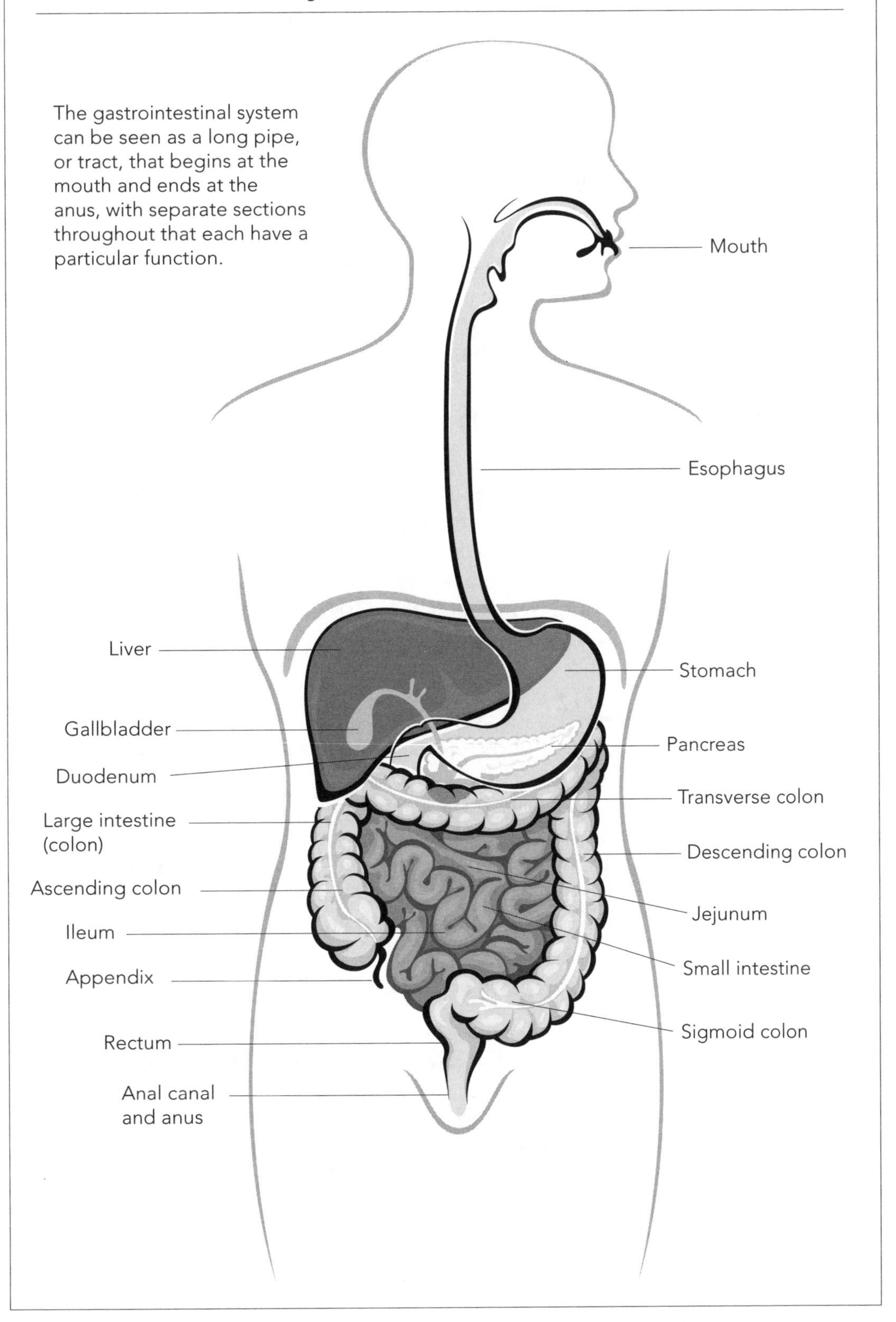

Esophagus

After being swallowed, food and saliva from the mouth are carried down through the esophagus to the stomach by muscle contractions, known as peristalsis.

Diaphragm

Although not strictly part of the GI tract, the diaphragm is a muscle wall that divides the chest area from the abdomen and assists in breathing.

pH Connection: Intense exercise may lead to a mild form of metabolic acidosis for many people. Under these circumstances, the diaphragm muscle appears to become fatigued due to increased and unmanaged carbon dioxide levels in the bloodstream.

Stomach

The stomach begins at the end of the esophagus with the lower esophageal sphincter and empties into the small intestine through the pyloric sphincter.

pH Connection: Cyclic vomiting due to any level of metabolic acidosis may reduce acid levels in the stomach, leading to metabolic alkalosis in that compartment of the GI tract.

Gut

The part of the GI tract between the stomach and small intestines is often called the gut.

pH Connection: Partial or complete blockage in the small intestine, as can be seen in IBD, may cause the loss of alkaline fluids and result in metabolic acidosis. A more acid environment in the gut can lead to fermentation in the gut, causing many health issues and poor digestion.

Pancreas

This long glandular organ is tucked in behind the stomach. The pancreas secretes pancreatic juice into the duodenum to aid absorption, as well as insulin, somatostatin and glucagon into the bloodstream to support other body functions.

pH Connection: Inflammation of the pancreas (pancreatitis) may lead to the breakdown of tissues and metabolic acidosis. Severe pancreatitis leads to nutritional deficiencies and, in some cases, can be fatal.

Liver

This organ is the largest gland in our bodies, with several lobes that make and secrete bile, produce urea and antibodies, synthesize enzymes and change sugars to glycogen. The liver is responsible for storing glycogen, vitamins and some other substances, removing wastes and toxins from the blood, managing blood volume and destroying old blood cells.

Gallbladder

This small organ is located beneath the liver. Bile is made and secreted by the liver and stored in the gallbladder. After a meal, the gallbladder releases bile into the small intestine to break down many foods, especially fats.

pH Connection: Normal pH for bile is around 7.6, which is important for digesting and absorbing fats. Bile also raises the pH in the intestines from the lower pH levels associated with the more acidic stomach area.

Bowel

This term is used collectively to refer to the small and large intestines.

pH Connection: Maintaining a healthy colon and having regular bowel movements are important factors for disease prevention and for removing toxic wastes, which tend to be acidic. The higher the burden of acid buildup, the higher the risk of chronic disease.

Duodenum

The duodenum is the first segment of the small intestine, between the stomach and the jejunum.

pH Connection: Metabolic acidosis has an impact on permeability and ion transport in the intestine cells that transport nutrients.

Jejunum

The jejunum runs from the duodenum to the ileum.

pH Connection: The pH of the inside of the jejunum, if not within a healthy range, may affect the ability of the intestines to absorb amino acids and water, and to recapture electrolytes.

Ileum

This segment of the small intestine runs from the jejunum to the colon.

Large Intestine

Collectively, this is the name for the cecum, the colon and the rectum.

Colon

Also called the large intestine, the average colon is about 5 feet (1.5 m) long and is located between the small intestine and the rectum.

pH Connection: Metabolic acidosis leading to oxidative stress has been identified as a cause of colon cancer. Diet and lifestyle changes are important for reducing cancer risk.

Rectum

This final segment of the large intestine ends at the anus, where the stool is stored until it is excreted.

pH Connection: Normal pH for the rectal fluid is between 7 and 8, slightly alkaline. People with ulcerative colitis were found to have a more acidic surface area (~6.9).

Anus

This sphincter muscle, located at the bottom of the GI tract, expels broken-down foods from which nutrients have been extracted.

pH Connection: Normal pH for the skin surface of the anus of healthy people is around 7.9, slightly alkaline. People with ulcerative colitis have been found to have a more acidic surface area (~6.9).

Kidneys

The two kidneys are lima-bean-shaped organs that sit just above the waistline at the back, one on either side of the spine. The kidneys filter our blood through nephron units, which remove waste products from the blood. The kidneys also regulate fluid, salts and body chemicals, and produce hormones that regulate blood pressure, bone health and red blood cell production.

pH Connection: The kidneys protect blood plasma against extremes in acidity or alkalinity by regulating the ions that shift the pH balance, making bicarbonate and recapturing buffers from the urine. About 7% of the total amount of carbon dioxide in the body is excreted by the kidneys.

Gastrointestinal Functions

The GI tract manages the fundamental functions of digestion, absorption, excretion and secretion.

Digestion

This function involves the combined mechanical and chemical breakdown of food to the three major components — proteins, fats and carbohydrates — that can be absorbed through the intestinal walls. The stomach has several functions. First, it stores food that has been chewed and swallowed, the first step in digestion. Second, the stomach churns the swallowed food (called chyme), mixing it with stomach acids to continue the digestion process. Finally, the stomach releases partially digested foods through the pyloric sphincter to the small intestine for further breakdown.

pH Connection: The stomach has the lowest pH reading of any of the "compartments" of our bodies, with hydrochloric acid being produced in special "crypts" in the stomach walls. A mucus lining protects the stomach walls from being broken down by the acid. In a healthy gut, the hydrochloric acid is confined to the stomach; the acid level is reduced immediately as food is moved to the intestine through the pyloric sphincter at the bottom of the stomach.

Absorption

As part of the digestion process, absorption helps move food molecules across the GI tract wall into the bloodstream.

pH Connection: Most of the nutrients from the food we eat are moved across the wall of the small intestine to the bloodstream. Electrolytes, such as sodium and potassium, in and outside of cells, work with energy pumps to move molecules across the wall barrier. If your electrolytes are out of balance, normal cell activity, including nutrient absorption, may not work properly. Vegetables and fruit are good sources of potassium.

Excretion

Indigestible foods and bacteria are excreted through the colon, rectum and anus. The colon processes alimentary food and bacterial waste into stool, from which water, salts and fat-soluble vitamins are removed. Waste from the colon is moved into

Did You Know?

Peristalsis and Motility

In the digestion process, peristalsis is the involuntary movements of muscles (longitudinal and circular) that help push food through the digestive system. Motility muscles mix contents and move digesting food along the gastrointestinal tract. Abnormal motility or extreme sensitivity in any of the gastrointestinal tract segments may indicate a health issue.

the anus and rectum through the peristalsis process. Excretion (defecation) helps maintain fluid levels and salt balance. Feces is the name used for the expelled waste products.

pH Connection: The typical pH of the colon ranges from 5.5 (mildly acidic) to 7 (neutral). A pH imbalance, antibiotic overuse or inflammation in the colon can lead to yeast or fungal growth. Keeping the prebiotic and probiotic colonies that live in our gut at healthy levels promotes a healthier digestive system overall.

Secretion

About one-sixth of the volume of fluids in the body is secretions from the gastrointestinal tract. Secreted substances (fluid, ions, digestive enzymes and mucus) are produced and then expelled from cells, organs or glands to enable the gastrointestinal tract to function, from food breakdown and digestion to excretion of waste from cells and from the body. Dehydration and electrolyte imbalance are two issues that can occur when secretions are not reabsorbed by the intestines. The release of secretions is stimulated by the presence of food.

pH Connection: The secretions from glands in the mouth, nose, throat and other body cavities are made from a combination of mucins, electrolytes, skin cells, leukocytes, bicarbonate and water. Mucus sticks to interior surfaces, is resistant to digestive enzymes, reduces acid levels and, because of its slippery, jellylike consistency, acts as a buffer between food particles and GI tissue. Mucus secretion is controlled by the enteric nervous system that lines the GI system, but also by messengers from the immune system. All of our interior surfaces (lungs, GI tract, bladder) have a mechanical barrier of mucus (mucous membrane) that is constantly replaced.

The main function of mucus is to protect and lubricate surfaces, but it is also involved in the inflammatory cascade. The mucus in the respiratory system traps small particles to prevent bacteria and other foreign invaders from entering the body, and they are then expelled from the body by sneezing or coughing. Mucus has antibodies that break down bacterial walls, so they can be destroyed, and protects tissue by preventing foreign particles from attaching to the interior walls. When mucous membranes are tacky, more fluid intake is required to overcome mild dehydration. If you have an infection in any tissue with a mucous membrane, inflammation changes the pH of mucus.

The pH of the stomach also changes during and following meals and at some points in digestion. Depending on the diet, the digestive enzyme pepsin may not be activated in a high-pH environment, allowing a higher concentration of bacteria to get to the stomach wall.

GI Secretions

- **Amylase:** Released from salivary glands in the mouth, this digestive enzyme starts the breakdown of carbohydrates. Mucus is released by salivary glands in the mouth to protect and lubricate the GI tract.
- **Bicarbonate ions:** These ions reduce acid levels formed by populations of bacteria.
- **Bile:** This substance is produced in the liver, stored in the gallbladder and released into the duodenum (small intestine) through the bile duct. Bile is slightly alkaline (pH from 7.0 to 7.7) and acts like soap to break down dietary fats.
- **Gastric juices:** These are a mixture of chemicals in the stomach, including the digestive enzymes pepsin and gastric lipase.
- **Gastric lipase:** This digestive enzyme is made in the same cells as pepsin — the chief cells in gastric glands — and breaks down some lipids.
- **Mucus:** This digestive aid is made in mucous cells in the stomach and in goblet cells in the small intestine (as many as one-quarter of the cell walls in the small intestine are goblet cells), and is secreted from the large intestine.
- **Pancreatic juices:** These juices are made up of digestive enzymes that break down every type of nutrient macromolecule: carbohydrates, lipids, proteins and nucleic acids. They include pancreatic amylase, pancreatic lipase, trypsinogen/trypsin, chymotrypsin, carboxypeptidase and nucleases. Three separate enzymes break down the 20 amino acids that build proteins. Bicarbonate is also released into the small intestine from the pancreas as part of pancreatic secretions and bile to reduce acid levels by capturing hydrogen ions to form water and carbon dioxide, which is absorbed into the bloodstream and released through the lungs.
- **Pepsin:** This digestive enzyme is secreted in an inactive form into the stomach by gastric glands. Once in the stomach, it is activated to break down proteins.
- **Peptidases (protein fragments), intestinal lipase (lipids), sucrose (carbohydrate molecules), maltase (carbohydrate molecules) and lactase (carbohydrate molecules):** These digestive enzymes are embedded in the microvilli that line the inside of the intestinal walls.

Did You Know?

Good Bugs, Bad Bugs

In the digestion process, as the stool is moved along the colon, bacteria act on the food debris to produce some important vitamins and necessary enzymes. These "good" bacteria also protect our bodies from harmful bacterial invaders.

Control of the GI System

The GI system is controlled by components of the enteric nervous system and the central nervous system. Like other body systems, the GI system is managed by electrical (nerve) and chemical (hormonal) processes. Nerves operating outside of the GI tract (extrinsic nerves) connect each of the organs along the gastrointestinal tract with the brain through the spinal cord. This nerve network releases chemicals that relax or contract the muscle layer that surrounds the GI tract, based on signals indicating that food is being digested. The action of food stretching the walls of the organs triggers the nerves inside the GI tract (intrinsic nerves). The intrinsic nerves release messenger substances (hormones) from cells along the inside of the GI tract that will increase or reduce the speed of the movement, or motility, of food through the GI tract, as well as the production and secretion of digestive juices in each GI compartment.

Nervous Systems

Central nervous system

Peripheral nervous system

- Somatic nervous system
- Autonomic nervous system
  - Sympathetic nervous system
  - Parasympathetic nervous system
  - Enteric nervous system

Central Nervous System (CNS)

Composed of the brain and spinal cord, the CNS integrates sensory information and provides feedback and situation-appropriate responses.

Peripheral Nervous System (PNS)

This system includes all the nerves outside of the brain and spinal cord. There are two subcategories of the peripheral nervous system: somatic (sensory) and autonomous.

Somatic Nervous System

Made up of any peripheral nerves involved in sending sensory-related information to the central nervous system, the somatic system includes the motor nerves that send information from the CNS to the skeletal muscles to initiate movement. Two networks, or plexuses, of nerve cells (neurons) are embedded in and run the full length of the wall of the GI tract. The myenteric plexus controls the motility of the GI tract, while the submucous plexus manages GI blood flow and epithelial cell function. Lesser plexuses are embedded within the circular smooth muscle, as well as in the mucosa. Sensory, motor and interneurons are part of the plexus networks, with more than five different kinds of sensory receptors in the mucosa for thermal, chemical, mechanical and osmotic information, and in the muscle to register stretch and tension. Receptors that are sensitive to glucose, acids and amino acids (chemoreceptors) relay information about gut contents. Motor nerve cells or neurons manage secretion and motility. Interneuron cells manage information from the sensory nerve cells to send back to the enteric nervous system.

Autonomic Nervous System (ANS)

This system manages the control of all muscles involved in internal organs (called viscera) and glands. The ANS is further broken down into three categories: sympathetic, parasympathetic and enteric.

Sympathetic Nervous System (SNS)

The sympathetic nervous system is responsible for managing our fight-or-flight response, an automatic, all-system reaction we go through when responding to an emergency. The reaction includes expansion of the pupils of the eyes, increased blood pressure and heart rate, and a slow-down of systems that are not essential to handling an emergency, including the digestive system. Specifically, the SNS communicates with the CNS, inhibits secretion or motor activity in the GI tract, and slows down or stops the movement of food by contracting blood vessels and sphincters along the GI tract, such as the lower esophageal sphincter and the pyloric sphincter.

Did You Know?

Disease or Syndrome?

Conditions with symptoms that affect several organs or body systems are called syndromes, and those with symptoms that affect a single organ or system are called diseases. IBS is a syndrome, but IBD is a disease.

Parasympathetic Nervous System (PNS)

This network of nerve cells has the opposite responsibility of the sympathetic nervous system: it manages the "rest and relax" response, in which the pupils constrict, the heartbeat slows down, blood vessels dilate and blood pressure drops. The PNS also regulates glandular functions (tears and saliva, for example) and, when it comes to the digestive systems, communicates with the CNS, stimulates secretion or motor activity in the GI tract, and begins or speeds up the movement of food by expanding blood vessels and sphincters along the GI tract.

Enteric Nervous System

Called the second brain, this mesh-like network of nerve cells lines the GI system, producing "gut feelings" or "butterflies" about challenging situations and affecting the movement of foods through the digestive system. The enteric neurons are responsible for secreting neurotransmitters, messengers that stimulate or inhibit digestion (while intense exercise is occurring, for example).

GI Diseases and Syndromes

The GI tract is prone to a wide range of medical conditions, listed alphabetically in the chart that follows. Among the various GI diseases and syndromes, three are the most common, arguably the most serious and the most closely connected to pH indications:

- GER and GERD
- IBS
- IBD (Crohn's disease and ulcerative colitis)

These three conditions, discussed in detail starting on page 54, are the focus of this book.

Medical Conditions of the GI Tract

Condition	Symptoms
Bloating	The feeling or actual symptom of having a swollen or distended abdomen; can be painful.
Constipation	Difficulties in having bowel movements, most often with associated hardened feces.
Cramps	Painful and involuntary contraction of abdominal muscles, often associated with a need to have a bowel movement or with menstrual periods, and sometimes both.
Diarrhea	Loose or watery feces expelled from the bowels more frequently than is typical. Often accompanied by cramps. Can be caused by food, stress, medication or a medical condition.
Distension	The process of expansion forced by pressure from the inside (typically associated with bloating).
Dyspepsia	Pain or discomfort in the stomach or upper abdomen; also called indigestion or upset stomach.
Dysphagia	Ranges from discomfort or difficulty when swallowing to not being able to swallow at all, thus taking longer and having to work harder to swallow food.
Gastroesophageal reflux (GER), gastroesophageal reflux disease (GERD)	A digestive disorder affecting the ring of muscle between the esophagus and the stomach, called the lower esophageal sphincter (LES). Heartburn and acid indigestion are two symptoms of GERD, which may be caused by a hiatal hernia.
Heartburn: Pyrosis, cardialgia, acid indigestion	A burning sensation in the chest, behind the breastbone and in the upper central abdomen (epigastrium). Pain is often felt in the chest and from there moves outward to the throat, neck or angle of the jaw.
Hiatal hernia	Protrusion of part of the stomach into the chest through an opening in the diaphragm, which may be caused by weaker supporting tissue, such as with people over 50 years old. A congenital version also exists.
Indigestion: Dyspepsia, heartburn, hyperacidity, stomachache	Discomfort or pain in the stomach area, typically associated with problems with the digestion of food.
Inflammatory bowel disease (IBD): Crohn's disease, ulcerative colitis	Recurring or chronic conditions with immune response and inflammation in the gastrointestinal tract.
Irritable bowel syndrome (IBS): Spastic colon	A collection of chronic symptoms, including abdominal pain, bloating, discomfort and a shift in bowel habits, with no known cause.

How Healthy Is Your Gastrointestinal System?

1. Do you have a dry cough that doesn't go away? YES or NO
2. Do you "wheeze"? YES or NO
3. Do you have asthma or recurrent pneumonia? YES or NO
4. Do you frequently feel sick to your stomach (nauseated) for no reason? YES or NO
5. Do you often throw up for no reason? YES or NO
6. Do you often have a sore throat, are you often hoarse, or do you frequently have laryngitis? YES or NO
7. Do you have problems swallowing or is swallowing painful? YES or NO
8. Do you have pain in your chest or abdomen? YES or NO
9. Are your teeth worn down and do you have bad breath? YES or NO
10. Do you have bowel movements more than 3 times per day? YES or NO
11. Do you have fewer than 1 bowel movement per day? YES or NO
12. Are your bowel movements watery or mushy, or hard and lumpy? YES or NO
13. Do you have abdominal pain? YES or NO
14. Does your abdominal pain stop when you have a bowel movement? YES or NO
15. Do you have diarrhea 3 or more times a day? YES or NO
16. Do you often feel that you're not "finished" with a bowel movement? YES or NO
17. Do you pass mucus with your bowel movement? YES or NO
18. Do you suffer from bloating? YES or NO
19. Do you have rectal bleeding? YES or NO
20. Have you lost weight (a significant amount) even though you are not trying? YES or NO
21. Do you have a fever with no known cause? YES or NO
22. Do you have anemia? YES or NO

Take this completed questionnaire to your next appointment to discuss your symptoms with your health-care provider.

Special Clinical Tests for GI Conditions

Several special tests may be used in the diagnostic workup of a gastrointestinal disorder.

- **Colonoscopy:** Designed to examine or assess the inside of the colon and rectum. Typically done to test for colon cancer symptoms or evaluate GI symptoms (abdominal pain, changes in bowel movements or rectal or abdominal bleeding).
- **Endoscopy:** Uses a thin, flexible tube with a light and a small camera at its tip to examine part of the body's interior, in this case the esophagus.
- **Gastroscopy:** Also called upper gastrointestinal endoscopy or esophagogastroduodenoscopy. An endoscope is inserted into the mouth to assess the esophagus, stomach and duodenum.
- **CT scans:** Used to detect tumors and abscesses.

Endoscopy

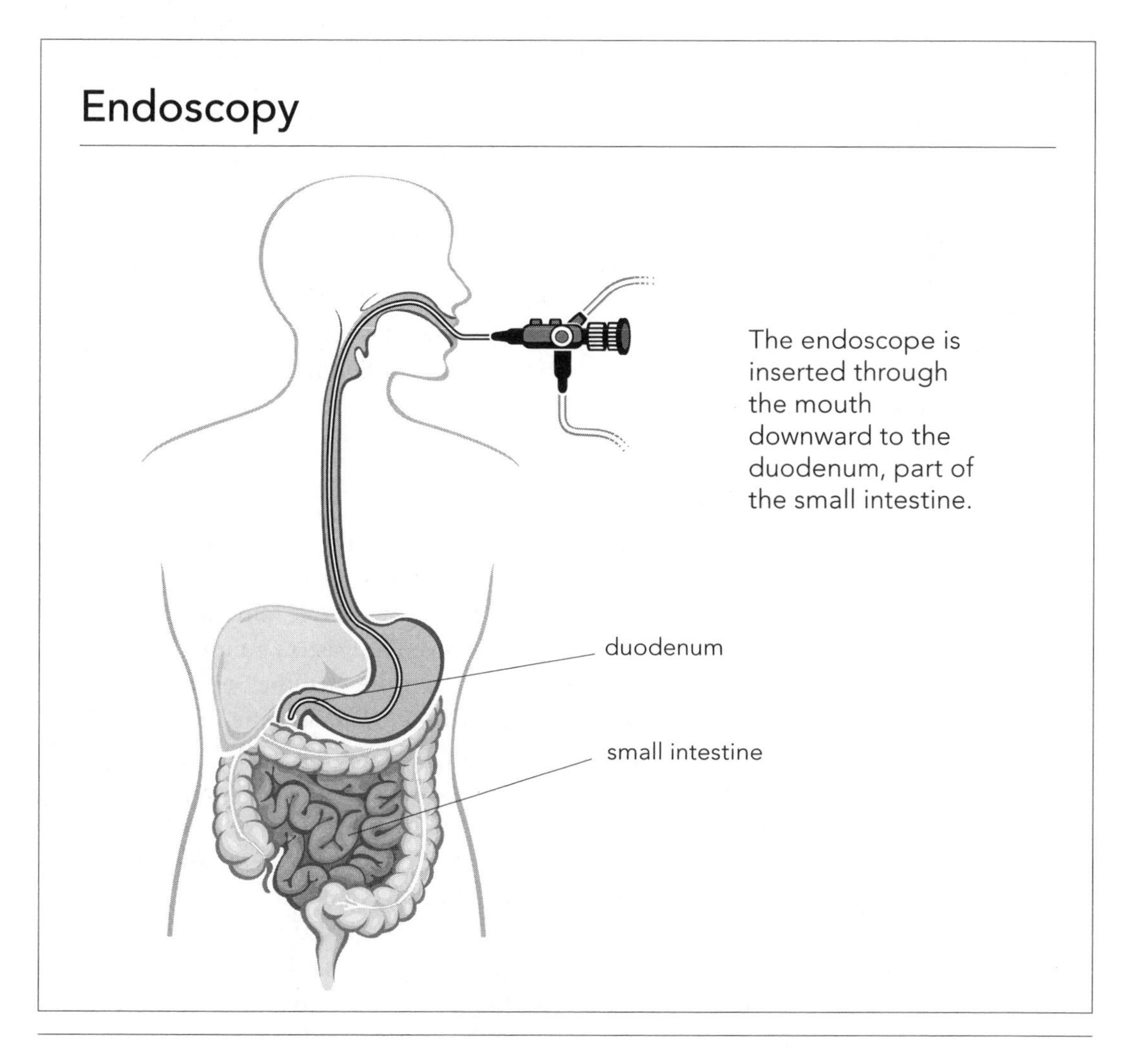

The endoscope is inserted through the mouth downward to the duodenum, part of the small intestine.

- **Ultrasound:** Designed to detect masses.
- **Radionucleotide imaging:** Used to find areas of increased or decreased metabolic activity, which is helpful in identifying tumors.
- **Barium X-rays:** Used to detect defects, strictures and tumors in the gut.
- **Urinary tests**: Indicate excess absorption of bowel toxins.
- **Scoping:** Used to view the interior of the GI tract and remove tissue samples to be tested. The tests most often conducted are the sigmoidoscopy, the gastroscopy, which is an upper endoscopy, and the colonoscopy.
- **Sigmoidoscopy:** Allows examination of the sigmoid colon through a flexible tube inserted into the anus.

Did You Know?

Medical Care

If you experience GER more than twice a week for a few weeks, this could indicate something more serious that could lead to other health problems if left untreated. If you suspect you may have GERD, discuss your concerns and symptoms with your health-care provider.

GER

Gastroesophageal reflux (GER), also called heartburn, acid regurgitation and acid reflux, occurs when the contents of your stomach, along with some digestive juices, move up into your esophagus. This stomach acid may leave a bad taste in the back of your mouth and cause a burning sensation. When the acid touches the esophagus lining, which is not protected by mucus, heartburn or acid indigestion may result. Most people experience GER at some point in their lives.

pH Connection: Often seen in babies under 2 years old, GER may be caused by milk curdling in the GI tract, which in itself could have an impact on the pH levels and prevent the digestive enzyme pepsin from being able to break down proteins. Regurgitation of the curdled milk and stomach acid could follow.

GERD

Gastroesophageal reflux disease (GERD) is a more serious long-term or chronic form of GER where the esophagus is affected by irritation and inflammation, leading to reflux of gastric acid into the esophagus. The gastric contents consist mostly of hydrochloric acid and the enzyme pepsin, which back up, or are refluxed, into the esophagus frequently or in an overwhelming amount. The pain of GERD can also be felt when the refluxed gastric acid prevents esophageal contractions from moving the contents to the stomach.

A more severe form of GERD is due to the esophageal lining becoming inflamed and ulcerated.

pH Connection: In a study published in the *Annals of Otology, Rhinology and Laryngology*, a small group of patients with reflux who did not respond to typical medication (proton pump inhibitors, or PPIs) found that a low-acid diet improved symptoms of gastroesophageal acid reflux.

Signs and Symptoms of GERD

If you have heartburn on a regular basis, you may have GERD, although some people who have been diagnosed with GERD do not experience heartburn. The most common symptoms are vomiting and difficulties with swallowing.

- Vomiting
- Difficulty swallowing
- Nausea
- Wheezing
- Dry, chronic coughing
- Sore throat and hoarse voice from irritation and swelling of the voice box
- Asthma and recurring pneumonia
- Bad breath and erosion of tooth enamel
- Chest pain
- Pain in the upper abdomen

Causes of GERD

GERD is a multifactorial condition with several possible causes.

- **Stomach acid excess or deficiency:** When acid is overproduced (often caused by *Heliobacter pylori* infection, alcohol, spicy foods or coffee), the risk for reflux is increased. If, however, stomach acid is underproduced, the process of emptying the stomach can be prolonged, leading to longer periods of churning in the stomach and possibly irritating the stomach walls and causing GERD symptoms.
- **Digestive enzyme deficiency:** Some people may not produce enough digestive enzymes, and this may be responsible for causing GERD symptoms.
- **Toxins:** Exposures to environmental toxins or food allergies, intolerances or sensitivities can also be factors.
- **Dysfunctional LES:** The lower esophageal sphincter (LES), which is the muscle or valve between the esophagus and the stomach, may become weak or fail to function properly, becoming relaxed and open in a way that allows movement of stomach contents at inappropriate times.
- **Hiatal hernia:** This happens when the upper part of the stomach pushes through the esophageal opening in the diaphragm into the chest area. Some people with hiatal hernias have GERD, but others have no symptoms at all.

Did You Know?

Disease Burden

Worldwide, it appears that the burden of GERD is increasing, with South Asia as the only region with fewer than 10% of the population affected. A 2012 systematic review reports that since 1995, a significant increase has been reported, especially in North America and East Asia.

- **Other factors:** These include pregnancy, smoking and exposure to secondhand smoke, medications (asthma medications, antihistamines, painkillers, calcium channel blockers, antidepressants and sedatives) and obesity.

Complications of GERD

If you think you may have GERD, see your health-care provider. Left untreated for a long time, GERD may cause more serious health conditions.

- Respiratory problems (trouble breathing).
- The muscles around the esophagus may tighten up (called strictures) and cause problems with swallowing.
- If the stomach acid has backed up into the esophagus, the esophagus lining could be damaged and cause bleeding or ulcers. For some adults who have long-term chronic esophagitis, precancerous changes in the esophagus may develop.
- Over time, the tissues that line the esophagus may become the same type as the intestine lining, a condition called Barrett's esophagus. For a small group of people who have Barrett's esophagus, the condition may develop into cancer of the esophagus (rare, but often fatal).

Who's at Risk?

People who are most at risk for GERD include infants and children, pregnant women and older people. GERD typically begins before the age of 30, and happens more often to women than to men. In Canada, five million people have heartburn or acid reflux once a week or more. In the United States, approximately seven million people have some symptoms of GERD. GERD is now known to be common in infants and children, with such symptoms as repeated vomiting, coughing and other respiratory issues or failure to thrive.

Region	Percentage of Population with GERD
North America	18.1% to 27.8%
Europe	8.8% to 25.9%
East Asia	2.5% to 7.8%
Middle East	8.7% to 33.1%
Australia	11.6%
South America	23.0%

Diagnosing GERD

If you are experiencing ongoing heartburn or acid reflux that occurs on a regular basis, or find that you are taking antacids frequently without seeing any relief, seek medical advice.

pH Connection: Mild metabolic acidosis may have an impact on the symptom severity of GERD and may also be a side effect of medication therapies, such as proton pump inhibitors (PPIs). It can also be worsened by the symptoms of IBD. Some GERD symptoms that may increase mild metabolic acidosis include increased acid production; acid indigestion; decreased ability of the kidneys to maintain acid balance, leading to a decrease in kidney acid excretion (because of lack of buffers); and loss of bicarbonate from the gastrointestinal tract and kidneys, which would set up a cycle of ever-increasing acidity.

Physical Examination and Medical History

When you visit your physician, you will likely be given a complete physical examination, and a comprehensive medical history will be taken, including any family history of gastrointestinal disease or colon cancer. Before your visit to your physician, it may help to write down details of your family's health history; if possible, contact relatives for details.

Measuring Acid Levels

GERD can be diagnosed by measuring levels of stomach acid, pH and betaine hydrochloride.

1. **Stomach acid levels:** Measure after a typical meal.
2. **pH sensitivity:** Measure fasting stomach pH after a stand challenge (a pH sensitivity telemetry capsule or gastro test). Better tolerated but may not be as sensitive, reliable or accurate.
3. **Betaine hydrochloride:** Supplementing with betaine hydrochloride with meals and monitoring symptoms provides indirect evaluations. Deficiency is suspected if symptoms improve; if symptoms are worse, then either excessive or normal stomach acid is indicated.

Source: Adapted with permission from El-Hashemy S, Downorowicz E, Rouchotas P, et al. *Family Medicine & Integrative Primary Care: Standards & Guidelines.* Toronto: CCNM Press, 2011. Gastroenterology, gastroesophageal reflux disease; p. 133–35.

Standard Tests for GERD

Test	Action	Possible Side Effects
Upper GI series Conducted at a hospital or outpatient center by an X-ray technician and explained by a radiologist (a physician who has specialist training in medical images).	Shows shape of the upper GI tract. A barium solution is inserted into the esophagus. The chalky barium that the patient is asked to swallow just before the test coats the esophagus, stomach and small intestine, allowing the health-care providers to see any physical issues that would explain symptoms such as a hiatal hernia or stricture (narrowing) of the esophagus, ulcers or sores that may result from GERD. Mild irritation will not show up.	A few days following the test, you may experience nausea and bloating, as well as light or white stools.
Upper endoscopy (esophagogastroduodenoscopy, EGD) Performed at an outpatient center or hospital using a scope. The tissue removed will be examined by a specialist (called a pathologist) who focuses on diagnosing disease. GERD is diagnosed if moderate to severe GERD symptoms have resulted in injury to the esophagus.	Assesses severity of GERD. A small, flexible, end-lit tube is inserted down the throat to view the upper GI tract and a biopsy taken of esophageal tissues. In some cases, sedation is delivered intravenously, and a liquid anesthetic may be sprayed or gargled to reduce any sensation in the back of your throat. Eating and drinking are not permitted for 8 hours before this test. Any over-the-counter medications should be stopped 7 days before the test. If you smoke, no smoking is permitted from midnight of the night before the procedure. Be sure to advise your physician of any health conditions or medications that may affect the procedure.	Effects from the medication given for this procedure usually wear off within an hour. You should not drive a car after this procedure. For the next 24 hours, some people experience a sore throat, bloating or cramping. You will be given instructions about how soon you may resume your normal eating and drinking activities. Contact your physician if you experience: • Trouble swallowing • Throat, belly or chest pain that continues to get worse • Vomiting • Blood in bowel movements (black stools have blood in them) • Fever
Esophageal pH monitoring This is the most accurate way to assess acid reflux. Conducted at a hospital or outpatient center. *(continued...)*	Measures liquid or acid present in the esophagus during daily activities, even while eating and sleeping. Sedation is used if required. A thin tube (nasogastric probe) that measures liquid or acid in the esophagus is inserted through *(continued...)*	Mild discomfort may occur at the back of the throat during the test, especially while swallowing. For most people, the test does not interfere with daily activities. *(continued...)*

Test	Action	Possible Side Effects
Esophageal pH monitoring *(continued)* A diet diary is helpful to assess any relationships between foods, times of day and symptoms. Any respiratory symptoms that may be triggered by acid reflux are also monitored by this procedure.	the nose or mouth, down the throat and esophagus, to the stomach. The tube is then pulled back into the esophagus and the tube taped to your cheek. Captured measurements are transmitted to a monitor attached to the end of the probe outside your body.	Some discomfort may be felt in the chest due to the capsule placement.
Esophageal manometry Performed in your doctor's office. Other disorders of the esophagus can be diagnosed using this method as well.	Measures esophageal muscle contractions and is often used to assess whether anti-reflux surgery is required. Anesthetic spray may be applied on the inside of your nostrils or in the back of your throat. A thin, soft tube will then be passed through your nose down into your stomach. You will be asked to swallow as the tube is pulled very slowly back into the esophagus from your stomach. To detect weak sphincter muscles, a computer measures and records muscle contraction along the esophagus through pressure on the tube.	For most people, this test does not affect regular activities, eating or medications, even immediately after the test.

Criteria for a GERD Diagnosis

1. Troublesome symptoms that affect the patient's quality of life, ranging from heartburn and reflux to severe damage to the esophagus and including associated complications, such as malignancy or airway-related disease.
2. Endoscopic visualization of any break in the mucosal tissue showing a damaged area that clearly stands out from the surrounding healthy tissue.
3. Peptic stricture, with malignancy having been ruled out through several biopsies.
4. Microscopic images of tissue showing evidence of Barrett's esophagus in damaged cells from the lower area of the esophagus, where the lining appears to be similar to the stomach lining.

Irritable Bowel Syndrome

Irritable bowel syndrome (IBS) is a common episodic gastrointestinal illness that involves severe abdominal pain and irregular bowel patterns as the result of problems with the movement of digested food through our intestines. IBS has mental and physical causes but is definitely not imagined. Other names that have been used for IBS include nervous colon, colitis, spastic colon and mucus colitis. Symptoms are described as being chronic and intermittent, going on for months to years. Although people who have IBS do have symptoms frequently, the GI system itself is not damaged. Since IBS symptoms occur because of changes in the way the GI tract works, it is called a functional gastrointestinal disorder. No physical abnormalities are found in patients complaining of IBS.

Bowel symptoms are often associated with the menstrual cycle for younger women, often involving more pain before and more diarrhea during menstrual cycles. When children under the age of 5 have IBS, they often have diarrhea with no pain. The most common symptom of IBS for men is diarrhea.

pH Connection: Mild metabolic acidosis may have an impact on the symptom severity of IBS and may also be a side effect of medication therapies, such as proton pump inhibitors (PPIs). It can also be exacerbated by the symptoms of IBS. Some IBS symptoms that may increase metabolic acidosis include increased acid production; acid indigestion; decreased ability of the kidneys to maintain acid balance, leading to a decrease in kidney acid excretion (because of lack of buffers); and loss of bicarbonate from the gastrointestinal tract and kidneys, which would set up a cycle of ever-increasing acidity. Health issues, such as diarrhea, which is associated with the loss of bicarbonate from the GI tract, may also lead to metabolic acidosis and affect pH.

Classifications of IBS

- IBS is classified as **IBS-C** when constipation is the main feature.
- IBS is classified as **IBS-D** when diarrhea is the main feature.
- IBS is classified as **IBS-A** when the two symptoms alternate.
- IBS is classified as **IBS-PI** when IBS begins after a bout of infection (post-infection).
- Another form of IBS is pain-predominant. Stress can also cause IBS.

Co-Existing Medical Conditions

Some people who are diagnosed with IBS have other GI-related medical conditions, such as GERD or dyspepsia. Other medical conditions that people with IBS are sometimes diagnosed with include:

- Chronic fatigue syndrome: tiredness that lasts a long time and limits ordinary daily activity
- Chronic pelvic pain
- Temporomandibular joint disorders: problems with the muscles responsible for chewing and the joints that connect the lower jaw and skull
- Depression
- Anxiety somatoform disorders: chronic pain and other symptoms with no known physical cause, thought to be due to psychological issues

Signs and Symptoms of IBS

IBS affects each person differently and cannot be cured. The most common symptoms are cramps and changes in bowel movements. Other known symptoms include:

- Abdominal bloating
- Constipation or diarrhea, or swinging from one condition to the other
- Mucus in or around stools
- Ribbonlike stools
- Immediate need to move your bowels on waking, or during or after meals
- Feeling of incomplete emptying after bowel movements
- Nausea or heartburn
- Rectal pain
- Loss of appetite
- Fatigue
- Depression
- Anxiety
- Headache
- Backache
- Difficulty concentrating

FAQ

Q. Is there a cure for IBS?

A. As yet, there is no single cure for IBS and the cause (or causes) is not known.

Causes of IBS

IBS is one of the most common complaints seen by family physicians. If an examination is done, no physical or biochemical reason can be found to explain the symptoms of IBS. Some medical experts suspect the brain of causing the condition, and others maintain that a lack or abnormal population of gut bacteria or flora is the cause of inflammation and problematic bowel function. Still others suggest that genetic or environmental factors, perhaps combined during the pre- or postnatal period, may cause changes in motor activity or increased sensitivity to function. These changes may lead to changes in the usual colonies of bacteria that live in our gut or may increase inflammation. In turn, any of these changes may negatively affect the quality of life of a person with IBS symptoms.

Main Known Factors

- Genes that increase susceptibility to IBS
- Dysfunction of the gut barrier that prevents undigested foods from getting into the bloodstream
- Problems with the immune system
- Bacterial and viral infections
- Environmental factors

Possible Contributing Factors

- Increased activity by the sympathetic nervous system
- Problems with the populations of bacteria that live in the gut
- Faulty digestion
- Excess consumption of proteins or sugars

Who's at Risk?

Research indicates that IBS affects 1 out of 10 people around the world (3% to 20% of the adult population, with only 5% to 7% diagnosed). In North America alone, 32 million Americans and 4 million Canadians are affected and IBS is the reason for 20% to 50% of visits to gastroenterologists in the United States.

Most of the time, IBS happens to people under the age of 45. Twice as many women as men get IBS, and they are more likely to suffer from pain, bloating and constipation. As children, boys and girls are diagnosed with IBS in equal numbers and have similar patterns of symptoms as adults. Symptoms may first appear after a stressful event (teething, flu, emotional stress). Knowing that IBS does not progress to Crohn's disease, ulcerative colitis or colon cancer is some comfort.

FAQ

Q. How can IBS symptoms be managed?

A. Symptoms can be alleviated through a combination of therapies. If your health-care provider has recommended lifestyle changes that have not resolved your IBS symptoms, medications may be prescribed for specific symptoms.

Diagnosing IBS

Visit your health-care provider if you have had pain or discomfort in your abdomen or changes in your bowel movements for more than 6 months and/or if you have had events more than 3 times per month over the last 3 months.

Diagnostic Criteria

At least two of the three following cardinal symptoms must be present to meet the diagnostic criteria for IBS:

1. More or less frequent bowel movements than is usual.
2. More watery, less solid stool than is usual or lumpier and harder stool than is usual.
3. Pain stops as soon as the stool is passed.

Diagnostic Procedures

A comprehensive physical exam and medical history will be taken, including:

- Rectal exam to assess for blood in the stool
- Record of family history of gastrointestinal disorders and any recent infections
- Record of medications being taken or recently taken before or during the time of your symptoms
- Record of stress that may be before or at the time the symptoms started

At this point, your health-care provider may conduct blood tests to rule out other possible health issues. These may include tests for:

- Anemia (low levels of red blood cells in the blood, which leads to low oxygen levels)
- Celiac disease
- Colon cancer
- Unexpected weight loss
- Rectal bleeding
- Unexplained fever

Standard Tests for IBS

Test	Action	Side Effects
Stool test Your health-care provider will give you a sealed package that includes step-by-step instructions and the kit necessary for catching and storing a small stool sample, along with instructions on where to return it.	Your stool sample will be analyzed at a laboratory. The analysis will include tests for parasites or blood in the stool.	None.
Lower GI series An X-ray technician, usually located in a hospital or at an outpatient center, will perform an X-ray and the results will be analyzed by a doctor with a specialty in medical imaging, called a radiologist.	X-ray to examine your large intestine. You may be given instructions to prepare your bowels for the test, such as following a clear diet for up to 3 days, or you may be given a laxative to soften the stool and speed up bowel movements — or even an enema (a squirt bottle or tube inserted into the anus flushes the lower intestine with water or a laxative). Barium is used to fill the large intestine, administered through a flexible tube inserted into the anus as you lie on a table. The barium helps expose any damage or health issues on the X-ray.	Enemas and loose, frequent bowel movements may lead to anal soreness. As the last traces of barium are excreted from the large intestine, the stools may be light-colored or even white. Your health-care provider will give you instructions about what to eat after the test.
Colonoscopy A gastroenterologist will perform the test at a hospital, outpatient center or clinic.	Test to view the rectum and full length of the colon. You may be asked to follow a clear diet for up to 3 days before the test, or you may be given a laxative or one or more enemas the night before. As well, enemas may be done a few hours beforehand to fully empty the colon. To help you relax and reduce any pain that may be experienced during this test, low levels of anesthesia and, in some cases, pain medication may be given. *(continued...)*	Cramps and possible bleeding for an hour or so after the procedure Risks include: • Bleeding • Hole or tear (called perforation) in the colon lining • Diverticulitis: small pouches in colon become irritated, swollen and infected. *(continued...)*

Test	Action	Side Effects
Colonoscopy (continued)	A flexible tube with a small camera and light on the end is inserted into the anus and a video of the intestinal lining is transmitted to a computer monitor screen, where it is analyzed for any problems in the lower GI tract, such as irritated and swollen tissue, ulcers or polyps (extra bits of tissue growing on the lining of the intestine). In some cases, the gastroenterologist may remove a small piece of intestinal lining that will be examined by a pathologist in a laboratory (called a biopsy). Driving a vehicle is not allowed for 24 hours following a colonoscopy.	Risks include: • Cardiovascular events: heart attack, low blood pressure, heart skipping beats or beating fast or slow • Severe abdominal pain • Death (rare)
Flexible sigmoidoscopy Similar to a colonoscopy.	Test to view the rectum and lower colon only. In some cases, you may be asked to follow a clear diet for up to 3 days before the test. You may be given a laxative or one or more enemas the night before. One or more enemas (water, laxative or mild soap solution flushed into the anus) are given about 2 hours before the procedure. A flexible, lighted tube is inserted into the anus and the scope inflates the colon with air for better viewing. A small camera mounted on the end of the scope transmits a video to a computer monitor screen. Biopsies may be taken during a flexible sigmoidoscopy. Driving a vehicle is not allowed for 24 hours following a flexible sigmoidoscopy. Discharge instructions should be closely followed.	After the tests, some cramping or bloating may occur for an hour or so. Risks include bleeding or punctures in the large intestine.

Did You Know?

IBD Management

Managing inflammatory bowel disease can be challenging because the cause is still not known. Infectious agents have been suggested, but more research needs to be done. For clinical purposes, any factor that initiates the inflammatory process needs to be identified and eliminated. Newer research has suggested that immune system factors that become sensitized to bacteria or other foreign invaders may damage the intestinal wall. A drug (cyclosporine) that reduces the activity of the specific immune system factor thought to be involved — T cells — has successfully reduced inflammation due to Crohn's disease.

Inflammatory Bowel Disease

Two conditions fall under the heading of inflammatory bowel disease (IBD): inflammation (called Crohn's disease), which causes redness and swelling; and ulceration (called ulcerative colitis), which causes sores or ulcers and sometimes holes right through the large or small intestines. Although Crohn's disease and ulcerative colitis appear to be different, the two GI conditions have many features in common. Five million people around the world have Crohn's disease and ulcerative colitis.

pH Connection: Mild metabolic acidosis may have an impact on the symptom severity of IBD and may also be a side effect of medication therapies, such as proton pump inhibitors (PPIs). It can also be exacerbated by the symptoms of IBD. Some IBD symptoms that may increase metabolic acidosis include diarrhea, with an associated decreased ability of the kidneys to maintain acid balance, leading to a decrease in acid excretion (because of lack of buffers), and loss of bicarbonate from the gastrointestinal tract and kidneys, which would set up a cycle of ever-increasing acidity. Health issues associated with the loss of bicarbonate from the GI tract may also lead to all levels of metabolic acidosis that affect pH levels in cases of colostomy, ileostomy, diarrhea or enteric fistulas (abnormal openings along the GI tract).

Crohn's Disease

Crohn's disease, also called ileitis or enteritis and at one time regional ileitis, may cause swelling, inflammation or irritation to any part of the GI tract — from the mouth through to the anus. The large and small intestine are most commonly affected, with the final segment of the small intestine (the ileum) the primary site. Symptoms shared with ulcerative colitis include diarrhea and abdominal pain.

Signs and Symptoms of Crohn's Disease

When inflammation is present, in some cases it may cut deeply into the intestine lining. If the inflammation is chronic, scar tissue may lead to a stricture being formed where the intestine walls are permanently pinched, slowing the movement of digested food or waste. Symptoms include:

- Nausea
- Diarrhea
- Abdominal pain, tenderness and cramping, often after meals
- General feeling of illness
- Fever
- Bloody stool
- Loss of appetite, sometimes leading to weight loss

- Irritation or swelling around the rectum
- Eye inflammation
- Difficulty concentrating
- Anxiety
- Depression
- Fatigue
- Canker-like sores in the mouth
- Possible delay in growth and sexual development in younger teens due to lack of nutrition

Causes of Crohn's Disease

Currently, the root cause of Crohn's is not known, but research is pointing to the immune system as the culprit, reacting inappropriately to foods, harmless bacteria or other molecules in our bodies rather than identifying, attacking and destroying harmful invaders like bacteria, viruses or other foreign substances. The normal immune system process brings white blood cells to the area under attack by foreign invaders. In Crohn's disease, when these white blood cells collect in the bowel walls, chronic inflammation results and may cause damage to the region, such as ulcers or sores.

Complications of Crohn's Disease

- Delayed growth for children
- Weight loss
- Nutrient deficiencies from the inability of the intestines to absorb nutrients
- Restless leg syndrome (disturbing leg discomfort when sitting or lying down)
- Arthritis
- Skin problems
- Weakness of the bones (which may be caused by the use of steroids as therapy for Crohn's disease)
- Liver function–related disease
- Decreased energy (anemia)
- Intestinal obstruction from narrowing or strictures
- Fistulas (openings from the interior of the large to the small intestine, the bladder or the anus, causing infection)
- Gallstones
- For some people, stress may cause inflammation flare-ups
- Kidney stones
- Inflammation in the eyes
- Canker sores (oral aphthous lesions)

Who's at Risk?

Crohn's disease often (90% of the time) starts in adolescence and the 20s, with women and men, girls and boys being equally affected. There appears to be a genetic component, since some form of IBD is also generally present in near relatives. Smoking increases the risk of getting Crohn's. A Jewish heritage also increases the chance of getting Crohn's, and an African-American heritage reduces the risk.

Did You Know?

Stress

Although stress does not cause UC, the daily trials of having this disease may be responsible for symptoms becoming worse. Specific sensitivities to foods and food products also do not cause UC but may act as a trigger for symptoms.

Ulcerative Colitis

Although ulcerative colitis (UC) is also an inflammation of the GI tract, it is different from Crohn's disease in many ways. If you are diagnosed with ulcerative colitis, your condition will not resolve quickly. For some people, ulcerative colitis is mild and may only flare up a few times, but UC is more often a long-term or chronic condition. The inflammation and ulcers from UC usually affect the lining of the large intestine (colon and rectum). Ulcerative colitis may impair the function of the large colon, which is absorbing water from the stool as it moves along and changing it from a liquid to a solid. In the more serious cases, a part of the colon may be removed.

People diagnosed with ulcerative colitis have abnormal immune system function. Some genetic factor is also involved.

Signs and Symptoms of Ulcerative Colitis

Most people with UC have mild to moderate symptoms, but around 10% have more severe symptoms, which may include:

- Bloody diarrhea
- Nausea
- Severe abdominal cramps
- Frequent fevers
- Joint pain
- Eye irritation
- Kidney stones
- Liver disease
- Osteoporosis (possibly the result of immune system–triggered general inflammation)
- Constant need to have a bowel movement
- Lesions in the mucus inner layer of the large colon and rectum, with lesions along the length
- Blood or pus in the stool
- Anemia
- Loss of appetite
- Weight loss
- Rectal bleeding
- Loss of nutrients and body fluids
- Skin lesions
- pH imbalance (as a result of other symptoms)

For children

- Failure to grow
- 10% also have symptoms of Crohn's disease
- Severe pain, high fever and constipation could indicate that UC has progressed to muscular layers

Microscopic Colitis

Collagenous colitis and lymphocytic colitis are two forms of colitis that are visible only with the use of a microscope. A milder form of IBD, microscopic colitis does not lead to cancer and very rarely needs surgery, but in no way does this lessen the impact of the considerable pain and discomfort that people with this condition suffer. The two forms have a different appearance under the microscope, with collagenous colitis showing a thicker layer of collagen (the structural protein that gives shape to body structures, bones and cartilage) below the inside lining of the large intestine. People with either form of microscopic colitis receive the same therapies.

Who's at Risk?

This form of IBD happens most often in people older than 45, with both men and women being affected, but women more often are diagnosed with collagenous colitis. Statistics show that approximately 9 out of 100,000 people are affected by this form of IBD.

Diagnosing IBD

If you are experiencing some of the symptoms of IBD, and if some of your family members have IBD, discuss your symptoms with your health-care provider because IBD can cause scar tissue and may raise your risk of colon cancer if left untreated.

Diagnostic Procedures

Diagnostic procedures for IBD include:

- Standard physical exam and medical history
- Blood tests
- Stool analysis

The blood tests will be analyzed at a laboratory for possible anemia (caused by bleeding) and may identify higher-than-normal white blood cell levels (a sign of inflammation or infection).

Stool tests will help rule out other possible causes of GI issues (infection, for example). The analysis, done in a laboratory, will also look for possible blood in the stool — a sign of bleeding in the intestines. Your health-care provider will give you a sealed kit that will provide step-by-step directions for collecting a stool sample along with instructions on where to return it.

Standard Tests for Crohn's Disease and Ulcerative Colitis

Test	Action	Side Effects
Colonoscopy Conducted by a gastro-enterologist at a hospital or outpatient clinic.	Designed to view the rectum and full length of the colon. You may be asked to follow a clear diet for up to 3 days before the test and be given a laxative or one or more enemas the night before the test. Enemas to fully empty the colon may be done a few hours beforehand. Low levels of anesthesia and, for some, pain medication may be given to help to relax and reduce possible pain. A flexible tube with a very small camera at the tip is inserted into the anus and video of the intestinal lining is transmitted to a computer monitor screen, then analyzed for issues in the lower GI tract. A small piece of the intestinal lining may be removed and examined by a pathologist in a lab (biopsy). Driving a vehicle is not allowed for 24 hours following a colonoscopy if any anesthesia has been given.	After the test, some cramping or bloating may occur for an hour or so. Risks include: • Bleeding • A hole or tear (called perforation) in the colon lining • Diverticulitis: small pouches in colon become irritated, swollen and infected • Cardiovascular events: heart attack, low blood pressure, heart skipping beats or beating fast or slow • Severe abdominal pain • Death (rare)
Flexible sigmoidoscopy Similar to a colonoscopy.	Test to view the rectum and lower colon only. In some cases, you may be asked to follow a clear diet for up to 3 days before the test and be given a laxative or one or more enemas the night before the test. One or more enemas (water, laxative or mild soap solution flushed into the anus) are given about 2 hours before the procedure. A flexible, lighted tube is inserted into the anus and the scope inflates the colon with air for better viewing. A small camera mounted on the end of the scope transmits a video to a computer monitor screen. Biopsies may also be taken. Driving a vehicle is not allowed for 24 hours following a flexible sigmoidoscopy.	After the tests, some cramping or bloating may occur for an hour or so. Risks include bleeding or punctures in the large intestine.

Test	Action	Side Effects
Computerized tomography (CT) scan Conducted at a hospital or an outpatient clinic by an X-ray technician, but the results are analyzed by a physician who has specialized as a radiologist.	Combination of X-rays and computer technology that creates 3-D images. You may be given a solution to drink and/or an injection of a special dye (a contrast medium). You will be asked to lie on a table that slides into a device that looks like a giant donut. The scans are analyzed to identify possible signs and symptoms of Crohn's disease. This test may be stressful. The taste of the medium may be unpleasant.	You may experience a sense of fullness in your abdomen from the medium. This procedure is not recommended for pregnant women.
Upper GI series Conducted at a hospital or an outpatient clinic by an X-ray technician, but the results are analyzed by a physician who has specialized as a radiologist.	An X-ray to examine your small intestine. You may be asked to not eat or drink anything for 8 hours before the test, then to drink a chalky liquid called barium as you stand or sit in front of an X-ray machine. The barium coats the small intestine to help identify signs and symptoms of Crohn's disease on the X-ray.	You may have nausea and bloating for a while following the test. As the last traces of barium are excreted, the stools may be light-colored or even white. Your health-care provider will give you instructions about what to eat after the test.
Lower GI series Conducted at a hospital or an outpatient clinic by an X-ray technician, but the results are analyzed by a physician who has specialized as a radiologist.	An X-ray to examine your large intestine. You may be given instructions to prepare your bowels for the test, such as following a clear diet for up to 3 days, or you may be given a laxative (to soften the stool and speed up bowel movements) or even an enema (a squirt bottle or tube inserted into the anus flushes the lower intestine with water or a laxative). The barium helps expose any damage or health issues on the X-ray.	Enemas and loose, frequent bowel movements may lead to anal soreness. As the last traces of barium are excreted from the large intestine, the stools may be light-colored or even white. Your health-care provider will provide diet instructions for after the test.

Complementary Diagnostic Procedures

In response to symptoms discovered during a physical examination and medical history, a complementary medical professional, such as a naturopathic doctor, may consider additional tests and suggest steps a patient may take to help in making a diagnosis and alleviating symptoms.

Symptom Patterns

Patient assessment discussions often reveal a pattern of symptoms, such as foods that commonly trigger symptoms, regularly occurring stressful situations that may relate to a set of symptoms, or regular intense exercise that is followed soon after by symptoms.

Total Load

Specific foods by themselves may not cause any GI upset, but some, if eaten together, may be aggravating to the GI system and overwhelm the body's defenses. And excess of sugar alcohols, such as malitol (found in low-carb sweets and chocolates), for example, can cause abdominal cramping and diarrhea. The cumulative effect may also have an impact on the level of damage over time when the aggravating foods are eaten frequently or on a daily basis. Eating a food you are allergic to will not likely damage the lining of the intestine in a day, except in cases of severe celiac disease, in which case 1 day of exposure to a gluten can affect the body. But wear and tear will emerge when this food is eaten every day for a decade. In the same way, one course of antibiotics may not cause an overgrowth of intestinal yeast (candida), but repeated antibiotic treatments, too much dietary sugar and a lack of naturally occurring probiotics in the diet can result in an overgrowth of yeast.

Diet Diary

Complementary medicine's diagnostic procedures may move more slowly than conventional procedures in the effort to see things in the long run. Patients are typically advised to keep a 7-day health journal and diet diary to evaluate food and beverage intake. In your diary, describe symptoms and any relationship to meals; for example, "Bloating after cow's milk." Record the time, intensity and duration of symptoms. Reactions to a potentially allergenic food can add to the diagnostic picture.

GI Health & Diet Diary Sample

DATE:	Gastrointestinal condition–related symptoms:	Time symptoms started: Time symptoms ended:	Level of pain experienced: 0 = no pain 10 = worst pain ever	Location of pain (left, right, just below belly button, rectum, etc.):	If pain shifted, indicate to where:
Medication name and dosage taken:	Time medication taken:	Time medication became effective (if ever):	Rate effectiveness: 0 = no difference 3 = helped somewhat 5 = pain totally gone	Any side effects and time when occurred. Use a level to indicate severity (1 is mild and 5 is severe):	Note any issues that you feel affect your symptoms:
Describe pattern of bowel movements (regular/irregular):	Changes in B.M. pattern, date started:	Changes in B.M. pattern, date ended:	Stress levels experienced: 0 = no stress 10 = worst stress ever	Note any possible stress triggers (external and internal, moods):	Menstrual cycle date and severity (note if related to gastrointestinal symptoms):
List all foods, including beverages and water	Time food was eaten:	Exercise description, length of time and level of intensity noted: 0 = low intensity 3 = medium intensity 5 = high intensity	What time did you go to bed?	What time did you get up?	Quality of sleep: 1 = restful 2 = restless 3 = insomnia

Stool Analysis

Analysis of the stool involves looking at the degree of undigested foods, the pH of the stool and other factors that reflect digestive function. Though not all cases of GI issues will require all the available tests, laboratory tests for parasites and for blood in the stool are part of an analysis. In an interview, a doctor can also collect information about stool frequency, consistency, incontinence, urgency, pain with bowel movements, blood in the stool, loose bowels, dryness or odor.

Bristol Stool Chart

Type	Description
Type 1	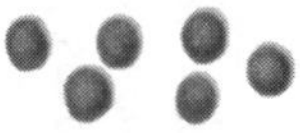 Separate hard lumps, like nuts (hard to pass)
Type 2	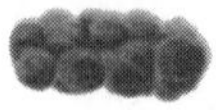 Sausage-shaped but lumpy
Type 3	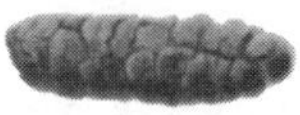 Like a sausage but with cracks on the surface
Type 4	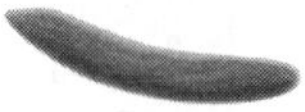 Like a sausage or snake, smooth and soft
Type 5	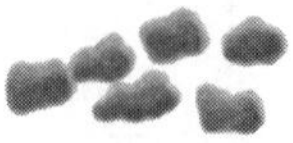 Soft blobs with clear-cut edges
Type 6	Fluffy pieces with ragged edges, a mushy stool
Type 7	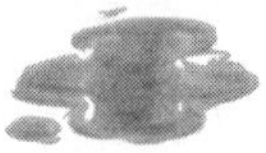 Watery, no solid pieces (entirely liquid)

Complications

Dysfunction of any of the organs or systems that make up the GI system can lead to disease elsewhere in the body. Some of the issues that may follow gastrointestinal disease states include:

- Increased allergies and hypersensitivities
- Vitamin and mineral deficiency due to reduced absorption
- Autoimmune disorders
- Protein, calorie and essential fatty acid malnutrition

Chapter 4

Lifestyle Modifications

CASE STUDY

Irritable Bowel Syndrome

Evan is tall, with wide shoulders, a thin build, a bit of a belly and a scraping kind of walk. He does web design at home, and his daily exercise consists of walking across the street to his post office box. He also goes down the street for tea with his buddies some days.

Evan has been suffering with a form of irritable bowel syndrome, his main symptom being constipation. He doesn't like to use medications for his constipation — he is concerned that he might become dependent on them, and he actually makes things worse because he worries a lot. Evan often has pain in his rectum, which makes it difficult for him to sit for any length of time.

It appears that Evan has an issue with slow transit — his meals may take 5 days to pass through his gastrointestinal tract, he feels bloated most of the time, and he wears suspenders so his pants are more comfortable. He also has headaches that may be related. But tests show that Evan is anatomically fine, with no medical issues that could be causing a problem.

Evan has decided to join a tai chi class because his naturopathic physician has suggested that it could help with many health issues, he didn't need special clothes and it wasn't high-energy, which might be uncomfortable for him. He has also been considering some group counseling where role playing is used to help people dealing with stress, as well as trying a pH-balanced diet for a month. He has already started keeping a health journal — it was a lot of work, but he'd found an app for his phone, so it was a bit like a game. He was tracking all foods and beverages, symptoms, mood and stress, and also testing the pH levels in his saliva and urine. It would be a gradual shift away from his usual luncheon meats on rye bread for lunch to vegetable soups and salads, with some meat, but roasted or slow cooked. He has a vegetarian friend who is going to help him with some recipes for vegetable dishes he has never tried before. Evan is feeling optimistic that life is going to get better soon.

The factors that cause pH imbalance in our bodies are also the factors that can bring balance back. Taking charge of certain lifestyle factors can improve your state of health overall, and depending on the severity of your symptoms, may provide enough relief that you won't need to resort to medications or

Lifestyle Factors

- Weight management
- Regular exercise
- Sleep hygiene
- Stress reduction

surgery. Restoring pH balance in the GI system can, for some people, help reduce GI tract symptoms such as reflux, diarrhea, constipation, pain and bloating seen in GERD, IBS and IBD.

Many GI conditions can be managed, even reversed, using conventional and complementary therapies; specifically, lifestyle modifications, mind–body strategies, pharmaceutical and botanical medications and a pH-balanced diet. A pH-balanced diet can also reduce the risk of hypertension and stroke and may improve cognition and memory. Reducing acidity through a more alkaline diet can remove built-up toxic waste and improve your body's ability to remove acid as it develops. If hormones are again balanced as a result of the pH diet, any issues related to disordered menstruation, such as cramps and diarrhea, will be reduced as well.

RESEARCH SPOTLIGHT

Low-Acid Relief

A 2011 research study of a small group of patients with reflux who did not respond to typical medication (proton pump inhibitors, or PPIs) found that a low-acid diet improved reflux symptoms. A 2014 systematic review of complementary and alternative medicine found some success for people with IBS who were tested for food sensitivities by assessing their immunoglobulin G (IgG) levels. Reducing food intakes associated with the results of the testing found that certain foods, such as milk, eggs, wheat, beef, pork and lamb, raised IgG levels. Excluding these more acidic foods from the diet reduced IBS symptoms in the gut.

Weight Management

If you are overweight, losing weight will help reduce physical stress on your esophagus and stomach and help regulate pH and stomach acids. Talk to a registered dietitian or your family physician to find out what weight is best for you and whether losing some weight might reduce any of your GI-related symptoms. Set realistic goals that don't raise your stress levels.

Counseling may be an important part of your weight-loss program, to keep you focused on the health benefits of losing just enough weight to reach your optimum point of wellness. There is no need to starve yourself to become skinny.

Tips for Changing Your Eating Habits

How you eat is as important as what you eat. Consider changing your eating habits.

- Avoid foods that commonly cause GI symptoms.
- Lose excess weight. Work with your health-care team to develop a long-term weight-loss plan that fits your goals and your lifestyle.
- Relax while eating to help digestion from the mouth down.
- Eat small meals with low fat content.
- Increase fiber intake.
- Do not overeat! Filling the stomach to excess, especially late in the day or before lying down to sleep, will exacerbate GI conditions. Overeating can lead to food retention in the stomach.
- For a healthier approach, upgrade your eating habits with a diet mentor who meets with you regularly and provides education, support and feedback.
- Avoid medications that aggravate the situation.
- Take bitters before eating high-protein meals.
- Take supplements that coat the insides of your intestines.
- Supplement with choline and lecithin.

More Tips for Modifying Your Lifestyle

- Wear loose-fitting clothes around your waist and stomach area to reduce reflux.
- Sit upright for at least 3 hours after any meal to help prevent reflux from the stomach.
- Securely attach 2- to 3-inch (5 to 7.5 cm) wood blocks under the bedposts at the head of your bed (or otherwise elevate the head of your bed) to reduce the amount of food that travels back up your esophagus.
- If you smoke, quit immediately (your primary health-care provider can help you meet this goal) and avoid exposure to secondhand smoke.

If a weight-loss program makes your health worse, talk to your health-care provider about other options, such as prescription weight-loss medications and bariatric surgery. Bariatric surgery reduces the size of the stomach or intestines, which can result in weight loss. This benefit needs to be weighed against some long-term side effects, such as loss of some ability to absorb essential nutrients.

Did You Know?

Rate of Reduction

Although everyone loses (and gains) weight at a different rate, losing between ½ and 2 lbs (0.25 and 1 kg) per week is a healthy approach and more likely to be maintained than weight lost from a very-low-calorie diet that may cause harm and requires constant monitoring.

Bona Fides

If you are considering a weight-loss program that has been promoted online, on your smartphone or on television, test the safety of the program by asking questions. Ask for written proof of results. If possible, speak to people who are on this program. Take the information away to share with family or friends before committing to any program. Remember the old saying: "If it sounds too good to be true, it likely is."

Energy Balance

If you consume more calories than your body "burns" from basal metabolism and physical activity, you will likely gain weight because the excess calories are stored in the body as fat. This is a state of energy excess. If you burn more calories than you consume, an energy deficit can occur and you will likely lose weight as your body burns those calories stored in body fat. Once you achieve your desired weight, you can maintain this weight by balancing the calories you consume with the calories you burn.

One lb (0.5 kg) of fat is equal to 3500 calories, so a daily calorie deficit of 500 should result in a total loss of 3500 calories or 1 lb (0.5 kg) of fat per week. However, our energy expenditure is not that predictable. Typically, energy use lessens as you lose weight until you reach a state where you are no longer losing weight (a plateau). During a plateau state, your weight will remain stable with the food intake that would previously have caused weight loss.

FAQ

Q. What do you mean when you say "burning calories"?

A. Calories are a unit of measure for the energy required to maintain our basal metabolic rate (breathing, sleeping and digesting, for example) and enable physical activity (walking, talking and writing, for example). Calories are expended, or "burned," during these unconscious and conscious metabolic activities. Analysis and calculation have determined the calorie content of most food items. These are available from a dietitian and on the Internet.

Energy Balance

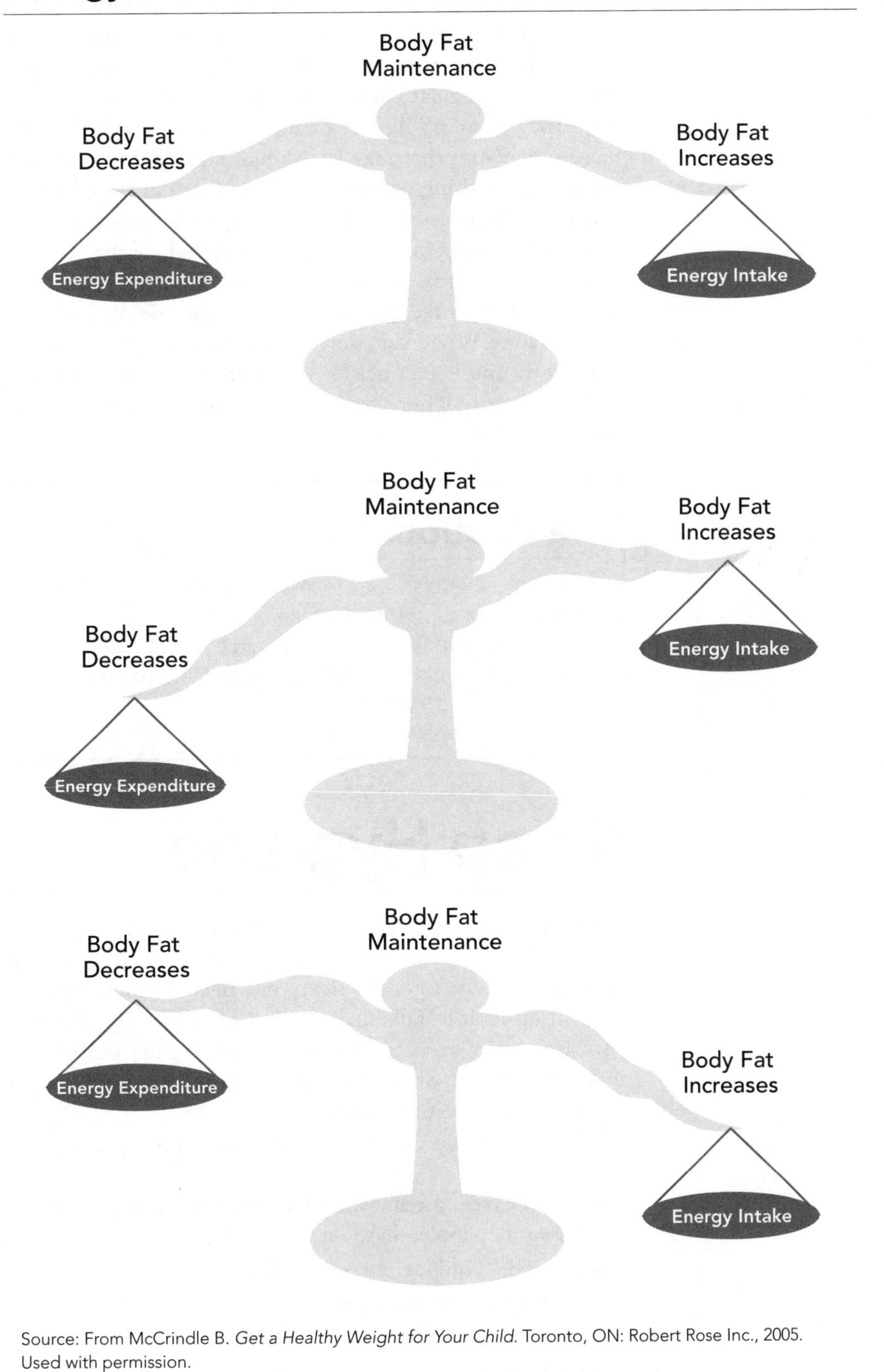

Source: From McCrindle B. *Get a Healthy Weight for Your Child.* Toronto, ON: Robert Rose Inc., 2005. Used with permission.

Regular Exercise

Exercise is the other side of energy balance. Regular exercise is helpful for balancing pH, improving digestion and preventing diarrhea, but regular exercise may be more difficult for people with IBD (Crohn's disease or ulcerative colitis) due to the painful flare-ups that may keep them close to the bathroom. Walking, breathing exercises, yoga and tai chi are all low-impact forms of exercise that are less problematic for people with IBS or IBD, but any exercise may reduce the stress that worsens symptoms. Choose a form of exercise that doesn't make symptoms like leakage worse — jogging may not work for everyone. Whatever exercise you choose, pay attention to your body and keep track of your experience in a diet diary to help identify when exercise works and when you need to take a breather.

✦ Caution

Extreme exercise may increase the risk of metabolic acidosis through the increase of low pH in body tissues (called lactic acid), caused by the body's inability to supply oxygen to muscles at the rate required. Moderation is key.

Sleep Hygiene

We are all different when it comes to how much sleep we need, but we all need some sleep to remain healthy. Unfortunately, many people don't get the sleep they need. Anxiety and stress make it difficult to fall asleep easily. Caffeine in the diet may also affect your sleep. Shift work or traveling across time zones may wreak havoc on your sleep health. Good sleep hygiene is critical for maintaining wellness.

Here are some tips to improve your sleep hygiene:

- Avoid excess mental stimulation before going to bed; for some people, that includes reading.
- Set aside a quiet time to be calm and restful for about an hour before going to bed.
- Take a warm bath.
- Listen to quiet, relaxing music.

- Seek help for dealing with the source of stress if you are suffering from anxiety or depression. Insomnia may be a sign that stressors are not being dealt with.
- Avoid caffeine and other stimulants: coffee, tea, cocoa, colas and sports drinks are sources.
- Maintain lower blood sugar levels (called hypoglycemia).
- Avoid excess simple carbohydrates during the evening — they can lead to a rapid rise in blood sugar, followed by an insulin surge to manage the blood sugar, which leads to a quick drop in blood glucose, often waking the sleeper to go in search of a snack.
- If you are experiencing sleep issues, seek help from your health-care provider. Although the suggested changes in lifestyle are the best solution for sleeplessness, conventional and complementary practitioners have effective therapies to help restore a normal sleep pattern and improve health. These remedies for sleep problems include vitamin and mineral therapies, melatonin and botanical medicines.

Stress Reduction

Stress has an impact on GI conditions, including GERD, IBS and IBD. Because the enteric nerve system lines the gastrointestinal system and connects with the brain, stress is known to cause cramps for people with IBS. Being overly responsive to slight conflict or stress causes painful contractions. Conversely, IBS symptoms may also increase stress.

For people with IBS who have been identified as experiencing extremely high levels of life-related stress, counseling may be of benefit. Stress related to a job, family, relationships and so on may worsen IBS symptoms. These emotions can affect the activity of the GI tract, and the chemical changes that occur in the body in long-term stress can make IBS worse. Learning to reduce stress responses to events or to change the environment is an important factor in preventing IBS.

It takes some work to identify your stressors and learn how to cope with them or eliminate them. Try using your health journal to monitor your stress levels. Rate your stress level between 0 for no stress and 5 as the most stress you have ever experienced. This will help you or your health-care provider find solutions. Healthy sleep patterns, exercise, counseling and mind–body treatments can all be successful means of reducing stress.

Mental and Emotional Health

Connections have been shown between mental illness and IBS. Several remedies have proven effective.

- **Mindfulness training:** This therapy helps people learn to focus on sensations in the moment, which helps them avoid needless worrying and anxiety.
- **Hypnotherapy:** This remedy helps you learn to relax muscles in the colon.
- **Talk therapy:** This form of cognitive behavior and interpersonal therapy (also called psychodynamic) is most effective. Cognitive behavioral therapy is a practical process that focuses on thoughts and actions, replacing dysfunctional actions, and interpersonal therapy uses relaxation and stress management tools to cope with emotions that affect IBS symptoms.

Mind–Body Therapies

Mind–body therapies are considered an excellent choice for managing stress, headache, muscle tension, insomnia, mood disorders and GI conditions, such as IBS. These therapies include biofeedback — such as thermogenic (heat) and muscular tension surface electromyography (sEMG) — as well as guided imagery, cognitive behavioral therapy, meditation, music therapy and relaxation training. All have been proven to be safe and effective. In addition, the use of these therapies in conjunction with medication has shown a synergistic improvement where all the therapies work together for a better outcome than each alone, reducing anxiety and depression in particular and increasing the sense of self-control in reducing stress levels.

Bodywork

Exercise, stretching, massage, manual therapy, manipulation and craniosacral therapy have been most effective when combined with biofeedback, relaxation training and exercise. An educational and physical program directed to your specific areas of concern from a qualified trainer may be most beneficial.

Therapeutic Touch

Therapeutic touch (TT) involves a therapist holding his hands a short distance from the patient's body (with no physical contact) to identify and correct any imbalances detected in the patient's energy field. Therapeutic touch follows a four-step protocol:

1. **Centering:** Focus attention on the patient and calm the mind.
2. **Assessment:** Evaluate the patient's energy flow for imbalances.
3. **Intervention:** Facilitate a symmetrical flow throughout the patient's energy flow.
4. **Evaluation and closure:** Verify the impact of the intervention and complete the therapy session.

Sessions can be as brief as 5 minutes or go as long as 30. Healing touch also focuses on patient empowerment, practitioner self-care and the practitioner–patient relationship as part of the healing process. Therapeutic touch has been used for pain, stress and anxiety, headache, well-being and depression but should not be used in place of therapies with proven effectiveness for severe conditions.

Meditation

Meditation is a complementary mind–body therapy for many health-related problems. The focus is on the quality of the breath during prescribed exercise and massage routines. The most popular forms of meditation and massage are yoga, tai chi and qigong.

- Yoga aims to calm the mind by adopting specific poses that stretch the body and relax the mind.
- Tai chi emphasizes fluid coordination of body movements and the mind.
- Qigong emphasizes the use of strength and force and is used for both physical training and therapy.

Other forms of meditation include mantra meditation (transcendental meditation, relaxation response, clinically standardized meditation), mindfulness meditation (Vipassana) and Zen Buddhist meditation (mindfulness-based stress reduction, mindfulness-based cognitive therapy).

Chapter 5
Medical Therapies

CASE STUDY ✍

IBD: Crohn's Disease

Richard sat on the side of the hospital bed and looked at the equipment at its head. It was all a little scary, but if it could change his life for the better, it was worth a try.

Richard had his first symptoms of Crohn's disease when he was in his late 20s — 8 years ago now. He had tried diet changes, antibiotics, steroids and immune system suppressors, but nothing had stopped the inflammation and bleeding, the pain that never stopped or the deepening scar tissue on his intestines, which he was sure he could feel, like a 2-lb (1 kg) dumbbell pressing on his intestines, deep in his belly. Finally, he had discussed surgery with his GI specialist and was at the hospital to have part of his bowel removed. The best he could hope for was remission, because there was no cure for Crohn's. He just wanted a rest from the severe pain, never-ending diarrhea and rectal bleeding that he found so frightening, feeling like his life was draining away.

The intestinal blockage that had happened 6 weeks ago, along with a new painful fistula — an opening from his inflamed bowel to the edge of his anus, an unbelievably painful affliction — brought on the discussion about surgery and the decision he had acted on right away. His wife was coming to the hospital as soon as her shift as a nurse at a nearby clinic ended, and she would be with him the following morning before surgery. Her knowledge and calmness around his symptoms had always been a blessing for Richard, and as he rubbed the back of his neck to relieve the strain, he thought that he couldn't have survived this long without her. Nodding grimly to himself, he got up and unpacked the few toiletry items he would need during his short stay, ready to move on with his life.

If the lifestyle modifications discussed in the previous chapter do not provide you with sufficient relief from your GI symptoms, it may be time to discuss medications and/or surgery with your physician.

Medications

Many medications designed to improve GI symptoms are available over the counter (without a prescription). If your symptoms persist for 2 weeks or more, be sure to visit your health-care provider. In some cases, your physician may prescribe a combination of medications.

First, Do No Harm

- Before you take any pharmaceutical medication, discuss possible risks and side effects with your physician or pharmacist.
- Read all information about side effects and warnings before taking any drug.
- Seek medical attention immediately if you experience any symptoms that indicate a severe allergic reaction: difficulty breathing, hives, blistering or peeling skin, or swelling of mouth or throat.
- Share your complete list of prescribed medications and any herbs or supplements with your health-care provider at every appointment.
- Contact your physician to discuss any concerns you may have about possible side effects.

Over-the-Counter Medications

Many common health conditions, including some GI conditions, can be treated using over-the-counter (OTC) medications. OTCs provide timely relief for symptoms (when directions are followed), reduce visits to physicians and help individuals manage their own health care. Risks come with the use of OTCs, though. Taking OTCs to relieve symptoms may mask more serious illnesses and may increase the risk of side effects if directions are not carefully followed. Sometimes OTCs increase the risk of interactions from other drugs you are taking. Some people may not consider OTCs serious drugs, but they can be harmful if misused or even abused.

✦ Caution

Do not self-prescribe any of the pharmaceutical and botanical medications presented in this book unless they are labeled for OTC use. With OTC medications, follow the instructions as closely as you would a prescription medication. Always discuss any OTC medication use with your health-care provider.

Standard Medications for GERD

OTC Medications

- Antacids (Alka-Seltzer, Maalox, Mylanta, Riopan, Rolaids)

Actions

- Used to make acids more neutral and reduce the irritation of sour stomach, heartburn, upset stomach or acid indigestion.
- Also effective for other symptoms, such as ulcer pain and excess gas, when simethicone is an ingredient.

Possible Side Effects

- Diarrhea, constipation.
- Excessive intake of calcium along with vitamin D can cause calcium deposits in the soft tissues and organs.
- Some antacids contain aluminum, which should not be consumed in large quantities.
- Excessive antacid use can throw off the pH of the body, making it too alkaline.

Did You Know?

Peppermint Problem

Peppermint is a component of many over-the-counter antacids, but beware — peppermint can relax the sphincter that holds acids back in the stomach and keeps it out of the esophagus.

H2 Blockers

OTC and prescription forms available, typically taken in oral form as tablets, liquids or capsules:

- Cimetidine (Tagamet, Tagamet HB)
- Famotidine (Pepcid AC, Pepcid Oral)
- Nizatidine (Axid AR, Axid capsules, nizatidine capsules)
- Ranitidine (Zantac, Zantac 75, Zantac Efferdose, Zantac injection, Zantac syrup)

Actions

- Short- and long-term relief from GERD symptoms.
- Decrease the amount of acid produced in the stomach.
- In some cases, H2 blockers will heal the esophagus.

Possible Side Effects

- Cimetidine: diarrhea, dizziness, rashes or headaches (all rare).
- Famotidine: headache.
- Nizatidine: side effects rare.
- Ranitidine: headache.
- Deletion of stomach acid may make protein digestion more difficult (acid helps with the initial breakdown of protein, especially meat).

Proton Pump Inhibitors (PPIs)

Generally available by prescription only (though generic, OTC versions of lansoprazole, omeprazole and pantoprazole are available), and should be taken on an empty stomach:

- Dexlansoprazole (Dexilant)
- Esomeprazole (Nexium)
- Lansoprazole (Prevacid)
- Omeprazole (Prilosec, Zegerid)
- Pantoprazole (Protonix)
- Rabeprazole (Aciphex)

Action

- More effective than H2 blockers for improving GERD symptoms quickly and may heal damage to esophagus for most people.

Possible Side Effects

- Mild headache, diarrhea (short-term use).
- Pneumonia, infection, fractures (long-term use).
- Deletion of stomach acid may make protein digestion more difficult (acid helps with the initial breakdown of protein, especially meat).

Did You Know?

Antacid Overload

Excessive use of antacids can throw off the natural pH homeostasis of the body, making it too alkaline. In some cases, combinations of medications may work better together and help manage your GERD symptoms. Antacids and H2 blockers work together, with the antacid coping with the stomach acid by neutralizing it until the H2 blocker is able to stop acid production.

Prokinetics

Used only for severe symptoms, because side effects are harmful. Cisapride and domperidone are not available in some regions.

- Bethanechol (Urecholine)
- Cisapride (Prepulsid, Propulsid)
- Domperidone (Motilium, Motinorm, Costi, Nomil, Molax)
- Metoclopramide (Reglan)

Actions

- Strengthen the lower esophageal sphincter.
- Empty the stomach at a faster rate.
- Bethanechol helps prevent nausea and vomiting.

Possible Side Effects

- Cisapride: irregular heartbeat.
- Metoclopramide: sleepiness, nervousness, anxiety, depression, fatigue, involuntary movements and muscle spasms; long-term use: tardive dyskinesia.
- Prokinetics can interact with medications prescribed for other medical conditions.

Antibiotics

- Erythromycin

Action

- Similar to prokinetics, emptying the stomach faster, but with fewer side effects.

Possible Side Effects

- All antibiotics may cause diarrhea.
- Antibiotics can disrupt the normal composition of bacterial flora in the gut.

✦ Caution

If you are taking more than one type of medication (prescription or over-the-counter), please be aware of possible drug interactions, which may include reduced effectiveness of a medication, an increase in a medication's effect or different side effects. Always read OTC labels carefully for possible side effects and interactions. Give your health-care provider a complete list of all medications you are taking, including prescription, OTC and complementary therapies, along with a list of your other medical conditions.

Standard Medications for IBS

Laxatives

Available over the counter as pills, capsules, powders that you mix with water and drink, or as a suppository you insert into your rectum, where it dissolves. Talk to your health-care provider about which laxative will help your specific symptoms. Be sure to stay well-hydrated when taking laxatives. Laxatives are meant for short-term use only.

- Bulk-forming: ispaghula (Fybogel, Regulan, Isogel), methylcellulose (Celevac), sterculia (Normacol)
- Stimulant: bisacodyl (Dulcolax), senna (Senokot)
- Osmotic: Movicol
- Stool softener: DulcoEase

Actions

- Soften stool and increase frequency of bowel movements.

Possible Side Effects

- Bulk-forming: bloating and gas.
- Stimulant: abdominal pain; over long term may cause lazy bowel.
- Osmotic: abdominal pain, bloating, gas.
- Stool softener: cramping, nausea, skin rash.
- Rare side effects: vomiting, dizziness, blood in stools, fainting.
- Excessive laxative use can lead to dehydration and loss of electrolytes.
- Some laxatives may be dangerous if you have Crohn's disease or ulcerative colitis.

Fiber Supplements

Fiber supplements should be taken with 8 oz (250 mL) of water, and plenty of water should be consumed throughout the day. Do not take fiber supplements if you have trouble swallowing.

Actions

- May reduce IBS symptoms, reduce diarrhea, improve constipation and improve stool frequency and consistency.

Possible Side Effects

- Insufficient water with the fiber supplement could lead to the fiber swelling in the throat.
- Can cause gas and bloating.
- May reduce or delay absorption of some medications.
- May interact with tricyclic antidepressants (Elavil, Sinequan, Tofranil).

> **✦ Caution**
>
> Do not take fiber supplements if you have impacted stool, unless you have your doctor's approval.

Antidiarrheals

- Loperamide (Imodium, Kaopectate, Maalox), along with rehydration therapy (fluids and electrolytes as directed by your health-care provider)

Actions

- For short bouts of IBS-related diarrhea, antidiarrheals reduce stool frequency and increase stool firmness by reducing speed of stool movement through colon.
- May reduce cramps; does not improve pain or bloating.

Possible Side Effects

- Possible burning or prickly sensation on tongue from quick-dissolve tablets, dry mouth, drowsiness, dizziness, gas, nausea, vomiting, headaches, fatigue.
- Rare side effects include abdominal or stomach pain, bloating, cramps, constipation or rash.

> **RESEARCH SPOTLIGHT**
>
> **Oral Cromolyn Sodium**
>
> In one study, oral cromolyn sodium (Gastrocrom), which reduces the breakdown of mast cells (which cause inflammation) in immune and stress responses, reduced IBS-related symptoms in 67% of patients.

Antispasmodics

- Hyoscine butylbromide (Buscopan)
- Cimetropium bromide
- Pinaverium bromide

Action

- Reduce IBS-related cramps and abdominal pain.

Possible Side Effects

- Hyoscine butylbromide: temporary blurred vision, constipation or diarrhea, decreased sweating, difficulties with urination, dizziness, flushing, nausea, fast heartbeat.
- Cimetropium bromide: dry mouth, pupil dilation and photophobia, flushing, dry skin, constipation, palpitations, erratic heartbeat.
- Pinaverium bromide: dyspepsia, epigastric pain, headache, nausea, rash, vertigo, dry mouth, abdominal bloating, constipation, diarrhea, fatigue, irritation of the esophagus.

✦ Caution

When taking hyoscine butylbromide, contact your physician if you have a skin rash and itching or changes in vision. Seek immediate medical attention if you have painful, red eyes with some loss of vision or any severe allergic reactions. Discuss all medication use with your physician or pharmacist, because interactions may be fatal.

Antidepressants

- Tricyclic antidepressants (TCAs), such as amitriptyline (Elavil), amoxapine (Asendin), desipramine (Norpramin), doxepin (Sinequan), imipramine (Tofranil), nortriptyline (Aventyl, Pamelor), protriptyline (Vivactil), trimipramine (Surmontil)

Actions

- Reduce sensitivity to GI pain.
- Restore normal GI motility and secretions.

Possible Side Effects

- Weight loss or gain, blurred vision, constipation, dry mouth, rash, hives, low blood pressure when first standing, increased heart rate.
- More serious side effects include difficulty urinating, abnormal heart rhythms, sexual dysfunction and narrow angle glaucoma.

Antibiotics

- Rifaximin (Xifaxan)

Action

- May reduce bloating by killing off bacterial overgrowth in small intestine (more research is needed).

Possible Side Effects

- Nausea, stomach pain, dizziness, excessive fatigue, headache, muscle tightening, joint pain.

✦ Caution

When taking rifaximin, contact your physician immediately if you experience watery or bloody diarrhea with stomach cramps and/or fever (while taking the medication or for the 2 months following), hoarseness, rash, itching, hives, swelling of the face, throat, tongue, lips, eyes, hands, feet, ankles or lower legs, difficulty breathing or swallowing.

Lubiprostone (Amitiza)

Actions

- Reduces abdominal pain or discomfort.
- Improves consistency of stools.
- Reduces straining and severity of constipation.

Possible Side Effects

- Nausea, diarrhea, stomach pain or bloating, gas, vomiting, heartburn, headache, dizziness, discomfort in chest, fatigue, swelling of the hands, feet, ankles or lower legs.

Linaclotide (Linzess)

Actions

- Reduces abdominal pain.
- Increases frequency of bowel movements.

Possible Side Effects

- Diarrhea, stomach pain, swelling or feeling of fullness or pressure in the stomach area, gas, headache.

> **✦ Caution**
>
> When taking linaclotide, seek medical attention immediately if you experience unusual or severe stomach pain, hives, bright red or black, tarry stools, or if you have other concerns.

Probiotics

Probiotics are bacteria and other live microorganisms similar to those populating the GI tract. Concerns have been raised about the quality and quality control of probiotic products. Discuss any alternative therapies, herbal products or nutritional supplements with your health-care provider.

Action

- Large amounts of probiotics may improve IBS symptoms (more research is needed).

Possible Side Effect

- Gas.

Did You Know?

Combinations

Combinations of medications have been used to treat some people with Crohn's disease because research suggests that synergistic combinations may be more effective in prolonging remission; however, the research results are divided.

Standard Medications for Crohn's Disease

Anti-Inflammatory Aminosalicylates

- Sulfasalazine or 5-aminosalicylic acid (5-ASA) agents (Asacol, Dipentum, Pentasa); patients unable to tolerate sulfasalazine are prescribed 5-ASA

Action

- Reduce inflammation.

Possible Side Effects

- Headaches, heartburn, vomiting, diarrhea, nausea.

Cortisone or Steroids (Corticosteroids)

In some cases, large doses of steroids are prescribed in early stages for severe symptoms, then dosage is lowered as symptoms improve, to reduce side effects.

- Prednisone
- Budesonide (Entocort EC)

Action

- Reduce inflammation.

Possible Side Effects

- Increased risk of infection and osteoporosis (weakened bones).

Immune System Suppressors (Immunosuppressants)

- 6-mercaptopurine (6-MP, Purinethol)
- Azathioprine (Imuran)

Action

- Block immune reaction that contributes to inflammation.

Possible Side Effects

- Vomiting, nausea, diarrhea, increased risk of infection.

Biologics

These are medications that are genetically engineered from proteins, genes and antibodies. Your physician will monitor you closely while you are taking a biologic medication.

- Adalimumab (Humira)
- Certolizumab pegol (Cimzia)
- Golimumab (Simponi)
- Infliximab (Remicade)
- Natalizumab (Tysabri)

Action

- Interfere with the body's inflammatory response by targeting specialized proteins associated with IBD and involved in increasing or decreasing inflammation.

Possible Side Effects

- Site of injection: redness, itching, bruising, pain, swelling.
- Headache, fever, chills, difficulty breathing, low blood pressure, hives.
- Stomach pain, back pain, rash, nausea, upper respiratory infection (cough and sore throat).
- Drug interactions are possible.
- Serious infections, such as tuberculosis (TB) and sepsis (a life-threatening blood infection).
- Increase in risk of infection.

Subcutaneous Injections

Prescribed for patients with moderate to severe Crohn's disease who have not responded to conventional therapy or immunosuppressants, this kind of medication is delivered at home by the patient or a family member who has been trained to give injections.

- Adalimumab (Humira)
- Certolizumab pegol (Cimzia)
- Golimumab (Simponi)

Action

- These synthetic proteins block inflammation-causing proteins.

Possible Side Effects

- Injection site: redness, itching, bruising, pain, swelling.
- Headache, fever or chills, low blood pressure, stomach pain, nausea, back pain, rash and hives, difficulty breathing, cough, sore throat.

Crohn's and Ulcerative Colitis Remission

The two goals of medical treatment for Crohn's disease and ulcerative colitis are first to improve symptoms to the point of remission (total lack of symptoms) and second to maintain remission by health management to prevent flare-ups. The overall treatment goal is to control ongoing inflammation in the intestine — the cause of IBD symptoms.

Depending on where you live, if you are diagnosed with Crohn's disease, your health-care provider will weigh the benefits and risks of your personal health (location, severity and any complications related to CD) and available therapies. Because there is no cure for Crohn's, the goal is to manage any inflammation, improve symptoms (abdominal pain, rectal bleeding or diarrhea, for example) and correct any nutritional deficiencies through diet and possibly supplements. Possible therapies may include medications, surgery, nutritional supplementation or some combination. It is important to be monitored by a health-care provider over the long term if you have Crohn's disease, even if your condition is under control, with less frequent recurrences. Though periods of remission may occur, symptoms can recur without warning and make it difficult to assess therapies. Keeping a health journal where you record symptoms, stress, sleep and diet even during remission periods may help you understand possible triggers of a recurrence.

Standard Medications for Ulcerative Colitis

Anti-Inflammatory Aminosalicylates

- 5-aminosalicylic acid (5-ASA)
- Sulfasalazine (Azulfidine) containing sulfapyridine with 5-ASA

Actions

- 5-ASA may control inflammation.
- Sulfapyridine carries the 5-ASA to the intestines.

Possible Side Effects

- Headache, vomiting, heartburn, nausea, diarrhea.

Other 5-ASA Agents

With fewer side effects than sulfasalazine, these 5-ASA agents may be effective for people who are unable to tolerate sulfasalazine.

- Olsalazine (Dipentum)
- Mesalamine (Asacol, Canasa, Lialda, Rowasa)
- Balsalazide (Colazal)

Action

- May control inflammation.

Corticosteroids

Prescribed for short-term periods for people with more severe UC symptoms and those whose condition does not improve with 5-ASAs. Available in oral, intravenous, enema, rectal foam and suppository forms.

- Prednisone (Cortan, Deltasone, Liquid Pred, Meticorten, Orasone, Panasol-S, Prednicen-M, Sterapred)
- Methylprednisolone (Medrol)
- Hydrocortisone (Cortef, Cortenema, Hydrocortone, Anusol-HC, Proctozone HC, Anucort-HC, Westcort)

Action

- Reduce inflammation.

Possible Side Effects

- Weight gain, facial hair, acne, diabetes, hypertension, loss of bone mass, mood swings, increased risk for infection.

> **✦ Caution**
>
> Steroids are not recommended as a long-term medication therapy.

Immunomodulators

Prescribed for some people whose UC symptoms do not improve with 5-ASAs. Slow-acting immunomodulators take 3 to 6 months for any impact to be seen. Because cyclosporine is toxic over time and has harmful side effects, it is only prescribed for severe UC.

- Azathioprine (Imuran, Azasan)
- 6-mercaptopurine (6-MP) (Purinethol)
- Cyclosporine (Neoral, Sandimmun, Sandimmune)

Action

- Suppress the immune system.

Possible Side Effects

- Fatigue, nausea, increased risk of infection, vomiting, pancreatitis, reduced white blood cell count, hepatitis.

> **Suppressing Dysfunction**
>
> When inflammatory bowel disease is severe and highly destructive, drug therapies to suppress symptoms, such as prednisone or azathioprine (Imuran, Azasan), are required to shut off the immune function. For some people, such therapy may prevent the loss of a section of intestine. For people who are unable to tolerate some of the medical therapies, however, surgery may be the best route to controlling inflammation. Strong antibiotic treatment could be recommended when gut permeability and infection into the peritoneum may put the patient at risk.

Biologics

Prescribed when people with UC do not show improved symptoms from other medications or are not able to tolerate 5-ASAs. Given as an IV drip over 2 hours, usually every 8 weeks. Immunomodulators are also prescribed with infliximab to avoid any allergic reactions. The protein (TNF) that is targeted by this medication causes inflammation in the intestines.

- Infliximab (Remicade)

Action

- Reduce inflammation.

Possible Side Effects

- Some people have experienced serious infections associated with infliximab, such as tuberculosis or a life-threatening blood infection called sepsis. A TB test will help identify anyone at risk for developing or reactivating TB.
- Biologics may also increase the risk of other infections. Your physician will monitor you closely while you are on biologic therapy. Inform your doctor immediately if you get infections easily or develop symptoms of infection (fever, fatigue, cough or flu) while taking these medications.

Did You Know?

Ulcerative Colitis Severity

A cure for UC does not yet exist, but current medications may improve symptoms. The level of severity determines the type of medication that might best improve symptoms of UC, and the form of medication may be dictated by the parts of the colon and rectum affected. Medications may also be prescribed for related emotional stress, to reduce pain, to improve diarrhea symptoms or for infections.

Botanical Medicines

Although botanical medicines may not act as quickly as pharmaceuticals, these medications have been used for IBD and IBS quite successfully. Antimicrobial botanicals, for example, have been used to reduce antigenic bacteria and yeasts and prevent flare-ups. And antispasmodics (Buscopan) can relieve IBS-related symptoms, although IBS is best treated through addressing deficiencies in lifestyle, exercise, digestion and immunity.

Glycyrrhiza glabra (Licorice)

Botanicals that are known to coat the intestine may be useful during flare-ups if no perforation is present. *Glycyrrhiza glabra* (licorice) is such a botanical, and also has compounds that are indirectly anti-inflammatory. In higher doses, this botanical may raise your blood pressure and should be avoided by anyone taking drugs that cause potassium excretion. Discuss any use of botanicals and all medications with your health-care providers.

Mentha piperita (Peppermint)

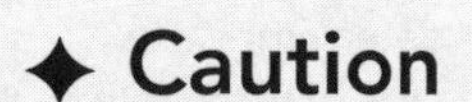

Caution

Avoid peppermint if you have gastritis or peptic ulceration.

Peppermint is effective in reducing IBS symptoms because one of its active compounds, menthol, has antispasmodic properties. Like a calcium channel blocker, menthol inhibits smooth muscle activity, relaxing the muscles of the colon and lessening the spasms that can make IBS worse. Using a coated form allows the peppermint to bypass the stomach, where it could cause an irritation. Possible side effects are heartburn, perianal burning, blurred vision, nausea and vomiting.

Althaea officinalis (Marshmallow) and *Ulmus fulva* (Slippery Elm)

Marshmallow and slippery elm bark may soothe the gut by coating an irritated colon. Antispasmodics, such as *Scutellaria lateriflora* (skullcap) may be used in combination with these botanicals.

Hospitalization

For some people, the symptoms of ulcerative colitis may be grave enough to require hospitalization. Severe bleeding or diarrhea may cause dehydration, and intravenous fluids will be given to treat diarrhea and loss of blood, fluid and mineral salts. Other care that may be required in this situation (such as a special colitis diet, tube feeding and corticosteroids) may become harmful, so surgery may be recommended. Other UC-related issues that may lead to surgery include rupture of the colon, massive bleeding, severe illness or increased risk of cancer. Recovery from surgery can take from 4 to 6 weeks following a hospital stay of 1 to 2 weeks.

Surgery

When lifestyle modifications, mind–body strategies and medications fail to manage severe GI symptoms, surgery may be the best option.

Standard Surgical Procedures

Be sure to weigh the benefits and risks of these procedures by consulting with your health-care providers and patient support groups.

Fundoplication

The standard surgical treatment for serious GERD is called fundoplication, and this procedure is known to lead to control of long-term reflux for most people. During surgery the upper stomach region (the fundus) is wrapped around the esophagus and sewn so that the lower esophagus passes through the small circle created by stomach muscle. This procedure increases the

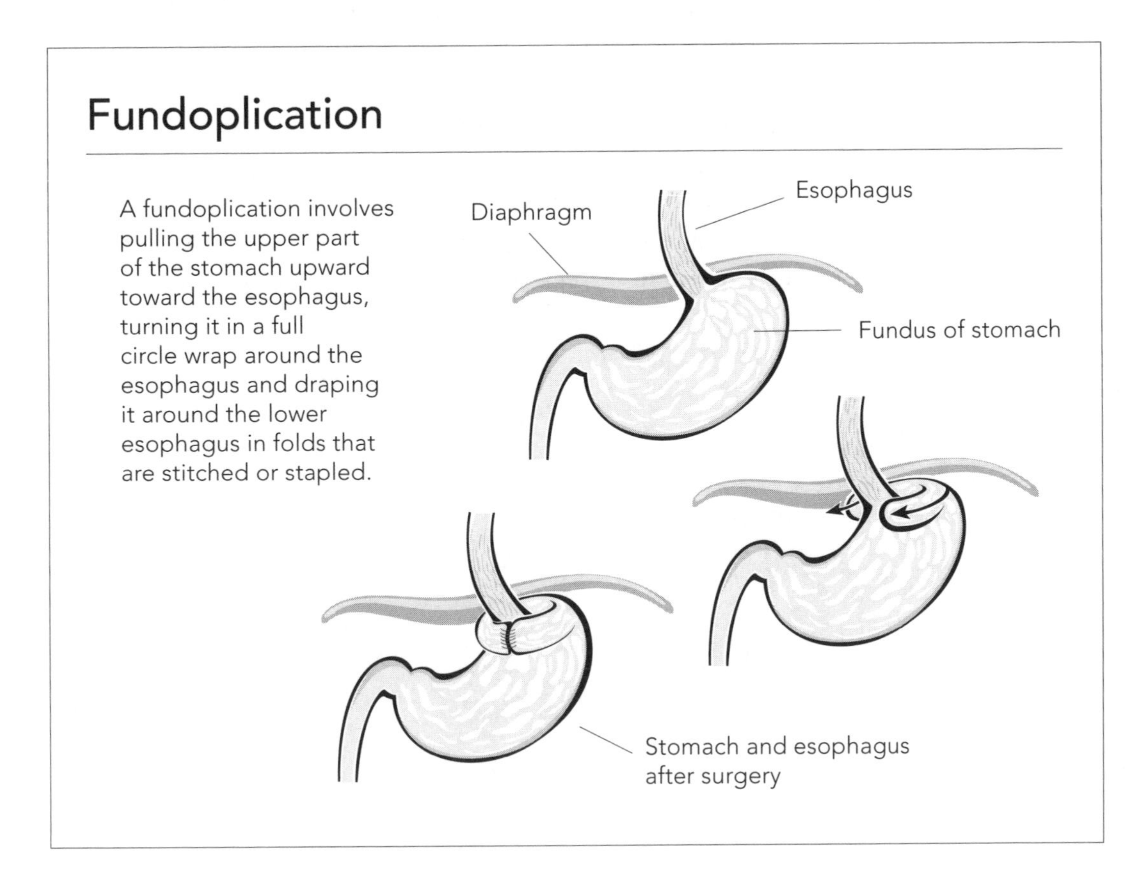

Did You Know?

Ileoanal Pouch Anastomosis

During this procedure, also called pouch surgery, the ileum is pulled through the remainder of the rectum and joined directly to the anus, creating a pouch where the stool is stored before being excreted through the anus. This surgical procedure helps people with ulcerative colitis have normal bowel movements by preserving part of the anus and avoids an ileostomy. Bowel movements may be more frequent and more fluid.

strength of the lower esophageal sphincter (LES), preventing stomach acid from moving up into the esophagus. Without acid present, the esophagus will heal.

Endoscopic techniques may also be used to treat GERD.

Proctocolectomy

The rectum and part or all of the colon are removed. Full recovery from this procedure may take 4 to 6 weeks after a 1- to 2-week stay in hospital.

Ileostomy

This procedure is used to improve Crohn's disease symptoms that do not respond to medical therapy or if infection causes perforation, bleeding, blockage or a swollen, extremely painful area caused by infection that may be filled with pus (called an abscess). During the procedure, the lower end of the small intestine (the ileum) is attached to an opening in the abdomen called a stoma, usually in the lower right side, where a belt would sit, and an ostomy pouch is attached to the stoma, outside of the body, to collect stool. The patient is taught how to maintain the ostomy pouch and protect the skin around the stoma. Most people with an ostomy pouch lead normal, active lives.

Intestinal Resection

Only the section of intestine that is affected by Crohn's disease is removed and the healthy intestine above and below the cut are connected during this surgical procedure. Full recovery may take 3 to 4 weeks following a hospital stay of several days.

Pelvic (Ileal) Pouch Procedure

Panel 1

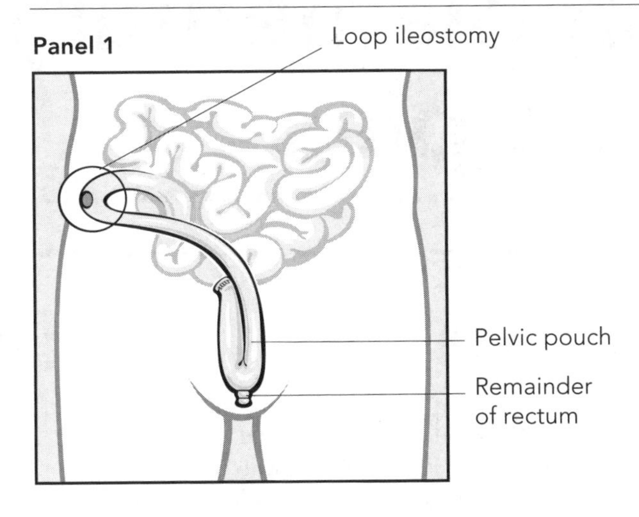

The pelvic pouch procedure is usually done in two or three stages. Initially, the pouch is formed by folding the small intestine (ileum) back on itself to make a "J" shape. The bottom of the "J" is opened and sewn to the small segment of remaining rectum (detail panel). The temporary loop ileostomy is created above the pouch (panel 1), and several months later the ileostomy is closed (panel 2), thus producing an intact digestive tract (panel 3).

Panel 2

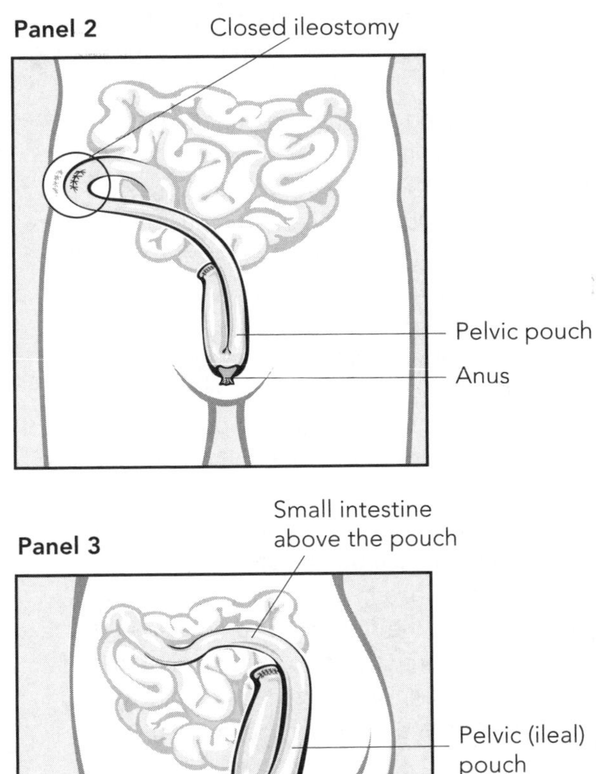

Panel 3

Detail Panel

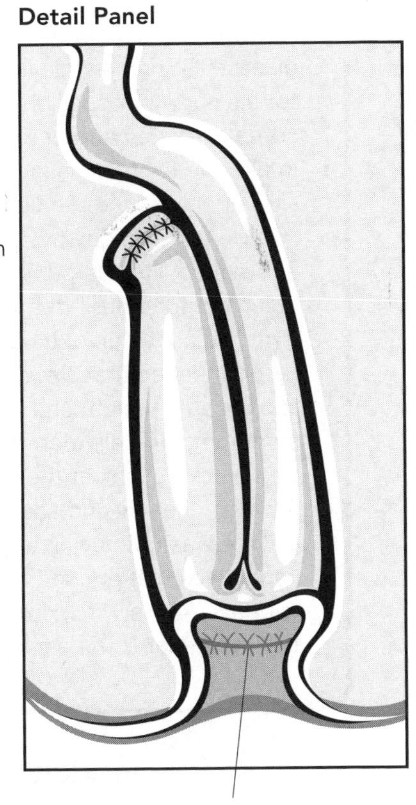

Chapter 6

Complementary Therapies

CASE STUDY

GERD

Detlev was going to his new in-laws' for dinner, and he was very nervous about the upcoming evening. He was having problems with food moving back up his esophagus, causing acid indigestion. Then the acid fluid in the back of his mouth made his throat sore and talking difficult, and he would start wheezing and coughing. He was also concerned about having bad breath.

Detlev had been tentatively diagnosed with gastroesophageal reflux disease (GERD) just days before. He was now waiting to have some tests to rule out other possible medical issues. The physician had suggested some over-the-counter medications, Maalox or Riopan, to reduce acid intake. Detlev had his fingers crossed that he wouldn't suffer the possible side effects of the medication — diarrhea.

He turned sideways as he put on his jacket, ready to go out the door, and sighed. He had put on weight in the last year; being happy and in love, going out for dinner frequently and making it to fewer appointments at the gym had added an extra couple of inches to his waist. His physician had recommended that Detlev begin to pay closer attention to his diet, consider losing some weight and keep a record of the foods he was eating and his symptoms, to help identify any specific foods that were an issue for him. Detlev took a look at the diet diary app he had downloaded to his phone earlier in the day and added the apple he had had for a snack to his food list. He was not having any symptoms at the moment and grinned at the happy face that popped up when he entered the zero in the symptoms window. As his wife came down the stairs, Detlev smiled at her, knowing that whatever came along, he would have the support he needed.

In addition to standard GI therapies, complementary therapies can be effective not only for treating GI conditions but also for restoring pH homeostasis. Specialized therapeutic diets and nutritional supplements can bring about lasting improvements for many gastrointestinal and metabolic conditions.

Clinical Nutrition

Modifications to the diet by increasing dietary fiber and eliminating allergenic foods can help prevent and treat GI conditions. High-soluble-fiber diets and elemental diets have proven to be effective. In addition, specific supplements can be added to a tool kit for managing GI conditions.

Specialized Diets

A nutrient-dense and easy-to-digest diet is fundamental for managing GI conditions. Poorly digested food is more likely to have a high load of antigens, which increases the likelihood of activating the immune system and more inflammation in the gut. Lack of digestibility may also prevent or reduce nutrient absorption. Anyone who has GI issues needs all the nutrients they can get.

High-Soluble-Fiber Diet

In some cases, improvement to GERD symptoms can be achieved by increasing the dietary fiber that is required for regular bowel function. Diets low in fiber can be irritating to the bowel. Insoluble fiber (wheat bran, for example) helps improve bowel transit and speeds up the movement of stool, as well as adding bulk to the stool, but can irritate the bowel. Oat bran soluble fiber offers the benefits without the irritation. Fruit pectins also provide beneficial fiber.

Bacterial fermentation of soluble fibers produces short-chain fatty acids (SCFAs), which are exactly what they sound like — fats that are simple and short in molecular structure compared to fats like omega-3 fatty acids. These SCFAs are important for bowel health and absorption of electrolytes and water in the colon. People with IBS have been found to have lower levels

Bowel Transit Time

This is the time needed for any food to travel through your gastrointestinal system and any wastes to be excreted. Your transit time is likely unique, but a general pattern emerges for most people. Transit time is affected by the kinds of foods you include in your diet, the amount (and kind) of fiber, the level of hydration and regular exercise. Other factors that may affect transit time include some drugs and some neurological conditions.

of SCFAs, acetate and propionate, along with less activity from bowel pro- and prebiotics. Supplementation with soluble fiber and probiotics (*Lactobacillus acidophilus*) is recommended.

FAQ

Q. What is a healthy bowel transit time?

A. A healthy bowel transit time is between 12 and 24 hours. Testing your transit time is a good idea, because having a bowel movement on a daily basis might lead you to believe that your GI system is working well, when, in fact your transit time may be longer than 2 days, putting you at risk. A transit time that is less than 10 hours suggests that the food in your diet is moving through your gastrointestinal system too quickly. Your intestines may not be getting the full benefit of the nutrients in your food because these nutrients are not being fully absorbed, which could lead to nutritional deficiencies. If you also have loose stools along with the fast transit, your risk increases for a weaker immune system, nutritional deficiencies, anemia, osteoporosis or electrolyte imbalance. People who have had gastric bypass or other forms of bariatric surgery may find that they have shorter transit times because the surgery allows food to literally "bypass" a certain length of the gut.

You can test your transit time by eating something that will show up in your stool, such as beets or corn. In your health journal, make a note of the time when you ate the food, then indicate when you have passed it in your stool. If your bowel transit time is longer than 2 days, your risk of disease (diverticulosis or cancer, for example) or overgrowth of intestinal bacteria or yeast (such as candida), which can reduce the ability of the immune system to protect you from foreign invaders, is increased.

Elimination Diet

In many cases, reactions to specific foods in the diet may promote IBS. Food intolerances can be diagnosed through an elimination diet, where suspected foods are excluded from the diet for a couple of weeks and then reintroduced. Foods that appear to be related to symptoms should be avoided.

Elemental Diet

This liquid preparation includes all the required nutrients in an absorbable form that does need to be digested. For example, amino acids rather than proteins are included. After the diet is finished, the gastrointestinal tract will have become unaccustomed to foods, so reintroduction will have to be done at a slow pace, beginning with broths and soups. Foods that are more difficult to digest (heavy proteins, such as meat and high-fat foods) should be avoided for some time. Serve food at room temperature because you may have cramps and diarrhea for a while.

Therapeutic Principles

In general, prepare food with these dietary principles in mind when treating GI conditions:

- Include high-biologic-value proteins
- Use appropriate cooking methods: bake, sauté or stew, but no deep-frying
- Include an abundance of fruits and vegetables — but cook them enough to permit breakdown in the gut
- Include food high in fiber, including soluble fiber
- Include iron from food sources
- Include plenty of vitamin C from natural sources
- Include foods that can support the growth of healthy colonic flora (foods that include probiotics)

> **Did You Know?**
>
> **Gut Dysfunction**
>
> When diet therapy doesn't help, look for gut dysfunction. Having a stool sample analyzed may help show whether there is gut dysfunction — a change in the populations of bacteria or yeasts, such as *Candida albicans*, that live in our gut and help us digest food and, in some cases, produce vitamins. If the balance of healthy to pathogenic bacteria leans more to the toxic variety, your immune system may cause inflammation to protect against what would be recognized as a foreign invader. The gut is a dynamic organ lined with nerves throughout, with a rapid turnover of surface cells. It can respond to treatment that stimulates healing.

Nutritional Supplements

If you have IBD, you may be deficient in specific vitamins and minerals because of malabsorption. Malabsorption will reduce the intake of all nutrients, but especially essential fatty acids, fat-soluble vitamins and protein. Damage to the small intestine can cause impaired absorption of vitamins (B_{12}, for example.) And ulcerative colitis can lead to severe anemia due to bleeding.

Treatment for these deficiencies needs to be in a highly absorbable, hypoallergenic form to restore healthy levels quickly. For some people, iron can be supplemented with iron citrate or iron picolinate, but you may react poorly to oral iron (it can cause inflammation). Iron-rich foods (peas, meats, green leafy vegetables) are a better source, but even iron-rich foods may not be enough to improve anemia.

Probiotics

Probiotics, such as lactobacilli (*Lactobacillus acidophilus* and *bifidus*), can be used for clinical nutrition therapy except during flare-ups, when added bacteria may increase inflammation levels. High-dose probiotic and prebiotic therapy is a safe and effective treatment for Crohn's disease, but it is important to discuss all varieties of probiotics you may be taking, including those that are diet-based (such as those in some yogurts), with your health-care team.

Antioxidants

Antioxidants are an important therapy for treating Crohn's disease. Ongoing inflammation of the intestines will increase oxidative stress (which is similar to the process of rusting in metals exposed to air), which can be helped with water-soluble and lipid- or fat-soluble antioxidants plus antioxidant minerals, such as selenium. Higher-level doses of essential fatty acids can reduce inflammation.

FAQ

Q. What is glutamine?

A. Glutamine is essential as fuel for regenerating small intestine wall cells — a constant rebuilding process — and is involved in mucosal repair and improvement of barrier function. Research has suggested that glutamine is associated with adapting the human gut to specific diets. Crohn's disease has been seen to impair the intestines' ability to take up glutamine from the circulation, thus reducing our ability to self-heal. Soluble fibers, such as oat bran, provide a main source of fuel (butyrate and acetate) to the large intestine and are also a rich source of glutamine. A single dose of NSAIDs (nonsteroidal anti-inflammatories, such as aspirin or ibuprofen) may cause damage to the gut that leads to increased permeability, increased antigen activity and inflammation.

Quercetin

Quercertin, a bioflavonoid that will stabilize mast cells (related to the immune response and stress) and decrease the release of histamine, may help calm the bowel. Even though quercetin is poorly absorbed from the GI tract, a local effect from quercetin in the GI tract is the point of treatment. An elimination diet with supplemental quercetin as recommended by your complementary health-care provider may help reduce IBS symptoms.

Homeopathy

Homeopathic remedies involve taking a word picture of a patient's symptoms and applying an appropriate remedy, which may include:

- ***Citrullus colocynthis* (bitter cucumber):** For abdominal pain that feels better with pressure or bending over double and worse with anger.
- ***Strychnos nux-vomica* (strychnine):** For abdominal pain with loose stools or difficulty completing stools (never feel done). Also for IBS that is worse with too much caffeine, tobacco, alcohol and rich or spicy foods and when angry or impatient.
- ***Arsenicum album* (white arsenic):** For a high-strung person with stress-induced IBS or if burning pain occurs as stools are passed.

Reducing Antigenic Stimulation

An effective therapy to reduce inflammation in the intestinal mucosal immune system will also reduce the stimulation of antigens.

1. Eliminate food antigens, which can be from foods to which you have an allergy, such as gluten from wheat (elimination or hypoallergenic diet).
2. Reduce undigested proteins in the gut. If protein digestion is poor, a high level of peptides (pieces of protein) will be present in the gut. These peptides may initiate an immune reaction or make an existing food allergy reaction worse. Low levels of acid (hydrogen chloride, or HCl) in the stomach may be one reason for poor digestion of proteins and may be caused by H2-inhibiting drugs.

Did You Know?

Hydrotherapy

Hydrotherapy is excellent for managing GI conditions, restoring good circulation and calming muscle contraction. This involves applying warm and cold compresses, usually in some alternating fashion, to the body (including the abdomen). It should be done by someone trained in this therapy, but when it is done well, it can promote feelings of well-being and relaxation.

Chapter 7

Complementary Treatment Plans

CASE STUDY ✍

IBD: Ulcerative Colitis

Dana sat quietly in the GI specialist's waiting room, wondering how long the appointment would take. She had a midterm for her kinesiology course in 3 hours and just wanted to take one more look at her notes.

Dana had been to several appointments in the past few months, ever since she'd had bloody diarrhea. Since then, she had lost weight. She wasn't trying, but she hadn't been at all interested in food and often felt sick to her stomach. She was even more tired than usual and she had some fevers that didn't seem to have any cause, but she was really worried about the bleeding from her rectum. Dana was in her final year of her master's program for kinesiology and was looking forward to finally beginning to work in her field. She was concerned that whatever was going on might interfere with her decision to work with disabled children...
(*continued on page 117*)

A good plan makes for a successful treatment. Here are several treatment plans for GI conditions from naturopathic and homeopathic perspectives. If your physician does not follow these complementary medical protocols, you might ask for a referral.

Treatment Protocols

These protocols indicate the pattern of clinical reasoning a naturopathic physician follows while managing a case, though the terminology may be somewhat obscure for many readers.

- **Protocol 1:** Assess fundamental health measures.
- **Protocol 2:** Promote self-healing processes.
- **Protocol 3:** Enhance physiological function.
- **Protocol 4:** Mitigate or suppress dysfunction.

How to Use Protocol 1 to Treat IBD

Assess fundamental health measures:

- Assess and address the root cause of the IBD.
- Assess the degree of inflammation. Is the destruction covering the entire wall of the intestine, has a fistula formed, or do any perforations exist? It is important to recognize crisis situations that may develop subtly, especially for anyone who is taking steroids.
- Assess degree of anemia. If present, treat in a specific manner.
- Assess for food hypersensitivities. Try to reduce the sheer number of allergenic proteins in the gut to help ease food allergies.
- Assess for lactobacilli, especially if there is a history of antibiotic use.

How to Use Protocol 2 to Treat IBS

Promote self-healing processes: If impediments to healing are removed or limited, the body has the capacity to self-heal. In the case of the gut, this dynamic organ is lined with nerves throughout and has a rapid turnover of surface cells. It can respond quickly to treatment that stimulates healing.

How to Use Protocol 3 to Treat Crohn's Disease

Enhance physiological function: Reducing antigenic stimulation enhances physiological function. An effective therapy to reduce inflammation in the intestinal mucosal immune system will impede the stimulation of the antigens.

- Eliminate food antigens, such as gluten from wheat, through an elimination or hypoallergenic diet.
- Reduce undigested proteins in the gut. A high level of peptides (pieces of protein) in the gut may initiate an immune reaction or worsen an existing food allergy.
- Low levels of hydrochloric acid in the stomach may be one reason for poor protein digestion and may be caused by drugs that inhibit H2.

How to Use Protocol 4 to Treat Ulcerative Colitis

Mitigate or suppress dysfunction: Some people with ulcerative colitis have a higher risk for colon cancer when the full length of the colon is affected for a long time. Colon cancer risk is higher for people who have had ulcerative colitis for 8 to 10 years and continues to increase as time goes by. Managing this condition with therapy combinations that maintain remission may reduce the risk.

Case Management

Complementary naturopathic and homeopathic physicians are likely to spend more time with you than conventional physicians do, working up not only a diagnosis but also a case management plan. In the case of a patient with GI conditions, a management plan might follow this pattern:

1. Manage pain.
2. Determine the extent of constipation and diarrhea.
3. Assess the degree to which life stressors are a factor.
4. Eliminate food sensitivities.
5. Address life challenges.
6. Reduce stress levels through whatever activity works for the patient.
7. Increase dietary fiber (mostly soluble fiber).
8. Supplement with *Lactobacillus acidophilus* or *bifidus*; quercetin; *Mentha piperita* (peppermint); *Althaea officinalis* (marshmallow) or *Ulmus fulva* (slippery elm).

GI Management Plans

The following plans are more precise and tailored to a specific GI condition.

Plan 1: Treating Gastroesophageal Reflux Disease

1. Avoid foods that commonly cause GERD symptoms.
2. Relax while eating.
3. Eat small meals with low fat content.

4. Increase fiber intake.
5. Avoid medications that aggravate the situation.
6. Take bitters before eating high-protein meals.
7. Examine coatings from inside your intestines.
8. Supplement with choline and lecithin.
9. If necessary, lose weight, the goal being a healthy body mass index, or BMI.
10. Stop smoking.

Source: List adapted with permission from El-Hashemy S, Downorowicz E, Rouchotas P, et al. *Family Medicine & Integrative Primary Care: Standards & Guidelines*. Toronto: CCNM Press, 2011. Gastroenterology, gastroesophageal reflux disease; p. 133–35.

Plan 2: Treating Irritable Bowel Syndrome

1. Investigate specific issues that aggravate the problem.
2. Recreate a normal microbial colonic environment.
3. Make lifestyle changes, including stress reduction, to reduce bowel spasm.
4. Use natural substances to relax the bowel.

Plan 3: Treating Crohn's Disease and Ulcerative Colitis

1. Establish short- and long-term plans for
    a) Gut and abdominal infections
    b) Electrolyte imbalances
    c) Nutrient deficiencies
    d) Neoplasm
2. Comanage with conventional drug therapies.
3. Be mindful of possible complications and quickly changing symptoms and severity, such as:
    a) Extreme anemia
    b) Peritonitis or abscess
4. Be prepared to work around steroidal treatment and new-generation anti-inflammatories (Imuran).
5. Pay attention to any worsening of symptoms and ask for a referral for appropriate care for:
    a) Abdominal tenderness with tensing of muscles to guard inflamed organs below
    b) Fever of unknown origin
    c) Dyspepsia, tachycardia, fatigue
    d) Mental confusion
    e) Failure to thrive not resolved by natural treatment

Plan 4: Treating Crohn's Disease

1. Assess and address the root cause.
2. Assess the degree of inflammation. Is the destruction covering the entire wall of the intestine, has a fistula formed, or do any perforations exist? It is important to recognize crisis situations that may develop subtly, especially for anyone who is taking steroids.
3. Assess the degree of anemia and, if present, treat.
4. Seek out food hypersensitivities and try to reduce the sheer number of allergenic proteins in the gut to help ease food allergies.
5. Use lactobacilli probiotics, especially if there is a history of antibiotic use.
6. If digestion is poor, address malabsorption with enzymes. Malabsorbed foods will only contribute to gut antigens.
7. Address nutritional deficiencies, including protein, minerals and fat-soluble and water-soluble vitamins.
8. Supplement with:
    a) Essential fatty acids (EFAs): fish oil or evening primrose oil
    b) *Glycyrrhiza glabra* (licorice), but be alert to risks with high blood pressure or of interaction with other therapies
9. In acute situations, follow an elemental diet until improvement is seen.
10. Use homeopathic remedies as indicated.

Plan 5: Treating Ulcerative Colitis

Follow a similar treatment process as for Crohn's disease, but recognize that anemia may dominate, more so than malabsorption.

1. Treat toxic megacolon as an emergency condition. Symptoms include constipation, fever and abdominal tenderness.
2. Assess whether digestion is poor and address malabsorption with enzymes. Malabsorbed foods will only contribute to gut antigens.
3. Address nutritional deficiencies, including protein, minerals and fat-soluble and water-soluble vitamins.

4. Supplement with:
    a) Essential fatty acids (EFAs): fish oil or evening primrose oil
    b) *Glycyrrhiza glabra* (licorice), but be alert to risks with high blood pressure or of interaction with other therapies
5. In acute situations, follow an elemental diet until improvement is seen.
6. Use homeopathic remedies as indicated.
7. Plan a regiment of nutritional supplements (see chart, below).

Nutritional Supplements

Consult your physician or pharmacist for safe and effective dosage.

Treatment	Comment
Protein supplement	Rice or whey protein
Vitamin C	Use buffered form (ester-C) if diarrhea occurs at lower doses
Glutamine	Use more in flare-up Specific to small intestine
Glycyrrhiza glabra (licorice)	
Iron	For anemia Caution against stimulating inflammation Take with vitamin C
Comprehensive meal replacement	Several kinds on market Combines whey, rice or soy protein with range of vitamins and minerals
Other antioxidants: Vitamin E Beta-carotene Selenium	Need increases with increased fatty acid intake
Essential fatty acids (EFAs): Fish oil with at least 50% of oil containing EPA or DPA	Take with meals and fortify with antioxidants

Part 3

The pH Balance Diet Program

Chapter 8

What Is a Well-Balanced Diet?

CASE STUDY (continued from page 110)

IBD: Ulcerative Colitis

Two weeks later, Dana received the results of her kinesiology midterm and results from the tests the specialist had set up for her — blood tests, stool tests and a colonoscopy/sigmoidoscopy. She did very well on her midterm and went to her follow-up GI appointment with a smile on her face.

The results of these tests were sobering. The blood tests indicated that she had a high white blood cell count, meaning that she had inflammation somewhere. She was also anemic, which she had suspected. The stool tests showed that she had some white blood cells in her colon. Finally, the uncomfortable colonoscopy confirmed for the specialist that Dana did have ulcerative colitis.

During the appointment, the specialist talked about possible medications for reducing symptoms and improving Dana's quality of life. She came away with information about the medication she was going to try and information about diet and nutrition, along with a referral to a registered dietitian (RD). Some diets are known to be successful at reducing inflammation and improving bowel health. The specialist had mentioned that, although he wasn't recommending the diet, some of his patients had experienced improvements in symptoms with a pH-balanced diet and suggested that she discuss the diet with the RD. The specialist ended the appointment by talking to Dana about how important it was for her to monitor her diet and health carefully because ulcerative colitis brought with it an increased risk of colon cancer.

Our general state of well-being can be improved by aiming to maintain a healthy body weight, eating a range of nutritious foods and practicing good eating habits — keeping a regular mealtime schedule, taking your time while eating, sitting down to a table to eat, chewing your food thoroughly, avoiding late-night meals and staying well hydrated through the day with non-caffeine, nonalcoholic and non-fizzy fluids. This state of health is commonly called well balanced, and the best way to get there is to eat a balanced diet. Most public health agencies, however, claim that the Western diet is deficient in fruits and vegetables and overly abundant in grains and meats. And most fruits and vegetables are alkaline on the pH scale; grains and meats are acidic.

Food Guides

Perhaps the two best guides to eating well for optimum health are the United States Department of Agriculture (USDA) Choose MyPlate diet program and Health Canada's Eating Well with Canada's Food Guide. If you follow the recommendations of these national food guides, you will be less likely to suffer from nutrient deficiencies and weight issues and more likely to maintain good health.

The focus of food guides is on achieving optimum health through good nutrition or, if needed, nutritional therapy. The recommendations in the national food guides will help you reach your optimum health. They support eating a diet rich in vegetables and fruit, whole grains and low-unsaturated-fat proteins that are high in omega-3 fatty acids (legumes, fish, lean meat). Pay special attention to the recommended number of servings per day from each food group to maintain optimum health.

Food Groups

Both food guides break the three macronutrients into four groups and seek to strike a balance in their consumption:

Macronutrients

- Carbohydrate
- Protein
- Fat

Food Groups

- Fruits and vegetables
- Grains and grain products
- Meat and alternatives
- Dairy and alternatives

A Balanced Diet

The food guides recommend eating a balanced, or proportioned, diet of macronutrients.

- **Carbohydrates:** 45% to 65% of your total calories for the day
- **Proteins:** 10% to 30% of your total calories for the day
- **Fats:** 20% to 35% of your total calories for the day

The food guides also show how to balance, or divide, the food groups on your plate:

- **Fruits and vegetables:** 50% of your plate
- **Grains and grain products:** 30% of your plate
- **Meat and alternatives:** 20% of your plate
- **Dairy and alternatives:** Optional

Did You Know?

Eating a Rainbow

Eating vegetables of different colors over the course of a day — all the colors of the rainbow — ensures you are consuming a wide range of nutrients, including folate, fiber, potassium and vitamins A and C. Many people don't eat enough fruits and vegetables for optimum health, however, leading to nutrient deficiencies.

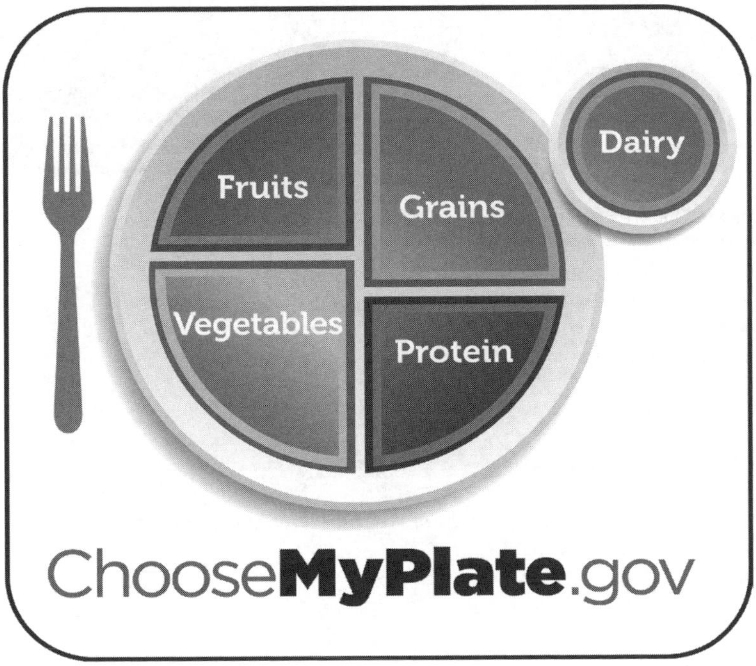

Servings and Portions

The national food guides also provide a guide to the recommended number of servings from each food group per day and directions for judging a portion. Eating small, more nutritious meals more often through the day may help you improve your metabolism, achieve better health and reach your optimum weight for wellness.

Fruits
Grains
Dairy
Vegetables
Protein
ChooseMyPlate.gov

Eating Well with Canada's Food Guide

*Recommended Number of **Food Guide Servings** per Day*

	Children			Teens		Adults			
Age in Years	2-3	4-8	9-13	14-18		19-50		51+	
Sex	Girls and Boys			Females	Males	Females	Males	Females	Males
Vegetables and Fruit	4	5	6	7	8	7-8	8-10	7	7
Grain Products	3	4	6	6	7	6-7	8	6	7
Milk and Alternatives	2	2	3-4	3-4	3-4	2	2	3	3
Meat and Alternatives	1	1	1-2	2	3	2	3	2	3

The chart above shows how many Food Guide Servings you need from each of the four food groups every day.

Having the amount and type of food recommended and following the tips in *Canada's Food Guide* will help:

- **Meet your needs for vitamins, minerals and other nutrients.**
- **Reduce your risk of obesity, type 2 diabetes, heart disease, certain types of cancer and osteoporosis.**
- **Contribute to your overall health and vitality.**

What is One Food Guide Serving?

Look at the examples below.

Fresh, frozen or canned vegetables
125 mL (½ cup)

Bread
1 slice (35 g)

Bagel
½ bagel (45 g)

MILK

POWDERED MILK

Milk or powdered milk (reconstituted)
250 mL (1 cup)

Cooked fish, shellfish, poultry, lean meat
75 g (2 ½ oz.)/125 mL (½ cup)

For the full guide, please contact Health Canada or visit their website (www.hc-sc.gc.ca).

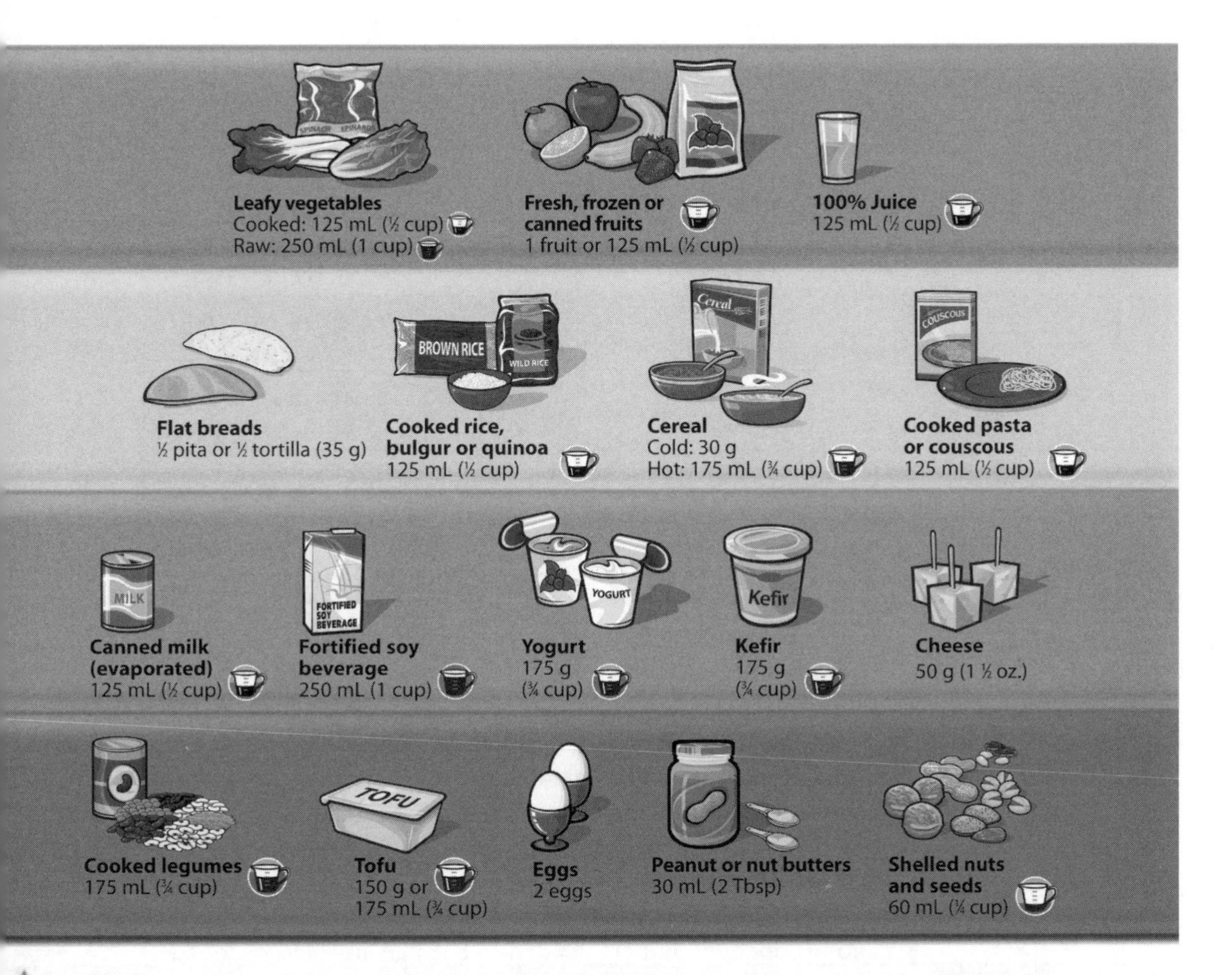

Oils and Fats

- Include a small amount – 30 to 45 mL (2 to 3 Tbsp) – of unsaturated fat each day. This includes oil used for cooking, salad dressings, margarine and mayonnaise.
- Use vegetable oils such as canola, olive and soybean.
- Choose soft margarines that are low in saturated and trans fats.
- Limit butter, hard margarine, lard and shortening.

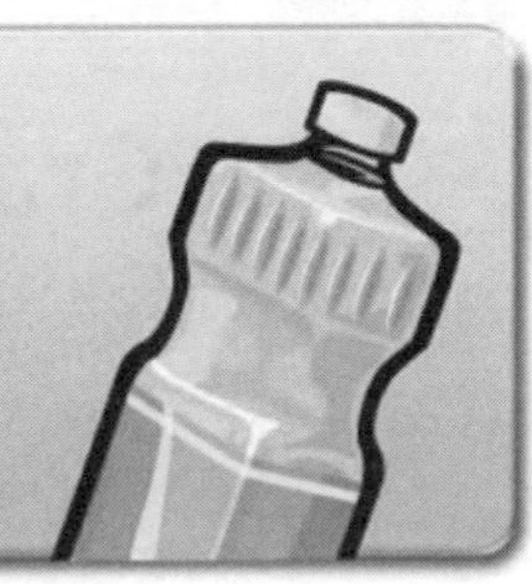

Daily Amounts and Portion Guidelines

Food Group	Women (Average)	Men (Average)	Serving Size	Portion Sample
Fruits	1½–2 cups (375–500 mL)	2 cups (500 mL)	½ cup (125 mL)	Rounded handful, 1 apple, 1 banana, 2 plums
Vegetables	2–2½ cups (500–625 mL)	2½–3 cups (625–750 mL)	½ cup (125 mL)	Rounded handful
Grains	3–6 oz (90–175 g)	3–8 oz (90–250 g)	1 oz (30 g)	Egg-sized potato, 1 slice of bread
Proteins	5–5½ oz (150–160 g)	5½–6½ oz (150–200 g)	1 oz (30 g)	Deck of cards, palm of your hand, 1 egg
Dairy	3 cups (750 mL)	3 cups (750 mL)	1 cup (250 mL)	1 small carton of milk
Fats & Oils	5–6 tsp (25–30 mL)	6–7 tsp (30–35 mL)	1 tsp (5 mL)	1 thumb tip, 1 dice

Adapted from the USDA MyPlate guide.

Did You Know?

Enriched Grain Products

Milling improves shelf life and gives grain a finer texture. At the same time, milling removes dietary fiber, iron and many of the B vitamins. Some B vitamins are added back to the milled grains (which are then called enriched); however, fiber is not added back. Also be aware that some products are combinations of whole and milled grains.

Fruits and Vegetables

On some days, it might not seem possible to eat the number of fruits and vegetables recommended by the food guidelines, but eating fruits and vegetables reduces the risk of cancer and other chronic disease states. Fruits and vegetables provide the essential vitamins and minerals, fiber and other disease-fighting substances that provide the building blocks for optimum health. Fruits and vegetables are also low-fat, have few calories and are filling.

pH Connection: Most fruits and vegetables are alkalizing and produce the buffers needed to balance any acid overload. Devote more than 50% of your meals to fruits and vegetables.

Grains and Grain Products

Grains are good sources of fiber, several B vitamins (thiamin, riboflavin, niacin and folate) and minerals (iron, magnesium and selenium). B vitamins are involved in your body's metabolism through their role in the release of energy from protein, fat and carbohydrates. B vitamins are also essential to support your nervous system. Whole grains are also sources of magnesium and selenium. Selenium protects your cells from oxidation (being broken down in the same way that metal rusts when exposed to air), supports your immune system and is safe in small amounts.

Whole Grains

Eating whole grains is more beneficial than eating processed and fortified grains. Whole grains contain the entire kernel (bran, germ and endosperm), whereas refined grains have gone through a milling process that removes the bran and germ and, along with them, most of the nutrients.

pH Connection: Quinoa, buckwheat and millet are alkalizing whole grains. Use them instead of other whole grains that are more acidic.

Fiber

Dietary fiber is known to reduce blood cholesterol levels and your risk of heart disease, obesity and type 2 diabetes. Fiber helps maintain healthy bowel function and reduces constipation and diverticulosis. This is not the case with refined or processed flour, however. Breads, rice, pasta and cereals made mostly from processed or refined white flours, as well as the refined sugars or corn syrup used in most cakes, cookies and candies, can cause poor digestion in your gut, disrupt your body's balance and lead to disease. Increase the nutritional value of your food by switching to whole grains with fiber and no added sugars wherever possible.

Meat and Alternatives

This group includes several sources of protein: meat and eggs, nuts and seeds, fish and seafood, and beans and peas (also part of the vegetable group), including soy products. Your age, sex and level of physical activity determine your need for protein.

These foods provide B vitamins, vitamin E, iron, zinc and magnesium. The proteins you eat are the building blocks

Did You Know?

Iron-Deficiency Anemia

Iron found in the meat and alternatives group helps carry oxygen in blood. Teenage girls and women in childbearing years who have iron-deficiency anemia should eat foods high in heme iron derived from meat or nonheme iron in combination with vitamin C, which will increase nonheme iron absorption. Poor iron status in adults can be due to diet issues but also from blood loss in the gut as the result of a stomach ulcer, a bleeding polyp or, in some cases, a colon tumor.

"Bad" Cholesterol

Meat products with high levels of saturated fats may raise the low-density lipoproteins (LDLs) in your blood. High levels of this "bad" cholesterol increase your risk of heart disease, and when blood levels of C-reactive protein (CRP) are also high, there may be increased risk of several major diseases. Saturated fats themselves are not the main culprit — overconsumption of carbohydrates can increase the risk for heart disease as well. The quality of foods and their preparation, including the use of saturated fats, does, however, count in the grand scheme of things. For example, saturated fat that has been burned over a flame or deep-fried in oil may be chemically different than the saturated fat from an avocado.

for your bones, muscles, cartilage, skin and blood. Enzymes, hormones and vitamins are built (metabolized) from proteins. Proteins also provide calories to fuel your body. A healthy diet includes at least 8 oz (250 g) of fish or seafood per week, unless you are vegetarian or vegan.

Magnesium-Rich Foods

Magnesium, found primarily in protein foods, is critical for building bones and releasing the energy from your muscles.

pH Connection: Magnesium-rich foods are excellent choices when you are working to keep your pH balanced.

Magnesium-Rich Foods

Food	Serving	Magnesium (mg)
Oat bran	½ cup (125 mL) uncooked	96.0
100% bran cereal	½ cup (125 mL)	93.1
Brown rice	1 cup (250 mL) cooked	86.0
Almonds	1 oz (30 g), about 23 almonds	78.0
Swiss chard, chopped	½ cup (125 mL) cooked	75.0
Molasses, blackstrap	1 tbsp (15 mL)	48.0
Okra, frozen	½ cup (125 mL) cooked	47.0
Hazelnuts	1 oz (30 g), about 21 hazelnuts	46.0
Milk, 1%	1 cup (250 mL)	34.0

Choosing and Preparing Protein-Rich Foods

Increase the nutritional value of foods containing protein by choosing leaner cuts of meat and skinless poultry. In addition, many foods in this group can spoil when not properly stored or refrigerated. Follow these guidelines for keeping your food fresh:

- Keep raw, cooked and ready-to-eat foods in separate containers.
- Store raw meats in containers that will not drip onto other foods.
- Do not wash or rinse your meat or poultry — washing is more likely to spread contamination around.
- Wash all cutting surfaces with warm soapy water after preparing each food item.

- To destroy microorganisms, cook foods to the correct temperature, tested using a meat thermometer, which will display the safe internal temperature for each kind of meat.
- Never defrost foods on the counter.
- Avoid raw or undercooked meats or eggs.
- Be aware of mercury content in some fish, especially for pregnant or nursing women or for children.

Dairy Products and Alternatives

Fluid milk and milk products are part of this food group, as are dairy alternatives such as soy milk and soy products. These products are often fortified with calcium.

Dairy Safety

- Avoid unpasteurized (raw) milk or milk products that have been made from raw milk.
- Put any dairy foods in the refrigerator right away.
- Do not defrost frozen dairy foods on the counter.
- Put any leftover food from meals that contain dairy products in the fridge immediately after serving.
- If dairy products have been left on the counter for 2 or more hours, throw them out.

FAQ

Q. What are the benefits and risks of eating dairy food?

A. The jury is out. Dairy foods are a good source of protein, and the calcium in dairy products — the primary source of calcium in some populations — leads to increased bone health and may reduce your risk of osteoporosis. Dairy products have been linked with reduced risk of cardiovascular disease and type 2 diabetes. These foods are also known to lower blood pressure in adults.

Calcium is most critical for bone health in the years when bones are being built (childhood and adolescence) and is used for building and maintaining bone mass, including your teeth. Dairy products that are fortified with vitamin D also help build and maintain bones and teeth by protecting the calcium and phosphorous levels. Yogurt, fluid milk and soy milk (soy beverage) also provide potassium, which can help maintain healthy blood pressure.

However, a high intake of dairy products may add to the level of saturated fats in your diet and thus contribute to a higher risk of elevated C-reactive proteins (CRPs) and increased risk of disease. Choosing low-fat or fat-free forms of dairy foods will add little or no fat to your diet.

Did You Know?

Sugar Names

Sugar has many names, based on what it is made from and the refining process, making it hard to identify. Some common types of sugar include fruit juice concentrates, nectars, malt syrup, cane syrup and juice, corn sweeteners, high-fructose corn syrup, honey and molasses.

Sugar

Sugar, natural or processed, is a simple carbohydrate that your body uses for quick fuel. Sources of carbohydrate, such as fruits, vegetables and dairy foods, all contain sugars. On food labels, "added sugars" refers to the sugars or syrups added during processing to increase the appeal of these foods. Sugar helps preserve foods (jellies, jams), adds bulk (baked goods, ice cream), gives baked foods texture and color and adds flavor to processed foods. It also balances the acidity of foods that contain vinegar and tomatoes.

Adding refined sugar to your diet, however, can have a significant impact on your health. Concerns about added sugars include:

- Tooth decay from bacterial growth around teeth combined with poor oral hygiene
- Possible weight gain from empty calories
- Increased triglycerides
- Replacing healthy food choices, which can lead to poor nutrition

Reading the information about sugar on food labels can be confusing. If you look at the ingredient list, ingredients that end in -ose are chemical names for many sugars (fructose, glucose, maltose, dextrose). The placement of the ingredient's name in the list — first, second or third — shows how much of that ingredient is in the product compared to the other ingredients.

How to Reduce Your Sugar Intake

- Drink water instead of sugary drinks.
- If you drink juice, drink 100% fruit juice, not fruit drinks. From a nutritional point of view, fruit is always better than fruit juice.
- Skip sugary cereals and choose sugar-free, whole-grain products only.
- Choose syrups, jams, jellies and preserves that have few ingredients and reduced sugar.
- Choose water-packed canned fruit.
- Choose fruits and vegetables; low-fat cheese; low-fat, low-calorie yogurt; and whole-grain crackers for snacks.

Artificial Sweeteners

Food additives, such as sugar substitutes, artificial sweeteners or intense sweeteners from natural sources, are carefully assessed by governmental regulatory bodies before they are approved for use in food products. These sweeteners include acesulfame potassium, aspartame, neotame, polydextrose, sucralose, thaumatin, steviol glycosides (a plant-based sweetener) and the sugar alcohols (called polyols): sorbitol, isomalt, lactitol, maltitol, mannitol and xylitol. Artificial sweeteners, along with other sugar substitutes, are common ingredients in:

- Soft drinks (soda pop)
- Ice cream
- Yogurt (sweetened)
- Juices (sugar added)
- Candy
- Chewing gum

Artificial sweeteners are popular because they have no calories and don't contribute to tooth decay and cavities. People with diabetes also use artificial sweeteners because they don't raise blood sugar levels. Even though these products are widely used, some health concerns exist, so recommendations are for limited use.

Beverages

In every cell of our bodies, water is essential for life and critical for maintaining good health every day. The water levels in your body maintain a normal temperature, keep joints lubricated and cushioned, protect the spinal cord by floating it in spinal fluid and manage your body's housekeeping system by getting rid of wastes through your urine, perspiration and bowel movements. Some of our water needs are satisfied through the foods we eat, such as celery, tomatoes, oranges, melons (foods that are 85% to 95% water) or prepared foods such as soups and casseroles. For optimum health, drink when you are thirsty, with meals and as appropriate, depending on your activities. As we age, our thirst does not always keep up with our true hydration needs, so it is important to somewhat overhydrate during hot days or after exercise, especially for the elderly.

Chapter 9

Balancing Dietary Fats

CASE STUDY ✍

IBD: Crohn's Disease

Denise sat back in her chair. She had just finished reading the information her naturopathic physician had given to her to review while she waited for him to return. Her recent attack of painful cramps and horrible diarrhea was causing her to lose time at work, and she had missed some family birthdays too. She had made an appointment after noticing blood in the toilet after a bowel movement. She held her stomach now, wondering just what was in store for her. She was slightly dizzy, perhaps from the fever that had swept over her first thing this morning, and she felt terrible. Reading the pamphlet certainly hadn't made her feel any better. It described the signs and symptoms of Crohn's disease, and some of the usual treatments.

Dr. Hendley bustled back into the room with the results of her tests showing on his tablet. He patted Denise's hand, knowing how bad she was feeling. He went through her symptoms, pointing out the data that showed how severe her Crohn's disease was. But she was lucky, he felt: she didn't have any ulcers breaking through her intestines. According to the results, food had been responsible for scraping the inflamed walls and causing the bleeding.

They talked about how stress was a strong factor in Crohn's disease and how, for some people, certain foods could make symptoms worse. Dr. Hendley explained that diet was one way she could help manage her symptoms, and that a pH-balanced diet, although not a cure for Crohn's disease, could improve her overall health. He referred Denise to a registered dietitian to talk about trying a pH-balanced diet.

They also discussed changes Denise could make to adopt a healthier lifestyle, making her physical, mental and spiritual health a priority. Dr. Hendley wanted her to try a mind–body therapy, such as yoga or meditation, to help manage stress. Gentle exercise was also very important. Denise didn't need to run marathons, but making a 15-minute walk part of her daily schedule would really help.

Dr. Hendley emphasized the importance of keeping a health journal, no matter what direction Denise took with any therapy. If she wasn't feeling better after trying a specific therapy, they would discuss other options.

Denise sighed deeply. She felt tired and ill, hardly in a state to take on new challenges. Dr. Hendley took her hand and reassured her that he would help her every step of the way.

According to the food guides, fats and oils are not a food group, but they do bring essential nutrients to the table and are therefore included in most diet programs. Fat is the major source of energy derived from food. Fat has 9 calories per gram, twice as many as either carbohydrates or proteins. Fat helps insulate your body organs. Fats also maintain healthy skin and hair. Some fats are essential to life — without them we would not survive. A diet high in fat, however, increases the risk of becoming overweight or obese.

Fatty Acid Chemistry

In nature, carbon, hydrogen and oxygen are single molecules that form many complex molecules. A fatty acid is a hydrocarbon (hydrogen + carbon) chain (different lengths have different names) with a common group at one end called a carboxyl group (COOH). The carboxyl group is made up of 1 carbon molecule with 2 links (bonds) to 1 oxygen molecule and a single bond to an oxygen molecule that is in turn linked to 1 hydrogen molecule. The COOH group has a positive and a negative end, which is why the molecule is an acid. Acetic acid, or vinegar, for example, has a COOH group.

Liquid Fats

Some plant-based and fish oils are liquid at room temperature:

- Canola oil
- Cottonseed oil
- Corn oil
- Soybean oil
- Sunflower oil
- Olive oil

FAQ

Q. What are essential fatty acids?

A. Fatty acids that are required by the body but cannot be synthesized in the body and therefore must be obtained from food are known as essential fatty acids (EFAs). There are two chief kinds of EFAs, omega-3 and omega-6, which must be properly balanced in the diet to ensure good health.

Triglycerides

A normal fat you would find in food is made up of three fatty acids bound together with glycerol to form a molecule called a triglyceride. The choice of fatty acid, which is determined by the length of the carbon chain, controls how the fat looks, whether it is solid or liquid at room temperature and how

Did You Know?

Heart Disease

Saturated and trans fats in your diet can increase your risk of developing heart disease. Choose healthier oils with little to no trans fats and reduce your intake of saturated fats.

healthy it would be in your diet. Some foods that are high in fatty oils include nuts, olives, avocados and some fish. Mayonnaise, some salad dressings and soft margarine (with no trans fats) are oil-based foods that are included in most diets.

Saturated Fats vs. Unsaturated Fats

When every possible link of the chain to the central line of carbon molecules is bonded to hydrogen molecules, the fat is called a saturated fat because the carbon molecules are saturated with hydrogen molecules. Saturated fats are solid at room temperatures.

In unsaturated fats, some of the bonds to the carbon molecules are not linked to hydrogen molecules and, as a result, stronger double bonds between two of the side-by-side carbon molecules are formed. If the carbon chain (known as an acid) is 1 hydrogen molecule short of being saturated, it is called a monounsaturated fatty acid. Polyunsaturated fatty acids have more than one double bond between carbon molecules and are liquid at room temperature.

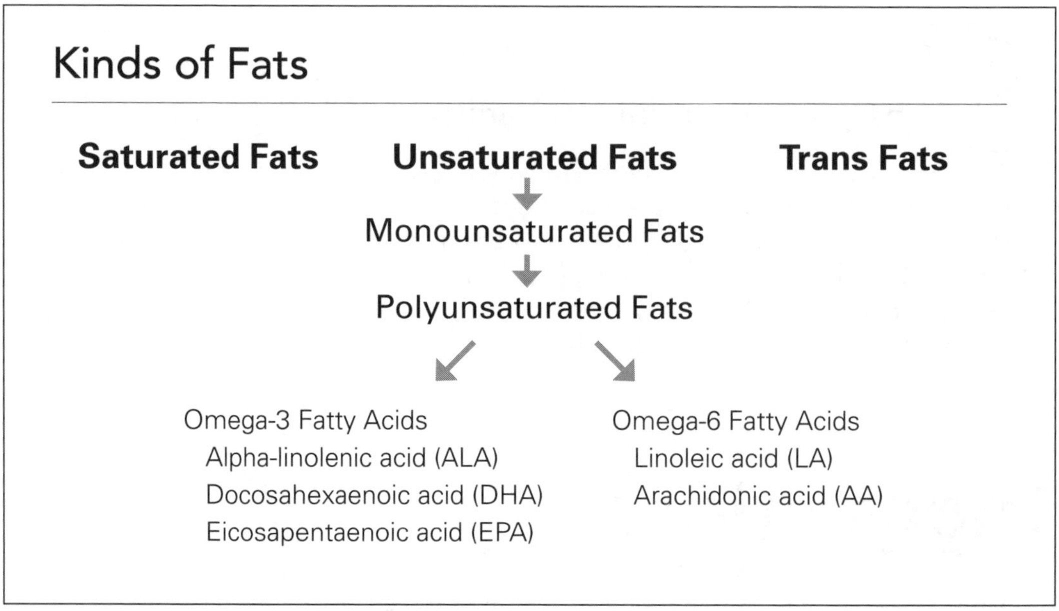

Kinds of Fats

Saturated Fats | **Unsaturated Fats** | **Trans Fats**

Unsaturated Fats → Monounsaturated Fats → Polyunsaturated Fats

Polyunsaturated Fats ↙ ↘

Omega-3 Fatty Acids
- Alpha-linolenic acid (ALA)
- Docosahexaenoic acid (DHA)
- Eicosapentaenoic acid (EPA)

Omega-6 Fatty Acids
- Linoleic acid (LA)
- Arachidonic acid (AA)

Trans Fats

A polyunsaturated fatty acid can be turned into a solid, such as margarine, by saturating it with hydrogen so that the double bonds are broken. The hydrogen molecules join to the carbon when heated and pressurized by hydrogen gas with a nickel catalyst (a catalyst helps the reaction occur at a lower temperature). The product of this reaction is called a partially hydrogenated vegetable oil (PHVO), or trans fat, and is the main ingredient of vegetable shortening and many margarines. Trans fats are also found in some animal fats used in cooking.

These trans fats are not healthy and should be avoided. They have been removed from the grocery shelf in most North American jurisdictions, but check food labels for trans fat and return the food to the shelf if you find trans fat listed.

Omega Fatty Acids

Two kinds of polyunsaturated fatty acids (PUFAs) are essential to our health: omega-3, or alpha-linolenic acid (ALA); and omega-6, or linoleic acid (LA). Both are essential fats that must be acquired from food and need to be balanced in your diet.

Once digested in your body, ALA is converted into two acids: eicosapentaenoic acid (EPA) and docosahexaenoic acid (DHA). LA is converted in our bodies to arachidonic acid (AA). EPA, DHA and AA are all metabolized through the same pathway.

Omega-3 fatty acids are known to decrease triglycerides and very-low-density lipoprotein blood levels but may not have an impact on low-density lipoprotein (LDL) levels. AA is involved in the body's responses to injury, infection, stress and certain disease states. EPA produces molecules (called eiconsanoids) that may protect you against heart attacks and strokes, as well as inflammation-based conditions like arthritis, lupus erythematosus and asthma. EPA also reduces cytokines, which are molecules that increase inflammation. DHA is the major PUFA found in the brain and plays a key role in signal transmission along neurons and inflammation response in the brain.

Omega-3 is found in leafy green vegetables, nuts, vegetable oils, flax seeds and flaxseed oil. Fish are good sources of EPA and DHA. LA is found in meat, vegetable oils (corn, sunflower, soy and safflower) and related processed foods.

Did You Know?

EFA-Fortified

Some foods may be fortified with omega-3 EFAs. For example, omega-3-fortified eggs are high in alpha-linolenic acid (ALA) because the hens are fed flaxseed meal. Any omega-3 is generally useful in a population where intake tends to be deficient or suboptimal, so there is a benefit here, but the process is not the most efficient and the effect is not as direct on the body as taking EPA or DHA as supplements.

Guidelines for Improving Your Omega-3 to Omega-6 Balance

- Eat less meat at a sitting.
- Use more olive and nut oils than safflower or corn oils.
- Eat fish more often.
- Eat more leafy vegetables on a daily basis.

Omega Fatty Acid Functions

AA and EPA are involved in many vital body functions, including:

- Cell division and growth
- Blood clotting
- Muscle activities
- Secretion of digestive juices
- Release of hormones
- Movement of calcium through the bloodstream

Without the involvement of these fatty acids, we would not survive.

Balancing Omega Fatty Acids

It is essential for optimum health to balance omega-3 and omega-6 fatty acids. The ideal ratio is not known, but is thought to be between 1:1 and 4:1. Some countries in the world have an average ratio of omega-3s to omega-6s of 10:1 and 30:1, which could lead to an imbalance in your body and raise the risk of disease.

pH Connection: Autoimmune diseases all have high levels of inflammation, known to be caused by omega-6 fatty acids. Several clinical trials have assessed the benefits of dietary fish oil supplementation in several inflammatory and autoimmune diseases, such as rheumatoid arthritis, Crohn's disease, ulcerative colitis, lupus erythematosus and psoriasis.

FAQ

Q. Which fats are good to eat and which ones should be avoided?

A. Trans fats should be avoided and saturated fats limited. Fats affect the cholesterol levels in the body. The saturated and trans fats raise bad cholesterol levels in your blood. Monounsaturated fats may decrease the total cholesterol as well as the bad cholesterol. Polyunsaturated fats cannot only decrease the total and bad cholesterol, but certain types of polyunsaturated fats may protect against heart disease and sudden death, and they have beneficial effects on the nervous system.

Chapter 10
Food Reactions

CASE STUDY ✍

A New Lifestyle

Jerry rubbed his chin, his face puzzled as he looked over the material the registered dietitian (RD) had given him. The information on how to balance pH through diet was a lot to take in, but Jerry was committed to achieving better health in the hopes of resolving his IBS symptoms. He sighed deeply, then leaned in to listen as she walked him through the steps of a pH-balanced diet.

A month later, Jerry sat back from the table, after a smaller dinner than he would have imagined would keep him satisfied. He was still working on cleaning out the acidic foods from his kitchen cupboards, but was starting to understand that cooking from the basics was much healthier than reaching for a packaged meal. He was filtering his water and adding half a teaspoon (2 mL) of sodium bicarbonate per gallon (4 L) to create alkaline water. (He still shook his head at the idea that adding a squeeze of lemon juice to a glass of distilled water would make it alkaline too. It just didn't make sense, even though the RD had explained that citrus, although acidic, was alkalizing once inside the body.) He was more conscious of drinking enough water throughout the day than he had been; he realized now that he had often been dehydrated, perhaps the source of some of his symptoms...
(*continued on page 138*)

Food additives, food poisoning and food allergies, intolerances and sensitivities impede good health by lowering resistance to antigens and pathogens.

Food Additives and Preservatives

Food additives and preservatives help make our food supply flavorful, nutritious, convenient, colorful and affordable. Fortification with vitamins and minerals and the enrichment of foods have also reduced malnutrition worldwide. Preservatives slow the process of food spoilage due to mold, air, bacteria,

Did You Know?

Food Poisoning

Food poisoning is an adverse reaction that happens only as a specific result of improper food storage, processing or contamination. You could eat the same type of food on other occasions and not have this reaction again.

fungi and yeast. They also help control the contamination that may cause food-borne illness (botulism, for example). Antioxidants help prevent fats and oils, and any foods that contain them, from becoming rancid or going "off" and are also responsible for preventing foods like apples from oxidizing and turning brown. Many consumers are concerned about the safety of food additives, however.

Functions of Food Additives

- Enhance the taste of food by adding spices, natural flavors and artificial flavors.
- Maintain or improve appearance by adding food colors.
- Create texture and consistency by adding emulsifiers, stabilizers and thickeners.
- Control the acidity and alkalinity of foods.
- Maintain the taste and appeal of foods, even those with reduced fat.
- Help baked goods rise through leavening agents.

Food Safety

There is no doubt that chemical additives to our food supply have created health hazards. For example, artificial sweeteners (such as aspartame), residues of antibiotics in animal proteins and agricultural fertilizer and pesticide residues in crops have all been shown to have an impact on human health.

Our foods have also been contaminated by soil and water pollution. Our fish supply, for example, is contaminated by mercury poisoning. In response to these and other concerns, agencies such as Health Canada and the U.S. Environmental Protection Agency (EPA) have been created to set food safety policies.

Food Allergy

A food allergy happens every time you eat a specific food or type of food that sets off a body-wide immune reaction that can be life-threatening. Food allergy reactions can range from a mild itch to acute swelling of the face and neck and difficulty with breathing. Such a severe allergic reaction is called anaphylaxis and is fatal if not treated urgently. People with serious food allergies carry injectable epinephrine (EpiPens) with them as a lifesaver and must avoid contact with their allergens for their entire lives. It is very important to be checked for food allergies if you suspect you have one.

> **Did You Know?**
>
> **Allergy or Intolerance?**
>
> Food allergies are caused by a direct reaction from the immune system in response to a particular protein in a food, whereas food intolerances may or may not be directly caused by an immune response.

Immune Functions

Our immune system functions through an intricate network of chemicals, proteins and cells, both in the blood and locally in various tissues. This system detects and destroys harmful organisms of various sizes, including bacteria, viruses, fungi and parasites — collectively known as pathogens, allergens and antigens — that constantly invade our body. The immune system also picks up and clears out our body's own cells that have become abnormal (that is, cancerous).

Normally, a state of dynamic balance, or homeostasis, exists within our immune system for us to enjoy a disease-free state. When our immune system deviates from the balance point, we can succumb to a state of hypoactive immunity (resulting in infections or cancer) or hyperactive immunity (resulting in autoimmune diseases or chronic pain).

Inflammation

Inflammatory chemicals are released when the immune system network is activated by the identification of a potentially harmful event (an infection, an irritant, a physical injury or an alien molecule). This pro-inflammatory action by the immune system has two goals: first, to enhance the odds of destroying the injurious agent, and second, to set the stage for the healing process.

> **Did You Know?**
>
> **Elimination and Limitation Diet**
>
> Food intolerances can be diagnosed through an elimination diet, where suspected foods are excluded from the diet for a period of time and then reintroduced. Foods that appear to be related to symptoms should be limited or avoided.

Food Intolerance and Sensitivity

We also need to distinguish a food allergy from a food intolerance or sensitivity. Some people think they have a food allergy when in fact they are suffering from a food intolerance or sensitivity. Food sensitivity, or intolerance, is an adverse reaction (such as an upset stomach) that happens every time you eat a particular food or type of food.

> **Did You Know?**
>
> **Food Sensitivity Tests**
>
> Some commercial tests make claims that they are able to diagnose food intolerances. These include the electrodermal (vega) test, the IgG blood test, kinesiology and even hair analysis. No convincing evidence exists that supports the results of any of these tests. The most reliable way to identify a food sensitivity is to eliminate foods and then reintroduce them after time has passed.

Testing for Tolerance

Although tests for food allergies generally produce positive or negative results, it is more difficult to test for sensitivities because often no allergic response is seen from testing the immune system. In addition, some people overcome their sensitivity to a particular food after gradual re-exposure over a period of time.

Antibodies

Three types of antibodies are typically linked to food sensitivity: IgE, IgA and IgG. Ig is the abbreviation for immunoglobulin, which is a protein made in our body to protect against foreign invaders (pathogens). Each Ig protein is specific for the pathogen it identifies. Finding immunoglobulins linked to specific foods in the bloodstream should make it easy to identify food issues, but sometimes foods cause inflammation even when no Ig proteins are found. One reason for this is that the reaction occurs inside the small intestine and not in the bloodstream.

Digestive Enzymes

A shortage of digestive enzymes or improperly working digestive enzymes may be the cause of many illnesses, including food intolerances. Enzymes are the driving force behind all metabolic activities in our bodies. Digestive enzymes break down all the foods we eat. The molecules that remain are used as nutrients to build, repair and replace tissues, as well as the source of the energy that drives our bodies. When our pH balance is on the acidic side, enzymes, which are protein molecules, unfold and lose their structure, leaving them unable to complete any activity.

Lactose Intolerance

Lactose intolerance is indicated by bloating, pain and gas every time you drink milk or eat milk-based products. Some people are unable to digest dairy products because they may not have sufficient amounts of the enzyme (called lactase) that breaks lactose down into glucose and galactose. Lactase enzyme deficiencies can be genetic, or they can be caused by injuries to the small intestine (diarrhea, chemotherapy, intestinal parasites or other environmental factors) or, more rarely, a complete lack of lactase. Symptoms of lactose intolerance include cramps, abdominal bloating, nausea, flatulence, diarrhea, rumbling stomach or vomiting. If you have these symptoms but no immune response to milk, you may have an allergy to the casein protein.

Lactose Substitutes

To ensure that you consume enough calcium, substitute lactose with other foods:

- Lactose-free dairy alternatives, such as almond milk
- Canned fish
- Soybeans and other soy products (tofu, soy yogurt, tempeh)
- Other beans
- Some leafy greens (collards, turnip greens, kale, bok choy)
- Calcium-fortified cereals and breads

Chapter 11

How Does This Diet Work?

CASE STUDY (continued from page 133)

A New Lifestyle

Jerry reached for his diary, a new habit he had to remind himself to follow. It helped that his diary was small enough to fit in his pocket. He'd last had a diary when he was a kid, in which he would record how many laps he could run and how many sit-ups he could do in a minute, along with the stats from his favorite baseball team. Now he was using a diary to record every bit of food he ate and how often he drank alkaline water, along with any symptoms he experienced, how severe they were, the medications he was taking and any side effects. He also recorded his sleep patterns and his stress levels, along with details about his exercise program. It was a lot of work, but his naturopathic doctor had told him it would really help both of them to see how well his therapy plan was working.

The pH-balanced diet wasn't so very different from how he usually ate, just more vegetables and less meat. The recipes he had been given were a big help, and remembering which foods to avoid or enjoy was starting to become more automatic. Jerry had always been someone who stuck to the familiar when it came to vegetables, but he was discovering that he really enjoyed the new flavors and textures of the different vegetables he was adding to his menu. He had more energy than he used to, and didn't feel quite so stressed.

He had a big smile on his face as he headed out the door for his nightly 15-minute stroll. An unexpected benefit from his new lifestyle was a slow loss of weight. He was looking forward to what the next month would bring.

There is no shortage of popular diet programs competing for your attention. Low-carbohydrate and high-fiber diets, high-protein and low-fat diets, South Beach and Mediterranean diets. The list goes on. Most of these diets are focused on weight loss, not on general good health or specific conditions. A pH-balanced diet, which is preventive in promoting general good health and therapeutic in addressing gastrointestinal conditions, could be readily adapted to other body systems — circulatory, renal and musculoskeletal, for example.

Preventive Practices

To prevent pH-related illness and maintain good health, consider these actions and review your outcomes from time to time with your health-care providers:

1. Eat a healthy balance of vegetables, fruits, seeds and nuts, as well as a variety of whole grains and proteins.
2. Include foods that increase levels of buffers to reduce existing acidity in the body.
3. Increase the amount of healthy fiber in your diet.
4. Stay properly hydrated.
5. Incorporate cooking methods that reduce the acidifying properties of foods.
6. Choose fresh whole foods over foods that are:
   - Processed
   - High in salt
   - Overly fatty or contain poor-quality fats
   - Laden with sugar

✦ Caution

Before adopting any new diet, it is important to discuss potential risks with your health-care team.

Therapeutic Practices

A pH-balanced diet can also be therapeutic and complementary to other dietary therapies. Take the case of chronic ulcerative colitis, where the short-term, or acute, goal is to relieve symptoms while the system is being restored to a state of homeostasis in the long term. In this case:

- A pH-balanced diet may help reduce the severity of your symptoms.
- A pH-balanced diet is critical for improving your ability to heal and recover from this gastrointestinal disease by countering low-level acidosis. Some of the health issues identified with low-level acidosis include fatigue, impaired endocrine functioning (but not in the thyroid) and increased risk of enzyme disruptions, which may lead to respiratory and urinary tract infections. Low-level acidosis may also cause premature aging from breakdowns in the cellular repair process, cognitive decline or increased breakdown of muscle to provide glutamine for acid detoxification.
- A pH-balanced diet can help buffer the nutrients lost during the balancing process. When our diet is regularly high in acidifying foods, our body attempts to bring the acid–alkaline balance back to normal, and in doing so may be using up our body's stores of essential minerals (magnesium, calcium, potassium and sodium), increasing the risk for disease.

- A pH-balanced diet can supplement the nutrients lost in the balancing process of homeostasis because of a dysfunctional GI system.
- A pH-balanced diet acknowledges that individual reactions to food may reduce your symptoms. As you follow the diet, continue to do pH readings of saliva and urine first thing in the morning. Once a healthy pH range is achieved, the ratio of alkalizing to acidifying foods can be shifted to 60% alkalizing and 40% acidifying foods.

Easing the Transition

All aspects of our diet are connected to our social and family structure, making any changes in our diet and eating habits extremely challenging. Does your partner bring you foods they know you love as a way of saying "I love you," even though these foods may be difficult for you to digest? Does every meal with your parents involve foods you struggled with as a child? Does every dinner party with your social circle involve high-fat, meat-focused meals that may set off an acidic party of your own?

Developing a strategy to respond to any situation you are faced with when changing your diet will ease the transition. We are all resistant to change, so along with fighting your own body's preference for those easy-to-prepare — and highly processed — foods from the box, you may also have to contend with family members missing their regular fix of high-carbohydrate pasta and meat dishes. Here are a few tips to help you move forward.

Guidelines for Handling Change

- Focus discussion about the new diet on your quality of life, not the quality of the new foods.
- Try setting up a romantic time to prepare some new acid–alkaline balanced foods that bring love to the table. Fruit and dip is always a delicious place to start.
- Talk to your family and friends about your health issues and how you are making changes to improve your health.
- For family gatherings, offer to bring a vegetable-focused dish that may be the main part of your meal, with smaller servings of meats or other foods served. Planning ahead for such events by increasing the alkaline-based percentage

of foods for a few days before special events may also help reduce any possible symptoms.

- If you are the chef, this is your opportunity to introduce just how delicious the acid–alkaline diet can be. Choose your favorite recipes from the selection offered in this book. Set out plenty of appetizers that focus on raw or lightly steamed vegetables with healthy dips and marinades. Provide smaller portions of any meats served, but with plenty of alkaline side dishes.
- If you are attending a party with friends, speak privately to them beforehand about your diet and explain how a pH-balanced diet is helping reduce your symptoms. Ask what they are planning to prepare and ask permission to bring a dish that will fit well with their planned menu. Again, taking smaller portions of the more acidic dishes and focusing more on the alkaline foods provided will see you through the evening. Reducing your intake of alcohol, soft drinks and caffeinated beverages will also help.
- If you are going to a restaurant, check the menu or call ahead of time to be sure you are comfortable with the food choices. Salads with broiled chicken or steamed vegetables are appropriate. Ask for salad dressings to be served on the side to permit dipping and using less dressing. Use any medications you find effective as soon as possible if you are having a dish that you know will cause symptoms.
- If you are attending a business function that may be stressful for you, try mind–body techniques such as yogic breathing, a series of yoga poses or tai chi to reduce your stress levels and help you cope with difficult events.
- Being up front about your health conditions and your decision to adopt a pH-balanced diet will ease your stress. Other people may have solutions for changing diets and will most likely congratulate you for making the effort to improve your health. Be proud of your efforts to attain a higher level of wellness.

✦ Caution

The acid–alkaline diet may be harmful for people with acute or chronic kidney disease, people with a pre-existing heart problem or anyone who is taking medications that affect potassium levels. Always discuss any alternative diet with your health-care team before making any changes.

12-Step Program

The pH Balance Diet is quite simply a plan that enables you to adjust your consumption of alkaline to acid foods to an average ratio of 60% alkaline-forming to 40% acid-forming foods. Reaching and maintaining this ratio is, however, easier said than done. Start by following these 12 steps slowly, one at a time.

Step 1: Eat More Alkaline-Forming Foods and Fewer Acid-Forming Foods

As a preventive measure for maintaining a healthy pH, most sources recommend eating a diet of foods with an alkaline to acid ratio of 60% to 40%, or 3 to 2, rather than the average 1 to 10 ratio eaten in North America. That is, for every 2 acidic food items you eat, eat 3 alkaline foods to balance them out. As a therapeutic measure to restore lost pH balance, the recommended ratio of alkaline to acid foods is 4 to 1 (80% to 20%). The pH balance point indicating good health and longevity reflects the normal pH range of our blood (7.35 to 7.45), which is slightly on the alkaline side. Use the PRAL list of foods showing their pH measure (see page 26) and the acidifying and alkalizing foods list on pages 149 to 153 to help select predominantly alkaline-forming foods. If you have a cafeteria at work, make a list of foods that are acceptable for your diet and stick to this list.

Step 2: Supplement Essential Buffering Minerals

To reduce existing acidity in your body, eat foods that increase the levels of buffers. When your diet is high in acidifying foods on a regular basis, your body attempts to bring the acid–alkaline balance back to normal and in doing so may use up your stores of essential minerals (magnesium, calcium, potassium and sodium), thereby increasing the risk for disease. Supplement your diet with these elements to restore a safe level.

Did You Know?

Detoxification

Another side effect of increasing alkaline-forming food and reducing acid-forming food is detoxification. Increasing alkalizing foods in the diet may also increase the excretion of toxins (and reduce acid levels) through the urine. Although severe alkalization of the urine is used in hospitals as a rapid treatment for poisoning through the excretion of pharmaceuticals and environmental toxins, smaller quantities of toxins may be excreted over a longer period using a slight alkaline shift of the urine based on alkaline-focused diet changes.

Step 3: Increase Plant Foods and Reduce Animal Foods

A diet that is low in plant foods (potassium-rich) and high in animal protein (acid-forming) may increase our body's overall acid load and could result in a low-grade level of metabolic acidosis. Anything outside of our normal acid range might put us at risk for disease, fatigue, impaired endocrine functioning (but not in the thyroid), enzyme disruptions, which may lead to respiratory and urinary tract infections, and premature aging.

Step 4: Stay Properly Hydrated

Water helps balance pH levels in every cell of the body. Pure water has a pH of 7, but the water we drink has a slightly alkaline measure that reduces acid in the body. The water in our bodies maintains a normal temperature, lubricates and cushions joints, protects the spinal cord and manages our body's housekeeping by getting rid of wastes through our urine, perspiration and bowel movements. If you wait until your lips are dry and you are really thirsty, your body is already in a state of dehydration. Manage your fluid intake with these tips:

- Carry a full water bottle with you.
- Freeze some water in a container that will not break down in the freezer (stainless steel or freezer-safe BPA-free plastic). The water will stay appealingly cold throughout your day.
- When you are having meals in restaurants, choose water rather than other beverages because juices, sports drinks and pop have added sugar and calories, and diet drinks have artificial sugars.
- Make your water more appealing by adding a squeeze of your favorite juice; you might drink more water than you would otherwise.

Be aware of how many cups of coffee or tea you drink during the day. Both coffee and tea (called diuretics) increase your urine output, which may lead to dehydration. Caffeine may also have an impact on your sleeping patterns. For optimum health, drink when you are thirsty, with meals and as needed, depending on your activities. And remember that some of our water needs are satisfied through the whole and prepared foods we eat.

Step 5: Increase the Amount of Healthy Fiber in Your Diet

Get plenty of fiber by choosing the right carbohydrates, including fruits, vegetables and whole grains. Avoid eating highly processed "white" carbohydrates: breads, baked goods and pastas made from white flour, as well as white rice and products with added sugars such as high-fructose corn syrup.

Step 6: Eat Good Fats

Use olive oil and omega-3 oils from fish and some plants (flaxseed, for example). Avoid animal-sourced saturated fats and any foods made with trans fats (which may include fried foods, commercial baked goods and some vegetable oils and dressings.)

Step 7: Choose Lean Animal and Plant Proteins

Avoid grain-fed, hormone-supplemented commercial beef, a source of saturated fat plus excessive omega-6 fatty acids.

Step 8: Eat Less

In a time where, for most people, food is abundant, most of us eat too much. Research has shown that people who consume less food live longer and are healthier in general. Measuring serving sizes, or even just removing a tablespoon (15 mL) of a serving from your plate, may help to reduce your weight, improve your health and increase your energy.

Step 9: Share Your Diet Plan with Family and Friends

Because you will be following an 80% to 20% or 60% to 40% alkaline-acid diet, an occasional unbalanced meal out or dinner with family or friends does not mean you have failed. Extra servings of healthy vegetables and smaller portions of dishes that are more acidic will help. Continuing to keep track of your meals in your health, life and diet diary will help you rebalance your diet in the days after consuming extra acidic foods.

Step 10: Make Changes to Your Diet Gradually

Add new vegetables one at a time, and try getting helpers in the kitchen to help cook and prepare new dips or salad dressings. Eventually, they will become converts. Offering a bite of an unknown vegetable to a child on several occasions rather than putting a whole serving on the plate may encourage them to add it to their regular fare. Having fun with food — making artwork, using it to build things or, if all else fails, an occasional food fight — may help.

Step 11: Make Sure Fresh Meats and Leftovers Are Stored Safely

Label all freezer items to be sure you don't let them sit there for too long. Look through your freezer on a regular basis as you prepare your shopping list and make decisions for lunches and dinners for the upcoming week.

Step 12: Savor Your Meals

If you're not accustomed to eating breakfast or lunch, following a pH-balanced diet will improve your health by providing steady levels of fuel for your brain and body. Take the time to arrange your meals attractively — pretend you're an internationally known chef at a world-famous restaurant preparing a meal for the VIPs in your life. Set the table and sit down for each meal, with the TV, computer and cell phone

Acidic Cooking Methods

Frying, barbecuing and broiling are acidifying cooking methods, while boiling, poaching and broiling are alkaline-forming. So put your frying pan and barbecue away. Instead, broil, poach or boil your meat, poultry or fish. Reduce the amount of meat-related fat you consume by draining off any fat from your meat before serving. Use herbs, spices and ground nuts for breading rather than bread crumbs, and pat or roll the mixture into the meat surface so you use less. Choose recipes that don't include sauces and gravies; use fresh or dried herbs for flavoring instead. Beans provide a lower-fat alternative to meats. Use nuts for snacks, in salads and in main dishes. Replace meat or poultry in recipes with nuts.

turned off. Take the time to enjoy each bite of your food and appreciate the decisions you have made to improve your health. Feed your soul as well as your belly!

Get Started

The time has come to switch your eating habits to balance the pH in your body to improve your general state of health and to treat any GI conditions you are experiencing. Before you begin meal planning, be sure to visit your physician for a physical to be sure that other medical conditions are not present and review the 12 steps for implementing the pH diet solution on page 143.

Don't start your new diet until you have reviewed your old eating habits and recorded them in a health journal. Take 2 weeks to complete this inventory. This creates a rough baseline for seeing outcomes once you implement your new diet regimen. Test your saliva and urine pH level first thing each morning.

1. Record your current diet and symptoms in a health, life and diet diary. Before making any changes to your diet, learn to observe your current dietary practice and to assess any symptoms you may be experiencing. Keep track of all the foods you eat throughout the day, recording the time the food was eaten, the method of cooking you used or the way food was prepared in a restaurant (asking questions about food preparation is appreciated!).
2. Keep track of any symptoms related to GI issues that you may be experiencing, including the time and duration of symptoms. Include your level of pain between 0 and 5, with 0 being no pain at all and 5 being the worst pain you have ever experienced.
3. Record any medications you are taking for GI symptoms, or any other medications, including when the medication was taken, any changes in symptoms and how long the medication provides relief.
4. Record your exercise habits, including what time of day, the exercises, the level of intensity (on a scale of 0 to 5 again), your weight and how you feel afterwards.
5. Record your sleep patterns, including your bedtime, whether you woke up during the night and when you woke up in the morning. Do you wake up on your own or with the help of an alarm? How do you feel in the morning — rested or like you could crawl right back into bed?

6. Record your mood and level of stress. If you are feeling stressed, record the source of your stress, if you know what it is. Just as for pain, record your level of stress between 0 and 5, with 0 being no stress at all and 5 being the worst stress you have ever experienced.

This diary, like most diaries, will be most effective if you can keep it private.

Clean Out Your Pantry

1. Use this 2-week period to list what foods you have in your cupboards, refrigerator and freezer, and use up those foods for preparing your meals. Meat-based protein will still be included in your diet, but red meat will be included only occasionally and portion sizes will be reduced. Assess your freezer and refrigerator to make use of any excess you may have.
2. Processed, preserved or packaged food products, crackers, chips and candies will no longer be on your grocery list. As you make your way through your current food supply, cook them up and carefully list any symptoms you may experience following this meal and over the next day or so. You may choose to pack some canned items in bins and put them away for emergency situations, but keeping packaged foods in the house makes it too easy to reach for them instead of preparing fresh whole foods.
3. Try making your own condiments. Whipping up a small batch of salad dressing, barbecue sauce, ketchup or mayonnaise is easy, and once you've tried the fresh, homemade version, you'll never go back!

Restock

Check out your local bulk food and natural food stores for whole food choices to restock your pantry. In conjunction with the PRAL food list (page 26) and the acidifying and alkalizing foods list (opposite), go shopping for:

- A variety of whole flours to use in recipes: soy, almond, coconut, spelt, millet, brown rice, oat, amaranth
- Alternative dairy products as options: almond, rice, coconut, soy, organic dairy milk from hormone-free cows
- Cold-pressed oils, coconut oil, organic butter for preparing clarified butter, healthy unsaturated-fat margarines
- Whole grains and whole-grain pastas: spelt, rice, corn, buckwheat/kasha, quinoa, teff, wild rice, basmati or brown (unprocessed) rice

- Nuts and seeds: almonds, cashews, chestnuts, pumpkin seeds, sesame seeds, sunflower seeds, macadamia nuts, cumin seeds, coriander seeds
- Sea salt (for necessary minerals) rather than iodized table salt, but use any salt sparingly

Acidifying and Alkalizing Foods

This list is an easy guide to balancing the pH in your diet. Simply eat more alkaline-forming foods than acid-forming foods — about 4 alkalizing to 1 acidifying to regain health, or 3 alkalizing to 2 acidifying to maintain good health. Use this as your shopping list. Photocopy it and pin it to your bulletin board, and keep a copy in the glove compartment of your car.

Note that the acidifying property of any food may be increased by frying, deep-frying or barbecuing. Save the barbecue for special occasions, and try steaming, roasting or slow-cooking your food as a healthy change from frying.

Vegetables

ALKALIZING

- Arugula
- Bamboo shoots
- Beets and beet greens
- Cauliflower
- Celery
- Fennel
- Kale
- Kohlrabi
- Lemongrass
- Peppers, all varieties (dried)
- Plantain
- Seaweed
- Shiitake mushrooms (dried)
- Spinach
- Sun-dried tomatoes
- Sweet potatoes
- Swiss chard
- Tomatoes and tomato products (canned)
- Turnip greens
- Wasabi
- Water chestnuts
- Watercress
- Yams

SLIGHTLY ALKALIZING

- Alfalfa
- Artichokes
- Asparagus
- Bell peppers (fresh)
- Broccoli
- Brussels sprouts
- Cabbage
- Carrots
- Cauliflower
- Celeriac
- Collard greens
- Dandelion greens
- Eggplant
- Fiddleheads
- Garlic
- Hearts of palm
- Horseradish
- Jicama
- Leeks
- Lettuce
- Mushrooms (fresh)
- Mustard greens
- Okra
- Onions
- Parsnips
- Potatoes
- Pumpkin
- Radishes
- Rutabaga
- Shallots
- Squash
- String beans, green or yellow
- Tomatoes, all varieties (fresh)
- Turnips
- Zucchini

SLIGHTLY ACIDIFYING

- Corn
- Peas
- Pickles
- Tomatoes (cooked)

continued...

Fruits

ALKALIZING

- All dried fruits
- Avocados
- Cantaloupes
- Dates
- Guavas
- Jackfruit
- Kiwifruit
- Prickly pears
- Tamarinds

SLIGHTLY ALKALIZING

- Apples
- Apricots
- Bananas
- Blackberries
- Casaba melons
- Cherries
- Clementines
- Coconut
- Cranberries
- Currants
- Elderberries
- Figs
- Gooseberries
- Grapefruit
- Grapes
- Honeydew melons
- Kumquats
- Lemons
- Limes
- Loganberries
- Lychees
- Mangos
- Mulberries
- Nectarines
- Oranges
- Papayas
- Passion fruit
- Peaches
- Pears
- Persimmons
- Pineapples
- Plums
- Quinces
- Raspberries
- Strawberries
- Tangerines
- Watermelon

NEUTRAL

- Blueberries

Grains, Flours and Breads

SLIGHTLY ALKALIZING

- Brown rice

NEUTRAL

- Arrowroot flour
- Brown rice
- Buckwheat groats and flour
- Bulgur
- Quinoa
- Rice noodles
- Tapioca
- Wild rice

SLIGHTLY ACIDIFYING

- Amaranth grain
- Bagels
- Barley
- Corn (flour, bran, meal)
- Cornstarch
- Couscous
- Hominy
- Kamut
- Millet
- Oat bran
- Pasta (homemade, egg-free)
- Quinoa
- Rice flour
- Rye
- Rye flour (light)
- Soba noodles
- Somen noodles
- Spelt
- Spinach-flavored egg noodles
- Teff
- Wheat bran (crude)
- White rice

ACIDIFYING

- Barley flour or meal
- Biscuits
- Bread
- Brown rice flour
- Cake
- Cookies
- Crackers
- Doughnuts
- Egg noodles
- French toast (recipe)
- Oat flour
- Pasta
- Pastry
- Rice bran
- Rye flour (dark)
- Sprouted wheat
- Wheat
- Wheat flour

Protein Foods

ALKALIZING

- Fava beans
- Lima beans
- Tofu, regular

SLIGHTLY ALKALIZING

- Adzuki beans
- Baked beans (homemade)
- Cowpeas
- Pigeon peas
- Pink beans
- Soybeans (roasted)
- White beans

NEUTRAL

- Black beans
- Chinese noodles (cellophane or mung)
- Egg whites
- Fish broth
- Fish oil
- Great Northern beans
- Navy beans
- Red kidney beans
- Split peas

SLIGHTLY ACIDIFYING

- Chickpeas
- Lentils
- Mung beans
- Oysters
- Peanut butter
- Soybeans (fresh)
- Tempeh
- Tofu, extra-firm

ACIDIFYING

- Anchovies (canned in oil)
- Bacon
- Beef
- Cod
- Chicken
- Cornish hen
- Crab
- Deli meats
- Duck
- Egg yolks
- Eggs, whole
- Goose
- Haddock
- Halibut
- Ham
- Herring
- Lamb
- Lobster
- Peanuts
- Pork
- Salmon
- Sausage
- Smoked fish
- Soybeans (dry-roasted)
- Trout (steamed)
- Tuna
- Veal

Dairy

NEUTRAL

- Buttermilk
- Cream
- Sour cream
- Goat milk
- Ice cream
- Low-fat yogurt
- Milk
- Soy milk
- Whipped cream

SLIGHTLY ACIDIFYING

- Cream cheese
- Cheese, full-fat soft
- Kefir

ACIDIFYING

- Camembert cheese
- Cheese substitute
- Cheese, fresh (Quark)
- Cheese, hard
- Cottage cheese
- Processed cheese
- Ricotta cheese

continued...

Nuts and Seeds

ALKALIZING

- Chestnuts
- Green pumpkin seeds (pepitas)

SLIGHTLY ACIDIFYING

- Almonds
- Pine nuts
- Hazelnuts

ACIDIFYING

- Cashews
- Pistachios
- Sesame seeds
- Sunflower seeds
- Walnuts

Fats and Oils

NEUTRAL

- Almond oil
- Avocado oil
- Butter
- Canola oil
- Fish oil
- Flaxseed oil
- Ghee (clarified butter)
- Lard
- Margarine
- Olive oil
- Peanut oil
- Safflower oil
- Sunflower oil
- Vegetable oil

Flavorings, Sweeteners and Condiments

ALKALIZING

- All herbs, fresh and dried
- All spices, fresh and dried
- Cocoa powder, unsweetened
- Molasses
- Tomato sauce

SLIGHTLY ALKALIZING

- Carob powder
- Cider vinegar
- Maple syrup
- Marmalades
- Sea salt
- Soy sauce
- Vanilla extract

NEUTRAL

- Agave syrup
- Dietetic syrup
- Honey
- Jams
- Mayonnaise
- Mustard
- Salt (except sea salt)
- Stock or broth
- Sugar
- Vinegars (except cider vinegar)

SLIGHTLY ACIDIFYING

- Artificial sweeteners
- Barley malt
- Gravy

ACIDIFYING

- Gelatin desserts
- Pudding desserts

Beverages

ALKALIZING

- Instant coffee

SLIGHTLY ALKALIZING

- Alcoholic beverages
- Cold chocolate beverages
- Coconut water
- Fruit juices
- Mineral water
- Wine, red or white

NEUTRAL

- Beer (draft, pale, bottled stout)
- Black tea
- Carbonated beverages (with caffeine)
- Coffee
- Herbal teas
- Hot cocoa
- Infused teas
- Tap water

SLIGHTLY ACIDIFYING

- Carob beverages

Source: Sampled from USDA Food lists, http://ndb.nal.usda.gov/ndb/foods.

Following a Meal Plan

Everyone's family has different needs, so develop a meal plan based on your normal schedule. Your meal plan should help you follow either the 60% alkaline-forming to 40% acid-forming food ratio for maintaining good health, or the 80% alkaline-forming to 20% acid-forming food ratio for improving health and reducing any GI-related symptoms.

Prepare grocery lists based on your meal plan — you will find that you buy and waste less food that way. Plan also for work meals, making some meals ahead of time on the weekend or days off (focus on days when you find it most difficult to find time to cook) and packing lunches as soon as dinner is cleaned up so you always have good food available. Preparing lunches and snacks will also save you money. Making a little extra for a meal, so you can set extra helpings aside to freeze for lunches, can produce huge savings.

If you choose to follow the meal plans in this book (page 159), be assured that they have been prepared by a registered dietitian and meet the recommendations from the USDA's MyPlate and Health Canada's Eating Well with Canada's Food Guide.

Part 4

Meal Plans for the pH Balance Diet Program

Introduction to the Meal Plans

The meal plans in this book are designed to support overall good health. They include nutrient-rich foods that, when eaten consistently, can provide the daily requirements the body needs.

An Alkalizing Bias

This diet tends toward an alkalizing effect. Although the bloodstream and body tissues do maintain a fairly narrow pH range (they never get too acidic or too alkaline), variations can occur due to dietary influences. One important aspect of this diet is that it attempts to correct an issue in the modern diet, which is the acidifying influences of processed food, excessive meat and a lack of plant foods. The diet is specifically designed to deliver a neutral or slightly alkalizing meal experience over the course of the day.

We have emphasized foods that can deliver important buffering minerals, such as magnesium and calcium, and have tried to keep sodium levels low. We have included ample whole grains, fruits and vegetables in a ratio to meat, sugar and white flour that helps to offset the acidity of the latter group. Many people eat way too much refined food and meat, which has a net acidic load on the body. The individual's metabolism must compensate and adapt to this acidity. We have found that some people express a variety of symptoms, or express symptoms more intensely, when their diet is thus out of balance. This diet can help to alleviate the gastrointestinal disorders that may result.

No Bans

This diet does not ban or exclude any particular food. For example, we have chosen many recipes that are gluten-free, but wheat and other gluten-containing foods do make an appearance in some recipes. Gluten can certainly aggravate the gastrointestinal distress of some individuals and cause other issues, but this diet is not aimed at those with a more severe gluten sensitivity or allergy, such as celiac disease. Many people eat 6 to 10 servings of gluten-containing foods per day: toast at breakfast, crackers for a snack, a sandwich at lunch, pasta and a roll at dinner, cake for dessert and so on. Rather than eliminating gluten from the diet entirely, we advocate limiting your intake of it.

Likewise, too much refined sugar has an adverse effect on GI conditions for some people because it encourages the growth of yeast in the gut, and simply because of the acidifying nature of pure sucrose in large amounts. But we have included some fun recipes that contain sugar. They do not, however, dominate the meal plans.

Individuality

Everyone's body is unique, and that includes slight (and sometimes marked) differences in the chemical pathways the body runs. Many patients with irritable bowel syndrome, for example, benefit over time from an increased intake of dietary fiber. But some patients, especially early in treatment, have their symptoms exacerbated by fiber, especially bran-type fiber.

We invite you to get all the benefit you can from these meal plans and from the 175 recipes that follow. But please pay attention to your own reactions to foods so you can make choices and fine-tune your diet. If, for example, you wish to alkalize your daily diet more than we suggest, simply add more fresh vegetables and/or cut down on the meat portions. Consult with a qualified health practitioner and take advantage of medical care from all the branches of medicine that you need. Build a team composed of health-care practitioners who will listen to your concerns, beliefs, symptoms and questions.

A Word About PRAL

Many nutritional factors were taken into consideration in formulating this meal plan. One important measurement we used was the potential renal acid load (PRAL) calculation. The PRAL is an attempt to estimate the impact of food on the buffering systems of the body. The kidney and a system of enzymes attempt to keep the pH of the body in balance. Some foods tend toward the alkaline side of the pH equation, and others are more acidic. Eating acidic foods does not instantly "acidify" the body, but they do make demands on the buffering system of the body. The PRAL looks at the likely demand on those systems. For example, a serving of kale will have a negative PRAL score of about –8, meaning that it is alkalizing. The PRAL of beef is about +7.8.

In looking at the impact of our meal plans, we examined each day's recipes and analyzed the foods that are components of the recipes. We found that the typical average PRAL score on many days was –4, which more than met our goals for providing a pH solution to the problem of acidifying diets. The overall effect of the day's meals tends to be gently alkalizing, so it does not make great demands on the body's buffering system.

There will be small variations in the PRAL of each day in the meal plans because of added components, recipe variations, slight differences between brands and so on. But the diet as a whole has an alkalizing effect on the body and, unlike the meat- and processed-food-heavy modern diet, does not place undue burden on the body's ability to absorb, neutralize and excrete acid and acid by-products.

Week 1 Meal Plan

Meal	Monday	Tuesday	Wednesday	Thursday	Friday	Saturday	Sunday
Breakfast	1 Home-Style Pancake* 1 banana 6 oz (175 mL) rice milk	1 cup (250 mL) Pear and Pumpkin Porridge* 1/2 cup (125 mL) blueberries 1/2 cup (125 mL) plain yogurt	1 Home-Style Pancake* 1/2 cup (125 mL) raspberries 6 oz (175 mL) nut milk	1 cup (250 mL) Pear and Pumpkin Porridge* 1/2 cup (125 mL) sliced strawberries 6 oz (175 mL) grape juice	Hot Millet Amaranth Cereal* 2 oz (60 g) low-fat cheese 6 oz (175 mL) nut milk	Hot Millet Amaranth Cereal* Tofu Quinoa Scramble* Orange Aid*	1 Hot Apple Crêpe* 1/2 cup (125 mL) plain yogurt
Morning snack	1/2 cup (125 mL) plain yogurt 1/2 cup (125 mL) blueberries	Cinnamon Apple Chips*	1/2 cup (125 mL) plain yogurt 1 banana	Cinnamon Apple Chips*	1 orange 1 oz (30 g) Swiss cheese	Almond Banana Smoothie*	1 slice Banana Walnut Oat Bread*
Lunch	Butternut Apple Soup with Swiss Cheese*	Sesame Noodle Salad*	Celery Root and Mushroom Lasagna*	Fast Egg Salad*	Tuna Avocado Salad*	Quick Quinoa Stir-Fry with Vegetables and Tofu*	Butternut Apple Soup with Swiss Cheese*
Afternoon snack	1/3 cup (75 mL) walnuts 1/2 apple 1/2 pear	1/3 cup (75 mL) hazelnuts 1/3 cup (75 mL) raisins	1/2 cup (125 mL) walnuts 1/2 apple 1/2 pear	1/3 cup (75 mL) hazelnuts 1/3 cup (75 mL) raisins	1/2 cup (125 mL) grapes 1/2 cup (125 mL) plain yogurt	1 Multi-Seed Energy Bar*	1 Multi-Seed Energy Bar*
Dinner	Veal Goulash* Old-School Collard Greens*	Celery Root and Mushroom Lasagna* Dandelion Salad with Balsamic Pepper Strawberries*	Sweet Potato, Apple and Raisin Casserole* Quinoa Salad*	Turkey Meatloaf* Cauliflower "Mashed Potatoes"*	Lentil Sloppy Joes* Sunny Lettuce and Avocado Salad*	Chicken Pot Pie* Roasted Root Vegetables with Wild Mint*	Poached Salmon* Swiss Chard Spring Rolls with Sesame Lime Dipping Sauce*
Evening snack	1/2 cup (125 mL) thawed frozen cherries	1 banana	The Ultimate Baked Apple*	1/2 cup (125 mL) thawed frozen cherries	1 banana	Chocolate Zucchini Cake*	Raspberry Custard Cake*

* The recipe is in the book; unless otherwise indicated, the amount is 1 serving.

Goals of the pH Balance Diet

You don't need to be ill to adopt a pH-balanced diet program. The diet is both preventive and therapeutic, general and specific, and it is not only for GI conditions but also for conditions in other body systems. Balancing your pH through diet may have some general effects on your health as well as effects specific to any medical condition you have. We are each individuals when it comes to the impact of the foods we eat.

pH Principles

The pH-balanced diet supports health and longevity when it reflects our blood's normal pH range (7.35 to 7.45), slightly on the alkaline side. Anything outside of our normal acid range might put us at risk for disease.

The aim is therefore to reach and maintain this balanced pH range. Depending on your personal goals, set your pH balance goal at 80% alkaline to 20% acid to regain health, or 60% alkaline to 40% acid to maintain good health.

Balanced Diet

In recommending a balanced diet, we are referring to five concepts of balance, or homeostasis:

- Balanced alkaline to acid pH measure: 80% to 20% during acute care, 60% to 40% during maintenance.
- Balanced among food groups: fruits (20%), vegetables (30%), grains (20%) and meats (30%).
- Balanced energy intake (calories) and energy expenditure (exercise) to achieve and maintain a healthy weight.
- Balanced omega-3 to omega-6 essential fatty acids: 1:1 to 1:4.
- Balanced chi, or energy, as conceived in traditional Chinese medicine (TCM). Traditional Chinese medicine recommends eating a diet high in alkaline-forming fresh vegetables and fruit — foods that raise our body's bicarbonate levels to achieve acid–alkaline balance in the body and promote longevity.

Week 2 Meal Plan

Meal	Monday	Tuesday	Wednesday	Thursday	Friday	Saturday	Sunday
Breakfast	½ cup (125 mL) Linda's Granola* Quick Quinoa Stir-Fry with Vegetables and Tofu*	1 Home-Style Pancake* Orange Aid* 6 oz (175 mL) nut milk	½ cup (125 mL) Linda's Granola* ½ cup (125 mL) plain yogurt ½ apple	1 Home-Style Pancake* 1 banana 6 oz (175 mL) rice milk	½ cup (125 mL) Linda's Granola* ½ cup (125 mL) plain yogurt ½ pear	Creamy Morning Millet with Apples* ½ cup (125 mL) plain yogurt 8 oz (250 mL) orange juice	Garden-Fresh Frittata* ⅓ cup (75 mL) applesauce 6 oz (175 mL) nut milk
Morning snack	Multi-Seed Energy Bar*	Cinnamon Apple Chips*	1 Strawberry Almond Muffin*	½ cup (125 mL) thawed frozen cherries ⅓ cup (75 mL) hazelnuts	1 Strawberry Almond Muffin*	Almond Banana Smoothie*	Cherries Jubilee*
Lunch	Fresh Vegetable Spring Rolls with Filipino Garlic Sauce*	Herbed Quinoa Deviled Eggs* 1 slice Old-Fashioned Cornbread* 1 tsp (5 mL) honey	Tuna Avocado Salad* 6 rice crackers	Red Beans and Red Rice* Dandelion Salad with Balsamic Pepper Strawberries*	Salad of Chicken and Peaches on Seedlings with Grilled Pepper Dressing*	Minestrone Soup* Hot Sweet Potato Salad*	Crispy Pecan Chicken Fingers* Salad of Fresh Spring Greens, New Potatoes and Asparagus *
Afternoon snack	1 Crispy Brown Rice Treat*	1 Crispy Brown Rice Treat*	½ cup (125 mL) walnuts ½ apple ½ peach	1 Strawberry Almond Muffin*	⅓ cup (75 mL) raisins ⅓ cup (75 mL) plain yogurt	¼ cup (60 mL) Sesame Ginger Cashews*	Strawberry Cheesecake Smoothie*
Dinner	Indian Chicken Kebabs* Fragrant Coconut Rice*	Turkey Meatloaf* Scalloped Potatoes with a New Twist*	Simple Chinese Steamed Fish* Sesame Noodle Salad*	Chickpea Herb Burgers* Nice 'n' Nutty Slaw*	Italian Sausage Patties* Red Beans and Red Rice*	Texas-Style Barbecue* Old-School Collard Greens* 1 slice Old-Fashioned Cornbread*	Minestrone Soup* Beef Tenderloin with Four-Peppercorn Crust* Yummy Asparagus* Horseradish Mashed Potatoes*
Evening snack	½ cup (125 mL) Grapey Pear Juice*	2 clementine oranges	½ cup (125 mL) thawed frozen cherries	1 apple	1 banana 1 scoop (2 oz/60 g) vanilla ice cream	Five-Minute Cheesecake Cups with Raspberries*	Chocolate Berry Pudding*

* The recipe is in the book; unless otherwise indicated, the amount is 1 serving.

Week 3 Meal Plan

Meal	Monday	Tuesday	Wednesday	Thursday	Friday	Saturday	Sunday
Breakfast	1 Home-Style Pancake* 1/3 cup (75 mL) applesauce 6 oz (175 mL) grape juice	Almond Ginger Apple Hemp Cereal* 1/2 pear 1/2 apple 6 oz (175 mL) nut milk	1 Hot Apple Crêpe* Cherries Jubilee*	Breakfast Rice* 1/2 cup (125 mL) plain yogurt Almond Banana Smoothie*	Almond Ginger Apple Hemp Cereal* 6 oz (175 mL) nut milk	Egg Cup Delight* 6 oz (175 mL) nut milk	Sweet Potato Omelet* 1 banana Orange Aid*
Morning snack	Cashew Scallion Cream Cheese* 8 rice crackers	1 slice Banana Walnut Oat Bread*	1 slice Banana Walnut Oat Bread*	1 Glazed Lemon Coconut Muffin*	1 Glazed Lemon Coconut Muffin*	1/4 cup (60 mL) Sesame Ginger Cashews*	3 Crispy Coated Veggie Snacks*
Lunch	12 Mediterranean Pizza Squares*	Salmon with Spinach*	Grilled Tuna with Roasted Pepper Sauce*	Chickpea Soup*	Macaroni and Cheese*	1 slice Thin Pizza Crust* 1/2 cup (125 mL) chopped pineapple 1 cup (250 mL) crumbled goat cheese	Sprouted Lentil and Spinach Soup*
Afternoon snack	2 tbsp (30 mL) Pumpkin Pepita Hummus*	1 tbsp (15 mL) Caramelized Onion Dip* 10 baked potato chips	1/4 cup (60 mL) Salty Almonds with Thyme* 1/2 cup (125 mL) Ginger Sun Tea*	1 Multi-Seed Energy Bar*	1/2 cup (125 mL) walnuts 1/2 apple 1/2 peach 1/2 cup (125 mL) Ginger Sun Tea*	1/3 cup (75 mL) raisins 1/3 cup (75 mL) plain yogurt	1/2 cup (125 mL) walnuts 1/2 apple 1/2 peach
Dinner	Simple Chinese Steamed Fish* Chinese Broccoli with Nori Mayonnaise* Speedy Weeknight Lo Mein*	Slow-Cooked Beef Stew* 1 cup (250 mL) torn romaine hearts 1 tbsp (15 mL) Apple Cider Vinaigrette*	Italian Meatballs with Chunky Tomato Sauce* 1 cup (250 mL) cooked gluten-free rotini	Baked Pork Chops with Vegetable Rice* Roasted Beets with Dill Sauce*	Slow-Cooked Chili Flank Steak or Brisket* Baked Summer Vegetable Layers*	Ribs with Hominy and Kale* Mushroom Pinwheels* Garden Pea, Butter Lettuce and Radish Salad*	Baked Ham with Citrus Glaze* Balsamic Roasted Fiddleheads* Cauliflower "Mashed Potatoes"*
Evening snack	1 Almond Flax Seed Energy Cookie*	1 banana	The Ultimate Baked Apple*	1/2 cup (125 mL) sliced peaches	1/2 cup (125 mL) raspberries	Pear Almond Torte*	Strawberry Rhubarb Pie*

* The recipe is in the book; unless otherwise indicated, the amount is 1 serving.

Week 4 Meal Plan

Meal	Monday	Tuesday	Wednesday	Thursday	Friday	Saturday	Sunday
Breakfast	Creamy Morning Millet with Apples* 1 banana 6 oz (175 mL) low-fat milk	1 cup (250 mL) Pear and Pumpkin Porridge* 6 oz (175 mL) grape juice	Creamy Morning Millet with Apples* 1/2 cup (125 mL) raspberries 6 oz (175 mL) low-fat milk	1 cup (250 mL) Pear and Pumpkin Porridge* 1/2 cup (125 mL) plain yogurt 6 oz (175 mL) rice milk	1 Hot Apple Crêpe* Breakfast Rice* 6 oz (175 mL) grape juice	1/2 cup (125 mL) Linda's Granola* 1/2 cup (125 mL) plain yogurt 1/2 cup (125 mL) raspberries	Garden-Fresh Frittata* 1/2 cup (125 mL) sliced strawberries 6 oz (175 mL) nut milk
Morning snack	1 slice Glazed Lemon Coconut Loaf*	1 slice Banana Walnut Oat Bread*	1 slice Glazed Lemon Coconut Loaf*	1 slice Banana Walnut Oat Bread*	1/2 pear 1/2 apple 1/2 cup (125 mL) grapes	Fruity Milkshake*	6 oz (175 mL) nut milk
Lunch	Cabbage Borscht*	Poached Salmon*	Butternut Apple Soup with Swiss Cheese*	Simple Chinese Steamed Fish*	Fennel-Scented Tomato and Wild Rice Soup*	Fast Egg Salad* 2 slices Seedy Brown Bread*	Green Pad See Ew*
Afternoon snack	1 Multi-Seed Energy Bar*	1/2 cup (125 mL) walnuts 1/2 apple 1/2 peach	1/4 cup (60 mL) Salty Almonds with Thyme*	1/3 cup (75 mL) raisins 1/3 cup (75 mL) cashews	1/4 cup (60 mL) Salty Almonds with Thyme*	6 oz (175 mL) nut milk	1/2 cup (125 mL) Apple Pear Lemonade*
Dinner	Apple Harvest Chicken* Mushroom Ragoût*	Jambalaya* Red Beans and Red Rice*	Dijon Ham Steaks* Cauliflower "Mashed Potatoes"*	Sweet Potato, Apple and Raisin Casserole*	Halibut with Beets and Beet Greens* Baked Parsnip Fries*	Leek, Onion and Garlic Tart* 1 Mini Crab Quinoa Cake* Salmon with Spinach* Scalloped Potatoes with a New Twist*	Roast Lamb with Marrakech Rub* Leafy Greens Soup* Vegetable Biryani*
Evening snack	1/2 cup (125 mL) Cinnamon Applesauce*	1 banana	1/2 cup (125 mL) grapes	1 apple	Raspberry Custard Cake*	Chocolate Zucchini Cake*	1 Maple Pumpkin Micro-Pie*

* The recipe is in the book; unless otherwise indicated, the amount is 1 serving.

Part 5

Recipes for the pH Balance Diet Program

About the Nutrient Analysis

The nutrient analysis done on the recipes in this book was derived from the Food Processor SQL Nutrition Analysis Software, version 10.9, ESHA Research (2011). Where necessary, data was supplemented using the USDA National Nutrient Database for Standard Reference, Release #26 (2014), retrieved June 2014 from the USDA Agricultural Research Service website: www.nal.usda.gov/fnic/foodcomp/search/.

Recipes were evaluated as follows:

- The larger number of servings was used where there is a range.
- Where alternatives are given, the first ingredient and amount listed were used.
- Optional ingredients and ingredients that are not quantified were not included.
- Calculations were based on imperial measures and weights.
- The smaller quantity of an ingredient was used where a range is provided.
- Reduced sodium broth, 1% milk, light mayonnaise, light cream cheese and light sour cream were used where these ingredients are listed as broth, milk, mayonnaise, cream cheese and sour cream.
- Calculations involving meat and poultry used lean portions.
- Canola oil was used where the type of fat was not specified.
- Recipes were analyzed prior to cooking.

It is important to note that the cooking method used to prepare the recipe may alter the nutrient content per serving, as may ingredient substitutions and differences among brand-name products.

Breakfasts, Breads and Muffins

Linda's Granola

Every time you make this granola, challenge yourself to add variety by trying coconut, soy nuts, walnuts, pistachios, macadamia nuts, pecans, buckwheat flakes, apricots, dates, dried apple slices, blueberries and pineapple. Keep your acid/alkaline food lists close at hand as you make your choices. Serve this granola for breakfast, as a snack or as a nibble on your next hike.

Makes 16 cups (4 L)

Tips

Vary the types of nuts and dried fruit you use; just keep the total volume at 4 cups (1 L).

Spray the large stirring spoon with cooking spray to prevent sticking.

Variations

Substitute an equal amount of liquid honey for the corn syrup.

For the GF multigrain cereal, substitute GF puffed rice.

- **Preheat oven to 300°F (150°C)**
- **Two 15- by 10-inch (40 by 25 cm) rimmed baking sheets, lightly greased**

1/2 cup	corn syrup	125 mL
1 tbsp	vegetable oil	15 mL
4 cups	GF multigrain cereal	1 L
2 cups	GF honeyed corn flakes cereal	500 mL
1 cup	mixed nuts	250 mL
1 cup	whole almonds	250 mL
1/2 cup	sunflower seeds	125 mL
1/2 cup	green pumpkin seeds (pepitas)	125 mL
3 cups	mixed dried fruit	750 mL

1. In a glass measuring cup, combine corn syrup and oil. Microwave, uncovered, on High for 45 seconds or until it can be easily poured.
2. In a very large bowl, combine multigrain cereal, corn flakes cereal, mixed nuts, almonds, sunflower seeds and pumpkin seeds. Pour in corn syrup mixture and stir to coat evenly. Spread in prepared pans.
3. Bake in preheated oven for 30 to 40 minutes or until toasted, stirring every 10 minutes. Add dried fruit. Stir gently to combine. Bake for 10 minutes more. Let cool in oven for 1 hour, with the oven turned off. Let cool completely on pans on a cooling rack. Store at room temperature in airtight containers for up to 3 months.

Health Tip

- If you are sensitive to gluten, check that all your ingredients are gluten-free. For optimum health, eat a variety of grains, rather than just one grain, such as wheat (in different forms), at mealtime.

Nutrients per 1/2 cup (125 mL)	
Calories	175
Fat	7 g
Sodium	59 mg
Carbohydrate	25 g
Fiber	3 g
Protein	3 g
Calcium	33 mg
Magnesium	34 mg
Potassium	106 mg

Almond Ginger Apple Hemp Cereal

This cereal, an aromatic, spicy, sweet and crunchy blend of apples, ginger, cinnamon and hemp seeds, is perfect for busy mornings when you're on the go.

Makes 1 serving

Tips

Royal Gala or McIntosh apples work well in this recipe because they have a higher sugar content. If you are watching your sugar intake, feel free to use Granny Smiths, but keep in mind that the cereal will taste a little more tart.

To remove the skin from fresh gingerroot with the least amount of waste, use the edge of a teaspoon. With a brushing motion, scrape off the skin to reveal the yellow root.

Use high-quality organic cinnamon. You will get the freshest flavor by grinding whole cinnamon sticks in a spice grinder.

Nutrients per serving	
Calories	382
Fat	17 g
Sodium	6 mg
Carbohydrate	48 g
Fiber	8 g
Protein	15 g
Calcium	72 mg
Magnesium	24 mg
Potassium	378 mg

- **Food processor**

2 cups	chopped peeled apples	500 mL
1/2 cup	whole raw almonds	125 mL
1/4 cup	chopped gingerroot	60 mL
1/4 cup	filtered water	60 mL
1 tsp	ground cinnamon	5 mL
1/4 cup	raw shelled hemp seeds	60 mL

1. In food processor, combine apples, almonds, ginger, water and cinnamon; process until roughly chopped (you want to retain some texture).
2. Transfer to a serving bowl and top with hemp seeds. Serve immediately.

Variations

For a creamier dish, substitute an equal amount of fresh Nut Milk (page 384) for the water.

Garnish with 2 to 3 tbsp (30 to 45 mL) each raw pumpkin seeds and raw sunflower seeds.

Health Tips

- Ginger has GI tonic and antinausea benefits that help support healing in people with gastrointestinal complaints.
- Keeping track of the foods you eat, the symptoms you experience, your stress levels, your exercise habits and your sleep patterns in your diary or journal may help you to understand how these factors relate to your health. For example, for some people with gastrointestinal conditions, seeds may worsen symptoms, but unless you are keeping track of the food you eat, you may not recognize the association.

Pear and Pumpkin Porridge

This porridge is alkalizing, heavily spiced and very stimulating for the digestive system.

Makes 6 cups (1.5 L).

Tips

To soak the cashews, pumpkin seeds and sunflower seeds for this recipe, combine them in a large bowl and add 1 cup (250 mL) water. Cover and set aside for 30 minutes. Drain and rinse under cold running water until the water runs clear.

To shred pumpkin or squash, remove the peel and use the large holes of a box grater or a food processor fitted with the shredding blade.

Variation

Try using various nuts and/or seeds in this recipe in the same quantities called for.

Nutrients per serving (1 of 6)	
Calories	228
Fat	10 g
Sodium	11 mg
Carbohydrate	33 g
Fiber	5 g
Protein	6 g
Calcium	42 mg
Magnesium	97 mg
Potassium	338 mg

- **Food processor**

½ cup	buckwheat groats, soaked (see box, below)	125 mL
¼ cup	raw cashews, soaked (see tip, at left)	60 mL
¼ cup	raw green pumpkin seeds (pepitas), soaked	60 mL
¼ cup	raw sunflower seeds, soaked	60 mL
2 cups	chopped pears	500 mL
1 cup	shredded pumpkin or squash	250 mL
½ cup	Nut Milk (page 384)	125 mL
3 tbsp	raw agave nectar	45 mL
1 tbsp	ground cinnamon	15 mL
¼ tsp	freshly grated nutmeg	1 mL
Pinch	ground cloves	Pinch
Pinch	fine sea salt	Pinch

1. In food processor, combine buckwheat, cashews, pumpkin and sunflower seeds and pears; process until slightly broken down but not completely smooth.
2. Add shredded pumpkin and nut milk and pulse three to four times to break down the squash. Add agave nectar, cinnamon, nutmeg, cloves and salt and pulse three to four times, until combined. Serve immediately, if possible, or cover and refrigerate for up to 2 days.

How to Soak Buckwheat

To soak ½ cup (125 mL) buckwheat, combine it with 1 cup (250 mL) water in a large bowl (it needs room to "grow"). Cover and set aside for 1 hour, changing the water once. Drain, discarding soaking water. Rinse under cold running water until the water runs clear.

Health Tip

- Cinnamon has a reputation as a good blood sugar regulator — which is useful for many people with diabetes or blood sugar control problems.

Breakfast Rice

Simple yet delicious, this tasty combination couldn't be easier to make.

Makes 6 servings

Tip

Made with this quantity of liquid, the rice will be a bit crunchy around the edges. If you prefer a softer version or will be cooking it longer than 8 hours, add ½ cup (125 mL) water or rice milk.

Variation

Use half rice and half wheat, spelt or Kamut berries.

- **Small to medium (1½- to 3½-quart) slow cooker, stoneware lightly greased**

1 cup	brown rice	250 mL
4 cups	vanilla-flavored enriched rice milk	1 L
½ cup	dried cranberries or cherries	125 mL

1. In prepared slow cooker stoneware, combine rice, rice milk and cherries. Stir well. Place a clean tea towel, folded in half (so you will have two layers), over top of stoneware to absorb moisture.
2. Cover and cook on Low for up to 8 hours or overnight or on High for 4 hours. Stir well and serve.

Health Tips

- Brown rice increases the alkalizing effect of this dish, as does the cooking method — slow cooking.
- Cranberries are one of the most potent antioxidant-containing foods available, and they help ward off the bacteria that cause urinary tract infections, an added bonus for those with this issue.

Nutrients per serving	
Calories	232
Fat	2 g
Sodium	62 mg
Carbohydrate	51 g
Fiber	2 g
Protein	3 g
Calcium	212 mg
Magnesium	46 mg
Potassium	89 mg

Creamy Morning Millet with Apples

If you're tired of the same old breakfast, perk up your taste buds and expand your nutritional range by enjoying millet as a cereal.

Makes 4 to 6 servings

Tips

Some millet may contain bits of dirt or discolored grains. If your millet looks grimy, rinse it thoroughly in a pot of water before using. Swish it around and remove any offending particles, then rinse under cold running water.

Use plain or vanilla-flavored rice milk. Vary the quantity to suit your preference. Three cups (750 mL) produces a firmer result. If you like your cereal to be creamy, use the larger quantity.

Nutrients per serving (1 of 6)	
Calories	230
Fat	3 g
Sodium	146 mg
Carbohydrate	48 g
Fiber	5 g
Protein	4 g
Calcium	150 mg
Magnesium	56 mg
Potassium	195 mg

- **Small (3½-quart) slow cooker, stoneware greased**

1 cup	millet (see tip, at left)	250 mL
3 to 4 cups	enriched rice milk or water (see tip, at left)	750 mL to 1 L
3	apples, peeled and chopped	3
¼ tsp	salt	1 mL
	Chopped pitted dates, fresh berries and toasted nuts (optional)	

1. In prepared slow cooker stoneware, combine millet, rice milk, apples and salt.
2. Cover and cook on High for 4 hours or on Low for 8 hours or overnight. Stir well, spoon into bowls and sprinkle with fruit and/or nuts, if desired.

Variations

Use half millet and half short-grain brown rice.

If you prefer a non-creamy version, substitute water for the rice milk.

Health Tips

- Iodized table salt is highly acidifying. Replacing table salt with sea salt in your diet will also increase your intake of trace minerals, which act to balance acids in our bodies.
- Apples are rich in pectin, a soluble fiber that supports GI function and health.
- Millet is an alkalizing food, making this a great start to your day.

Hot Millet Amaranth Cereal

Here's a great way to start your day and add variety to your diet. Both millet and amaranth are relatively quick and easy to cook — and as long as you keep the temperature low, they don't need to be stirred. Use a sweetener of your choice and add dried fruit and nuts as you please.

Makes 6 servings

Tips

For best results, toast the millet and amaranth before cooking. Stir the grains in a dry skillet over medium heat until they crackle and release their aroma, about 5 minutes.

If you're having trouble digesting grains, try soaking them overnight in warm non-chlorinated water (about 2 parts water to 1 part grain) with a spoonful or so of cider vinegar. Drain, rinse and cook in the morning.

Nutrients per serving	
Calories	123
Fat	2 g
Sodium	5 mg
Carbohydrate	23 g
Fiber	3 g
Protein	4 g
Calcium	30 mg
Magnesium	60 mg
Potassium	114 mg

$2\frac{1}{2}$ cups	water	625 mL
$\frac{1}{2}$ cup	millet, toasted (see tip, at left)	125 mL
$\frac{1}{2}$ cup	amaranth, toasted	125 mL
	Honey, maple syrup or raw cane sugar	
	Milk or non-dairy alternative	
	Dried cranberries, cherries or raisins (optional)	
	Toasted chopped nuts (optional)	

1. In a saucepan over medium heat, bring water to a boil. Add millet and amaranth in a steady stream, stirring constantly. Return to a boil. Reduce heat to low. Cover and simmer until grains are tender and liquid is absorbed, about 25 minutes.
2. Serve hot, sweetened to taste and with milk or non-dairy alternative. Sprinkle with dried fruit and nuts, if desired.

Health Tips

- To achieve a healthy balance of acid and alkaline, you can include low-fat milk in your diet as the more acidic part of your meal, but if you begin to use nut milks or other non-dairy milks, you may quickly find that you no longer prefer the flavor of regular milk.
- Raw or organic whole cane sugar is the most alkalizing form of sugar; most are slightly acidic (maple syrup or honey), but granulated sugar is highly acidic. More important than the form of sugar is to reduce the amount of sugars in the diet, being aware that some fruits are also high in sugars, so best eaten in moderation.
- Adding raisins to this dish is a great idea. Raisins are one of the most alkalizing foods, and they're also rich in iron and other nutrients.

Egg Cup Delight

This is an attractive and interesting way to prepare a special breakfast. It will even win over guests who aren't egg lovers. Serve with a leafy green salad, steamed broccoli or other greens, even at breakfast.

Makes 4 servings

- **Preheat oven to 350°F (180°C)**
- **Muffin pan, 4 cups lightly greased**

4	slices deli meat, preferably ham (8 if sliced very thin)	4
3	mushrooms, thinly sliced	3
1/4	bell pepper (any color), finely chopped	1/4
	A few leaves of spinach, chopped	
1 cup	shredded Cheddar, Swiss, feta or Gouda cheese	250 mL
4	large eggs	4
1 tbsp	freshly grated Parmesan cheese (optional)	15 mL
Pinch	salt	Pinch

1. Line the 4 prepared muffin cups with deli meat. Add about 2 tsp (10 mL) vegetables (mushrooms, bell pepper and spinach) on top of the meat in each cup. Add 1/4 cup (60 mL) cheese on top of the vegetables in each cup. Crack 1 egg into each cup and prick yolk with a fork. Sprinkle each egg with Parmesan (if using) and salt.
2. Bake in preheated oven for 12 to 15 minutes or until egg is cooked to desired texture. To remove from pan, slide a spoon around the underside of the deli meat and lift out.

This recipe courtesy of dietitians Heidi Piovoso and Kristyn Hall.

Health Tips

- Eggs are a complete protein and a great dietary source of all the essential amino acids.
- The combination of eggs, cheese and deli meat will make this your most acidifying meal of the day. Add leafy salads or steamed greens to help rebalance your pH.
- Hard cheeses are acidifying foods, so consume only small servings on an occasional basis. Soft cheeses are less acidic, but it's still best to consume them rarely rather than regularly. You may find that as you eat cheese less often, you crave it less frequently, and will prefer other foods.

Nutrients per serving	
Calories	199
Fat	14 g
Sodium	367 mg
Carbohydrate	1 g
Fiber	0 g
Protein	15 g
Calcium	232 mg
Magnesium	16 mg
Potassium	136 mg

Sweet Potato Omelet

This delicious and unusual omelet is reminiscent of potato pancakes. Your tummy will be smiling!

Makes 2 servings

Variation

Substitute sliced green beans, chopped bean sprouts, diced bell pepper, diced mushrooms or any combination of your favorite vegetables for (or with) the sweet potatoes.

Nutrients per serving	
Calories	209
Fat	12 g
Sodium	205 mg
Carbohydrate	18 g
Fiber	3 g
Protein	8 g
Calcium	60 mg
Magnesium	27 mg
Potassium	358 mg

2	large eggs	2
1 cup	shredded peeled sweet potatoes	250 mL
1/2 cup	chopped onion	125 mL
1	clove garlic, chopped	1
1 tsp	salt or reduced-sodium soy sauce (GF, if needed)	5 mL
1 tbsp	vegetable oil	15 mL

1. In a small bowl, beat eggs with a fork. Stir in sweet potatoes, onion, garlic and salt until well combined.
2. Heat a medium skillet over medium-high heat. Add oil and swirl to coat the pan. Pour in egg mixture; cook, turning once, until lightly browned on both sides, about 2 minutes per side.

This recipe courtesy of dietitian Nena Wirth.

Health Tips

- Sweet potatoes are rich in carotenoids, compounds that have a high antioxidant value and can be converted by the body to vitamin A, if needed.
- The more acidifying eggs in this recipe are balanced nicely by the highly alkalizing sweet potato and garlic.
- Soy sauce is an alkalizing food, but it's often high in sodium. Choose sodium-reduced soy sauce to reduce sodium load.

Garden-Fresh Frittata

A frittata, which can be described as a Spanish-Italian omelet or a crustless quiche, makes a quick and easy any-time-of-day meal.

Makes 4 to 6 servings

Tips

To ovenproof a nonstick skillet with a nonmetal handle, wrap handle in a double layer of foil, shiny side out.

To prevent your cast-iron skillet from rusting, set it on a warm stove element to completely dry before storing. Be careful: the handle gets hot.

- **Preheat broiler**
- **9- to 10-inch (23 to 25 cm) ovenproof nonstick or cast-iron skillet**

1 tbsp	extra virgin olive oil	15 mL
2	leeks (white and light green parts only), coarsely chopped	2
2	cloves garlic, minced	2
1/2	red bell pepper, cut into 1/2-inch (1 cm) squares	1/2
2 cups	thickly sliced mushrooms	500 mL
1	small zucchini, cut into 1/4-inch (0.5 cm) slices	1
8	large egg whites (1 cup/250 mL)	8
4	large eggs	4
1 tsp	Dijon mustard	5 mL
1/4 cup	snipped fresh chives	60 mL
2 tbsp	snipped fresh parsley	30 mL
2 tsp	dried tarragon	10 mL
1/2 tsp	salt	2 mL
Pinch	freshly ground white pepper	Pinch
1 cup	broccoli florets, steamed	250 mL
1 1/2 cups	shredded Swiss cheese	375 mL

1. In skillet, heat olive oil over medium heat; add leeks, garlic, red pepper and mushrooms. Cook, stirring frequently, for 5 minutes or until tender. Add zucchini and cook, stirring, for 2 to 3 minutes or until vegetables are softened. Remove skillet from heat and reduce heat to medium-low.
2. In a large bowl, whisk together egg whites, eggs, Dijon mustard, chives, parsley, tarragon, salt and pepper. Add broccoli and Swiss cheese, stirring to combine.
3. Pour into skillet over vegetables. Cook, without stirring, for 9 to 11 minutes or until bottom and sides are firm yet top is still slightly runny.

Nutrients per serving (1 of 6)	
Calories	230
Fat	13 g
Sodium	399 mg
Carbohydrate	10 g
Fiber	2 g
Protein	18 g
Calcium	271 mg
Magnesium	40 mg
Potassium	400 mg

Variation

Use different varieties of mushrooms for a more intense flavor.

4. Place under preheated broiler, 3 inches (7.5 cm) from the element, until golden brown and set, 2 to 5 minutes.
5. Cut into wedges and serve hot from the oven or at room temperature. Refrigerate, covered, for up to 2 days. Reheat individual wedges, uncovered, in microwave on Medium (50%) for 1½ to 2 minutes, just until hot, if desired.

How to Clean Leeks

Trim roots and wilted green ends. Peel off tough outer layer. Cut leeks in half lengthwise and rinse under cold running water, separating the leaves so the water gets between the layers. Trim individual leaves at the point where they start to become dark in color and course in texture — this will be higher up on the plant the closer you get to the center.

Health Tips

- Broccoli and other *Brassica* family vegetables have a regulatory effect on thyroid hormone production. (If you have low thyroid hormone levels, the cooked broccoli in this dish will not cause further thyroid dysfunction.)
- Fresh herbs increase the alkalizing effect of this recipe.
- The Swiss cheese in this recipe raises the acidifying effect of this dish. Serve with a leafy green salad to help balance the pH level. For the meal before or after, choose more alkalizing dishes.

Hot Apple Crêpes

This make-ahead breakfast can be assembled at the last minute the next time you have brunch guests. Or serve these crêpes as an elegant dessert.

Makes nine 6-inch (15 cm) crêpes

Tips

For 6 cups (1.5 L) sliced apples, you'll need about 1½ lbs (750 g) of apples.

Apple filling can be stored in the refrigerator in an airtight container for up to 4 days. To reheat, microwave on Medium (50%) for 2 to 4 minutes.

Nutrients per crêpe	
Calories	239
Fat	10 g
Sodium	165 mg
Carbohydrate	37 g
Fiber	3 g
Protein	3 g
Calcium	61 mg
Magnesium	11 mg
Potassium	144 mg

- **6-inch (15 cm) crêpe pan or nonstick skillet, lightly greased**

Crêpes

¼ cup	amaranth flour	60 mL
¼ cup	chickpea flour	60 mL
2 tbsp	potato starch	30 mL
2 tsp	granulated sugar	10 mL
½ tsp	xanthan gum	2 mL
½ tsp	salt	2 mL
2	large eggs	2
⅔ cup	milk	150 mL
⅓ cup	water	75 mL
1 tbsp	melted butter	15 mL

Apple Filling

⅓ cup	butter	75 mL
¾ cup	packed brown sugar	175 mL
6 cups	thickly sliced apples	1.5 L
1½ tsp	ground cinnamon	7 mL
	GF vanilla-flavored yogurt	

1. *Crêpes:* In a large bowl or plastic bag, mix together amaranth flour, chickpea flour, potato starch, sugar, xanthan gum and salt.
2. In a small bowl, whisk together eggs, milk, water and melted butter. Pour mixture over dry ingredients all at once, whisking until smooth. Cover and refrigerate for at least 1 hour or for up to 2 days. Bring batter back to room temperature before making crêpes.
3. Heat prepared pan over medium heat; add 3 to 4 tbsp (45 to 60 mL) batter for each crêpe, tilting and rotating pan to ensure batter covers entire bottom. Cook for 1 to 1½ minutes or until edges begin to brown. Turn carefully with a nonmetal spatula. Cook for another 30 to 45 seconds or until bottom is dotted with brown spots. Transfer to a plate and repeat with the remaining batter.

Tips

You can also prepare the apple filling in the microwave: In a large microwave-safe bowl, microwave butter, uncovered, on High for 1 minute or until melted. Add brown sugar, apples and cinnamon and microwave, uncovered, on High, for 2 to 4 minutes, stirring once or twice, until apples are just tender.

Substitute 2 cups (500 mL) of your favorite prepared GF fruit pie filling for the apple filling.

Substitute whipped cream, GF frozen yogurt or GF ice cream for the GF yogurt.

4. *Filling:* In a saucepan, melt butter over medium heat. Add brown sugar, apples and cinnamon and simmer gently for 4 to 6 minutes or until apples are just tender.
5. Spoon an equal portion of hot apple filling down the center of each crêpe. Roll and serve seam side down, topped with GF vanilla yogurt.

Health Tips

- Amaranth contains phytosterols, which have a positive effect on cholesterol levels.
- This dish is slightly acidic, so serving it with a leafy green salad or steamed greens, or choosing more alkaline dishes for other meals, will help to maintain your pH balance.
- Drinking alkaline beverages between meals will help support pH balance. Prepare your own alkaline water by squeezing a bit of fresh lemon or lime juice into filtered water, or drink non-fizzy mineral water that comes from a natural source. Some brands of water are truly alkaline. Avoid chlorinated water as much as possible. Read labels carefully.

Home-Style Pancakes

Serve these fantastic pancakes topped with fruit and drizzle with maple syrup.

Makes 7 pancakes

Tips

Choose your favorite GF non-dairy milk, such as soy, rice, almond or potato-based milk, or, if you can tolerate lactose, use regular 1% milk.

Combine the dry ingredients and store in an airtight container for up to 2 weeks.

Cook the pancakes the night before and store them in the refrigerator. Toast them in the morning.

Cooled cooked pancakes can also be placed in an airtight container, with parchment paper between each one for easier separation, and stored in the freezer for up to 4 weeks. Toast to serve.

Nutrients per pancake	
Calories	140
Fat	3 g
Sodium	160 mg
Carbohydrate	24 g
Fiber	4 g
Protein	4 g
Calcium	93 mg
Magnesium	19 mg
Potassium	172 mg

½ cup	sorghum flour	125 mL
½ cup	brown rice flour	125 mL
2 tbsp	psyllium husks	30 mL
1 tsp	GF baking powder	5 mL
¼ tsp	baking soda	1 mL
¼ tsp	salt	1 mL
1	large egg	1
1 cup	fortified GF non-dairy milk or lactose-free 1% milk	250 mL
1 tbsp	liquid honey, pure maple syrup or agave nectar	15 mL
2 tsp	grapeseed oil	10 mL
1 tsp	GF vanilla extract	5 mL
	Butter or grapeseed oil	

1. In a large bowl, combine sorghum flour, brown rice flour, psyllium, baking powder, baking soda and salt.
2. In another bowl, beat egg, milk, honey, oil and vanilla. Pour into flour mixture and whisk for about 1 minute or until smooth.
3. On a griddle or in a nonstick skillet, melt 1 tsp (5 mL) butter over medium heat. For each pancake, pour in ¼ cup (60 mL) batter. Cook for 1 to 2 minutes or until bubbles start to form and edges are firm. Flip over and cook other side for 1 to 2 minutes or until bottom is golden. Transfer to a plate and keep warm. Repeat with the remaining batter, greasing griddle and adjusting heat between batches as needed.

Variation

Applesauce Pancakes: Add ½ cup (125 mL) unsweetened applesauce to the batter. The pancakes may take a minute or two longer to cook. Serve sprinkled with chopped walnuts and ground cinnamon, then drizzled with maple syrup.

Health Tip

- Psyllium is a super source of dietary fiber, so make sure to drink plenty of water the morning that you eat this dish — psyllium will absorb it like a sponge.

Orange French Toast

The best part of this vibrant way to start the day is that you can prepare it the night before. The sunny orange flavor raises an ordinary recipe to the sublime.

Makes 6 servings

Tips

This lazy person's French toast is made even easier if you use a rasp to grate the orange zest. Rasps are available at cookware stores and have very sharp edges ideal for grating zest, Parmesan cheese and fresh nutmeg.

If bread is already sliced thinly, use two slices stacked on top of each other.

One medium orange will yield about 1½ tbsp (22 mL) zest, so you'll likely need two for this recipe. Although the recipe uses fortified orange juice for added calcium, don't waste the flesh of the oranges after you zest them. Orange slices would taste terrific as a garnish.

Nutrients per serving	
Calories	298
Fat	5 g
Sodium	251 mg
Carbohydrate	54 g
Fiber	1 g
Protein	11 g
Calcium	158 mg
Magnesium	22 mg
Potassium	219 mg

- **13- by 9-inch (33 by 23 cm) baking dish, greased**

6	large eggs	6
2 tbsp	grated orange zest	30 mL
1 cup	fortified orange juice	250 mL
2 tbsp	granulated sugar	30 mL
1 tbsp	orange-flavored liqueur (optional)	15 mL
1 tsp	vanilla extract (GF, if needed)	5 mL
6	slices (1 inch/2.5 cm thick) French bread	6

Orange Marmalade Sauce

½ cup	orange marmalade	125 mL
¼ cup	fortified orange juice	60 mL
2 tbsp	liquid honey	30 mL
1 tbsp	orange-flavored liqueur (optional)	15 mL

1. In a medium bowl, beat together eggs, orange zest and juice, sugar, orange-flavored liqueur (if using) and vanilla.
2. Arrange bread, cutting to fit, in single layer in prepared baking dish. Pour egg mixture over top; cover and refrigerate overnight.
3. Preheat oven to 350°F (180°C). Bake, uncovered, for 25 to 30 minutes or until firm to the touch and no longer soggy.
4. *Sauce:* Meanwhile, in a small saucepan, bring marmalade, orange juice, honey and orange-flavored liqueur (if using) to a boil over high heat; reduce heat to medium and simmer, stirring, for about 5 minutes or until slightly thickened. Serve with French toast.

Health Tip

- Replacing the granulated sugar in this recipe with dried organic cane sugar will reduce the acidifying effect.

Chocolate Berry Pudding

This rich, chocolaty, nutritious breakfast takes only a few minutes to prepare.

Makes 1 serving

Tip

Cacao powder is powdered raw chocolate. It is similar to cocoa powder but tastes even better, with a deeper, richer flavor. Cacao powder is available in well-stocked supermarkets, natural foods stores and online. If you can't find it, substitute a good-quality cocoa powder.

- **Blender**

1¼ cups	filtered water	300 mL
3 tbsp	chia seeds	45 mL
2 tbsp	raw agave nectar	30 mL
2 tbsp	raw cacao powder (see tip, at left)	30 mL
¼ tsp	raw vanilla extract (GF, if needed)	1 mL
¼ cup	fresh blueberries, strawberries or raspberries	60 mL

1. In blender, combine water, chia seeds, agave nectar, cacao powder and vanilla. Blend on high speed until smooth.
2. Transfer to a serving bowl and top with fresh berries. Serve immediately or cover and refrigerate for up to 2 days.

Variations

For a sweeter dish, substitute freshly squeezed orange juice for the water.

Banana Cinnamon Pudding: Substitute 2 tsp (10 mL) ground cinnamon for the cacao powder and ½ cup (125 mL) chopped banana for the fresh berries.

Health Tip

- Alkalizing chia seeds and fresh berries balance the more acidifying cacao powder in this recipe. Enjoy this as an occasional treat.

Nutrients per serving	
Calories	428
Fat	16 g
Sodium	43 mg
Carbohydrate	64 g
Fiber	21 g
Protein	12 g
Calcium	210 mg
Magnesium	5 mg
Potassium	80 mg

Cocoa Quinoa Breakfast Squares

The intense flavor of cocoa powder and the natural sweetness of plump dates combine with quinoa for a power-packed breakfast. Wrap the cooled squares in parchment or plastic wrap for a perfectly portable, make-ahead breakfast.

Makes 9 squares

Tips

To prepare 3 cups (750 mL) cooked quinoa, combine 1 cup (250 mL) quinoa and 2 cups (500 mL) water in a medium saucepan. Bring to a boil over medium-high heat. Reduce heat to low, cover and simmer for 12 to 15 minutes or until water is just barely absorbed. Cover and let stand for 8 to 10 minutes.

Store the cooled quinoa squares tightly covered or in an airtight container in the refrigerator for up to 3 days. Serve cold or at room temperature.

Nutrients per square	
Calories	191
Fat	5 g
Sodium	113 mg
Carbohydrate	32 g
Fiber	5 g
Protein	7 g
Calcium	99 mg
Magnesium	71 mg
Potassium	265 mg

- **Preheat oven to 350°F (180°C)**
- **Blender or food processor**
- **8-inch (20 cm) square metal baking pan, lined with foil (see box, below) and sprayed with nonstick cooking spray**

1 cup	pitted soft dates (such as Medjool)	250 mL
1/3 cup	unsweetened cocoa powder (not Dutch process)	75 mL
1/4 tsp	fine sea salt	1 mL
2 cups	milk or plain non-dairy milk (such as soy, rice, almond or hemp)	500 mL
1 tsp	vanilla extract (GF, if needed)	5 mL
3 cups	hot cooked quinoa (see tip, at left)	750 mL
1/2 cup	ground flax seeds (flaxseed meal)	125 mL

1. In blender, combine dates, cocoa, salt, milk and vanilla; purée until smooth.
2. Transfer date mixture to a large bowl and stir in quinoa and flax seeds. Spread evenly in prepared pan.
3. Bake in preheated oven for 55 to 60 minutes or until firmly set. Let cool completely in pan on a wire rack. Using foil liner, lift mixture from pan onto a cutting board; peel off foil and cut into 9 squares.

How to Line a Pan with Foil

Lining a pan with foil is easy. Begin by turning the pan upside down. Tear off a piece of foil longer than the pan, then mold the foil over the pan. Remove the foil and set it aside. Flip the pan over and gently fit the shaped foil into the pan, allowing the foil to hang over the sides (the overhang ends will work as "handles" when the contents of the pan are removed).

Health Tip

- A good source of omega-3 fat, ground flax seeds are an anti-inflammatory food, and in ground form, might be better tolerated.

Seedy Brown Bread

A sandwich bread with a rich color and added crunch — what a treat!

Makes 12 slices

Tips

You can purchase buttermilk powder in bulk stores and health food stores. Store it in an airtight container to prevent lumping.

For a nuttier flavor, toast the seeds.

Tent the loaf with foil partway through the baking time to prevent the top crust from becoming too dark.

Nutrients per slice	
Calories	198
Fat	9 g
Sodium	277 mg
Carbohydrate	25 g
Fiber	4 g
Protein	8 g
Calcium	91 mg
Magnesium	56 mg
Potassium	107 mg

- **9- by 5-inch (23 by 12.5 cm) loaf pan, lightly greased**

1 cup	sorghum flour	250 mL
½ cup	whole bean flour	125 mL
⅓ cup	tapioca starch	75 mL
¼ cup	rice bran	60 mL
⅓ cup	buttermilk powder	75 mL
1 tbsp	xanthan gum	15 mL
1 tbsp	bread machine or instant yeast	15 mL
1¼ tsp	salt	6 mL
¼ cup	green pumpkin seeds (pepitas)	60 mL
¼ cup	raw unsalted sunflower seeds	60 mL
¼ cup	sesame seeds	60 mL
2	large eggs	2
1 cup	water	250 mL
2 tbsp	vegetable oil	30 mL
2 tbsp	liquid honey	30 mL
1 tbsp	light (fancy) molasses	15 mL
1 tsp	cider vinegar	5 mL

1. In a large bowl or plastic bag, combine sorghum flour, whole bean flour, tapioca starch, rice bran, buttermilk powder, xanthan gum, yeast, salt and pumpkin, sunflower and sesame seeds. Mix well and set aside.
2. In a separate bowl, using a heavy-duty electric mixer with paddle attachment, combine eggs, water, oil, honey, molasses and vinegar until well blended. With the mixer on its lowest speed, slowly add the dry ingredients until combined. Stop the machine and scrape the bottom and sides of the bowl with a rubber spatula. With the mixer on medium speed, beat for 4 minutes.

Variations

Substitute brown rice flour, raw hemp powder or ground flax seeds (flaxseed meal) for the rice bran.

Replace the sesame seeds with flax, hemp or poppy seeds.

For a milder-flavored bread, substitute packed brown sugar for the molasses.

3. Spoon into prepared pan. Let rise, uncovered, in a warm, draft-free place for 70 to 80 minutes or until dough has risen to the top of the pan. Meanwhile, preheat oven to 350°F (180°C).
4. Bake for 35 to 45 minutes or until loaf sounds hollow when tapped on the bottom. Remove from the pan immediately and let cool completely on a rack.

Health Tip

- This recipe contains several kinds of seeds and may not be suitable for those with some GI conditions.

Pumpernickel Loaf

With all the hearty flavor of traditional pumpernickel, this version is great for sandwiches. Try it filled with sliced turkey, accompanied by a crisp, garlic dill pickle.

Makes 12 slices

Tips

Remember to thoroughly mix the dry ingredients before adding to the liquids because they are powder-fine and could clump together.

For a milder flavor, omit the coffee and unsweetened cocoa powder.

Variation

If yellow pea flour is unavailable, use chickpea or garbanzo bean flour. This recipe can either be made from any variety of bean flour or half pea and half bean flour.

- **9- by 5-inch (23 by 12.5 cm) loaf pan, lightly greased**

3/4 cup	whole bean flour	175 mL
3/4 cup	yellow pea flour	175 mL
1/2 cup	potato starch	125 mL
1/4 cup	tapioca starch	60 mL
2 tbsp	packed brown sugar	30 mL
2 tsp	xanthan gum	10 mL
1 tbsp	bread machine or instant yeast	15 mL
1 1/4 tsp	salt	6 mL
2 tsp	instant coffee granules	10 mL
2 tsp	unsweetened cocoa powder	10 mL
1/2 tsp	ground ginger	2 mL
1 1/4 cups	water	300 mL
2 tbsp	light (fancy) molasses	30 mL
1 tsp	cider vinegar	5 mL
2 tbsp	vegetable oil	30 mL
2	large eggs	2

1. In a large bowl or plastic bag, combine whole bean flour, yellow pea flour, potato starch, tapioca starch, brown sugar, xanthan gum, yeast, salt, coffee granules, cocoa and ginger. Mix well and set aside.
2. In a separate bowl, using a heavy-duty electric mixer with paddle attachment, combine water, molasses, vinegar, oil and eggs until well blended.
3. With the mixer on lowest speed, slowly add the dry ingredients until combined. With a rubber spatula, scrape the bottom and sides of the bowl. With the mixer on medium speed, beat for 4 minutes.
4. Spoon into prepared pan. Let rise, uncovered, in a warm, draft-free place for 60 to 75 minutes or until the dough has risen to the top of the pan. Meanwhile, preheat oven to 350°F (180°C). Bake for 35 to 45 minutes or until the loaf sounds hollow when tapped on the bottom.

Nutrients per slice	
Calories	162
Fat	4 g
Sodium	260 mg
Carbohydrate	27 g
Fiber	4 g
Protein	6 g
Calcium	25 mg
Magnesium	2 mg
Potassium	91 mg

Old-Fashioned Cornbread

This traditional favorite is the perfect accompaniment to soups, stews and chilis with a down-home feel. Use leftovers to make cornbread stuffing or, for a great snack, enjoy with salsa.

Makes 8 squares

- **Preheat oven to 400°F (200°C)**
- **8-inch (20 cm) square baking pan, lightly greased**

1 cup	stone-ground yellow cornmeal	250 mL
1/2 cup	sorghum flour	125 mL
1/4 cup	brown rice flour	60 mL
1/4 cup	tapioca flour	60 mL
2 tbsp	granulated sugar	30 mL
4 tsp	GF baking powder	20 mL
1 tsp	xanthan gum	5 mL
1/2 tsp	salt	2 mL
2	large eggs	2
1 1/4 cups	milk (see tip, at left)	300 mL
2 tbsp	melted butter	30 mL

1. In a bowl, combine cornmeal, sorghum, brown rice and tapioca flours, sugar, baking powder, xanthan gum and salt. Whisk to blend and make a well in the center.
2. In a separate bowl, beat eggs. Add milk and butter and beat well. Pour into well and mix with dry ingredients just until blended. Spread in prepared pan and bake in preheated oven until top is golden and springs back, about 30 minutes. Let cool in pan on wire rack for 5 minutes. Serve warm.

Tips

This recipe also works well when you replace the milk with brown rice milk, which qualifies as a gluten-free whole grain and is alkalizing rather than acidic. If you're limiting your intake of dairy products, give it a try.

As with other quick breads, when making cornbread, one key to success is not to overmix the batter.

Health Tip

- Try clarified butter instead of melted butter for an improved acid profile.

Nutrients per square	
Calories	193
Fat	4 g
Sodium	205 mg
Carbohydrate	36 g
Fiber	2 g
Protein	5 g
Calcium	158 mg
Magnesium	18 mg
Potassium	365 mg

Thin Pizza Crust

This version of right-to-the-edge thin-crust pizza is the perfect base for Roasted Vegetable Pizza (page 332).

Makes two 12-inch (30 cm) crusts, 6 slices each

Tip

This dough is thin enough to pour onto the pizza pans. It can be quickly spread to the edges with a moist rubber spatula.

Nutrients per slice	
Calories	125
Fat	4 g
Sodium	196 mg
Carbohydrate	20 g
Fiber	2 g
Protein	5 g
Calcium	12 mg
Magnesium	1 mg
Potassium	8 mg

- **Two 12-inch (30 cm) pizza pans, lightly greased**

1 cup	whole bean flour	250 mL
1 cup	sorghum flour	250 mL
1/3 cup	tapioca starch	75 mL
1 tsp	granulated sugar	5 mL
1/2 tsp	xanthan gum	2 mL
1 1/2 tsp	bread machine or instant yeast	7 mL
1 tsp	salt	5 mL
1 tsp	dried oregano	5 mL
1 3/4 cups	water	425 mL
1 tsp	cider vinegar	5 mL
2 tbsp	vegetable oil	30 mL

Bread Machine Method

1. In a large bowl or plastic bag, combine whole bean flour, sorghum flour, tapioca starch, sugar, xanthan gum, yeast, salt and oregano. Mix well and set aside.
2. Pour water, vinegar and oil into the bread machine baking pan. Select the Dough Cycle.
3. Gradually add the dry ingredients as the bread machine is mixing, scraping with a rubber spatula while adding. Try to incorporate all the dry ingredients within 1 to 2 minutes. Allow the bread machine to complete the cycle.

Mixer Method

1. In a large bowl or plastic bag, combine whole bean flour, sorghum flour, tapioca starch, sugar, xanthan gum, yeast, salt and oregano. Mix well and set aside.
2. In a separate bowl, using a heavy-duty electric mixer with paddle attachment, combine water, vinegar and oil until well blended.
3. With the mixer on the lowest speed, slowly add the dry ingredients until combined. With a rubber spatula, scrape the bottom and sides of the bowl. With the mixer on medium speed, beat for 4 minutes.

Tip

Don't worry about the cracks on the surface of this crust after 10 minutes of baking. Expect slight shrinkage from the edges.

For Both Methods

4. Immediately pour onto prepared pans. Spread evenly with a water-moistened rubber spatula. Allow to rise in a warm, draft-free place for 15 minutes. Bake in 400°F (200°C) preheated oven for 12 to 15 minutes or until firm.

5. Spread with your choice of toppings. Return to oven and bake according to recipe topping directions.

Health Tip

- Replacing the granulated sugar in this recipe with dried organic cane sugar will reduce the acidifying effect.

Banana Walnut Oat Bread

This moist and flavorful bread makes a delicious occasional snack. Try freezing individual slices for convenience.

Makes 8 slices

Tips

This bread can be made in almost any kind of baking dish that will fit in your slow cooker. A small loaf pan makes a traditionally shaped bread; a round soufflé dish or a square baking dish produces slices of different shapes. All taste equally good.

To ease cleanup, mix the dry ingredients on a sheet of waxed paper instead of using a bowl.

Nutrients per slice	
Calories	269
Fat	15 g
Sodium	206 mg
Carbohydrate	29 g
Fiber	3 g
Protein	7 g
Calcium	111 mg
Magnesium	39 mg
Potassium	372 mg

- **Large (minimum 5-quart) oval slow cooker**
- **Greased 8- by 4-inch (20 by 10 cm) loaf pan or 6-cup (1.5 L) soufflé or baking dish**

1⁄3 cup	butter, softened	75 mL
2⁄3 cup	demerara or evaporated cane juice sugar	150 mL
2	large eggs	2
3	ripe bananas, mashed (about 1 1⁄4 cups/300 mL)	3
3⁄4 cup	all-purpose flour (unbleached, if possible)	175 mL
3⁄4 cup	large-flake (old-fashioned) rolled oats	175 mL
2 tbsp	ground flax seeds (flaxseed meal)	30 mL
2 tsp	baking powder	10 mL
1⁄2 tsp	salt	2 mL
1⁄4 tsp	baking soda	1 mL
1⁄2 cup	finely chopped walnuts	125 mL

1. In a bowl, beat butter and sugar until light and creamy. Add eggs, one at a time, beating until incorporated. Beat in bananas.
2. In a separate bowl (see tip, at left), combine flour, oats, flax seeds, baking powder, salt and baking soda. Add to banana mixture, stirring just until combined. Fold in walnuts.
3. Spoon batter into prepared pan. Cover tightly with foil and secure with a string. Place pan in slow cooker stoneware and pour in enough boiling water to come 1 inch (2.5 cm) up the sides. Cover and cook on High for 3 hours, until a tester inserted in the center comes out clean. Unmold and serve warm or let cool.

Health Tip

- Oats are high in soluble fiber — a food to add to your menu when diarrhea symptoms occur.

Cinnamon Raisin Flax Bagels

The key to making these bagels perfect is to dehydrate them as long as possible to remove all moisture from the dough. They can be stored in an airtight container for up to a month, which makes them a perfect anytime snack. They are delicious served with almond butter.

Makes 8 bagels

Tips

When making raw breads in the dehydrator, you have options in terms of texture. For crispier, firmer bread, dehydrate until all of the moisture has been removed. This will make storing the bread easy, as it can't spoil without moisture. For softer, more chewy bread, dehydrate for less time, retaining moisture in the middle of the bread. Make sure to store breads that contain moisture in the refrigerator, because bacteria can grow when water is present.

When spreading out raw breads on a dehydrator sheet, have a small bowl containing room-temperature water handy. Use this to wet your hands intermittently to prevent the dough from sticking.

Nutrients per bagel	
Calories	261
Fat	18 g
Sodium	353 mg
Carbohydrate	22 g
Fiber	18 g
Protein	12 g
Calcium	114 mg
Magnesium	4 mg
Potassium	46 mg

- **Electric food dehydrator**

4 cups	ground flax seeds	1 L
3 tbsp	ground cinnamon	45 mL
1 tsp	fine sea salt	5 mL
2 cups	water	500 mL
1/4 cup	raisins	60 mL

1. In a large bowl, combine flax seeds, cinnamon and salt. Add water and raisins and mix well.
2. Using an ice cream scoop or a small ladle, drop 8 equal portions of dough onto a nonstick dehydrator sheet, distributing evenly, and shape into rounds. Using your index finger, make a hole in the center of each bagel.
3. Dehydrate at 105°F (41°C) for 4 to 5 hours, until firm enough to handle. Flip and transfer to the mesh sheet. Dehydrate for 3 to 4 hours or until dry throughout. Serve warm or allow to cool. Transfer to an airtight container and store for up to 1 month.

Variations

Sesame Garlic Bagels: Substitute 1/2 cup (125 mL) white sesame seeds, 1/4 cup (60 mL) shredded yellow onion and 4 cloves garlic, minced, for the raisins and cinnamon.

Lemon Dill Poppy Seed Bagels: Replace the ground cinnamon and raisins in this recipe with 3 tbsp (45 mL) each freshly squeezed lemon juice and poppy seeds and 1 tbsp (15 mL) dried dillweed.

Glazed Lemon Coconut Muffins or Loaf

Brown rice flour gives this loaf — a delightfully sweet tea bread — a warm creamy color. Bake ahead and freeze it, so it's ready the next time a friend drops in.

Makes 12 muffins or slices

Tip

Use either desiccated or shredded coconut in this recipe. If using a sweetened coconut, decrease the sugar by 1 or 2 tbsp (15 or 30 mL).

- **Preheat oven to 350°F (180°C)**
- **12-cup muffin tin or 9- by 5-inch (23 by 12.5 cm) loaf pan, lightly greased**
- **Instant-read thermometer**

1 cup	brown rice flour	250 mL
1/3 cup	potato starch	75 mL
1/4 cup	tapioca starch	60 mL
1 cup	granulated sugar	250 mL
1 1/2 tsp	xanthan gum	7 mL
1 tbsp	GF baking powder	15 mL
1/4 tsp	salt	1 mL
2 tbsp	grated lemon zest	30 mL
3/4 cup	unsweetened coconut	175 mL
3/4 cup	milk	175 mL
1/4 cup	vegetable oil	60 mL
2	large eggs	2
1/4 cup	freshly squeezed lemon juice	60 mL

Lemon Glaze

1 cup	GF sifted confectioners' (icing) sugar	250 mL
1/4 cup	freshly squeezed lemon juice	60 mL

1. In a large bowl or plastic bag, stir together brown rice flour, potato starch, tapioca starch, sugar, xanthan gum, baking powder, salt, zest and coconut. Set aside.
2. In a separate bowl, using an electric mixer or whisk, beat milk, oil and eggs until combined. Add lemon juice while mixing. Add dry ingredients and mix just until combined.

Nutrients per muffin or slice	
Calories	235
Fat	9 g
Sodium	72 mg
Carbohydrate	37 g
Fiber	2 g
Protein	3 g
Calcium	83 mg
Magnesium	23 mg
Potassium	233 mg

Variation

Orange zest and juice can replace the lemon, for a slightly sweeter and more mild-flavored loaf.

For Muffins

3. Spoon batter into each cup of prepared muffin tin. Let stand for 30 minutes. Bake in preheated oven for 35 to 40 minutes or until firm to the touch.

For a Loaf

3. Spoon batter into prepared loaf pan and bake for 55 to 65 minutes or until an instant-read thermometer registers 200°F (100°C).

For Both Methods

4. *Glaze:* In a small bowl, stir together confectioners' sugar and lemon juice. With a wooden skewer, poke several holes through the hot muffins or loaf as soon as the pan is removed from the oven. Spoon the glaze over the hot muffins or loaf. Let the muffins or loaf cool in the pan on a rack for 30 minutes. Remove from the pan and let cool completely on a rack.

Health Tip

- To achieve a healthy acid and alkaline balance, you can include low-fat milk in your diet as the more acidic part of your meal, but if you begin to use nut milks or other non-dairy milks, you may quickly find that you no longer prefer the flavor of regular milk.

Strawberry Almond Muffins

These fruity, nutty muffins are great for a morning snack or breakfast on the go.

Makes 10 muffins

Tip

Choose your favorite non-dairy milk alternative, such as soy, rice, almond, coconut or potato milk.

- **Preheat oven to 350°F (180°C)**
- **12-cup muffin pan, 10 cups lined with paper liners**

1/2 cup	sorghum flour	125 mL
1/2 cup	amaranth flour	125 mL
2 tsp	GF baking powder	10 mL
1/2 tsp	ground cinnamon	2 mL
1/4 tsp	salt	1 mL
1/2 cup	granulated raw cane sugar	125 mL
1/4 cup	butter or hard vegan margarine, softened	60 mL
1/4 cup	cream cheese or soy cream cheese alternative, softened	60 mL
1	large egg	1
1/4 cup	lactose-free 1% milk or fortified GF non-dairy milk	60 mL
1 cup	chopped strawberries	250 mL
1 cup	slivered almonds	250 mL

1. In a medium bowl, combine sorghum flour, amaranth flour, baking powder, cinnamon and salt.
2. In a large bowl, using an electric mixer, cream sugar, butter and cream cheese. Beat in egg until well combined. Beat in milk. Stir in dry ingredients until just combined. Gently fold in strawberries and almonds.
3. Spoon batter into prepared muffin cups, dividing equally. Bake in preheated oven for 20 to 25 minutes or until a tester inserted in the center comes out clean. Let cool in pan on a wire rack for 5 minutes. Transfer muffins to rack to cool.

Health Tip

- To achieve a healthy balance of acid and alkaline, you can include low-fat milk in your diet as the more acidic part of your meal, but if you begin to use nut milks or other non-dairy milks, you may quickly find that you no longer prefer the flavor of regular milk.

Nutrients per muffin	
Calories	223
Fat	13 g
Sodium	90 mg
Carbohydrate	23 g
Fiber	3 g
Protein	5 g
Calcium	104 mg
Magnesium	33 mg
Potassium	229 mg

Snacks and Appetizers

Multi-Seed Energy Bars

You've never had an energy bar quite like this one: a medley of seeds — quinoa, sunflower and sesame — fuse into a crisp-chewy base. Stow one away for a mid-morning energy boost.

Makes 12 bars

Tips

Any dried fruit, or a combination of dried fruits, may be used. Try raisins, cranberries, blueberries, cherries and/or chopped apricots.

If you're not following a gluten-free diet, try other puffed grain cereals, such as wheat or barley, in place of the puffed rice.

Store cooled bars in an airtight container at room temperature for up to 5 days. Or wrap them in plastic wrap, then foil, completely enclosing them, and freeze for up to 6 months. Let thaw at room temperature for 1 hour before serving.

Nutrients per bar	
Calories	190
Fat	8 g
Sodium	83 mg
Carbohydrate	26 g
Fiber	2 g
Protein	4 g
Calcium	42 mg
Magnesium	25 mg
Potassium	134 mg

- **Preheat oven to 350°F (180°C)**
- **Large rimmed baking sheet**
- **8-inch (20 cm) square metal baking pan, lined with foil (see box, page 181) and sprayed with nonstick cooking spray**

1 cup	quinoa flakes	250 mL
½ cup	sunflower seeds	125 mL
3 tbsp	toasted sesame seeds	45 mL
1 cup	unsweetened puffed rice or millet cereal	250 mL
1 cup	chopped dried fruit	250 mL
¼ cup	natural cane sugar or packed dark brown sugar	60 mL
¼ tsp	fine sea salt	1 mL
⅓ cup	tahini or sunflower seed butter	75 mL
¼ cup	pure maple syrup or brown rice syrup	60 mL
1 tsp	vanilla extract (GF, if needed)	5 mL

1. Spread quinoa flakes, sunflower seeds and sesame seeds on baking sheet. Bake in preheated oven for 8 to 10 minutes, shaking halfway through, until golden and fragrant.
2. Transfer quinoa mixture to a large bowl and stir in cereal and fruit.
3. In a small saucepan, combine sugar, salt, tahini and maple syrup. Heat over medium-low heat, stirring constantly, for 2 to 4 minutes or until sugar is dissolved and mixture is bubbly. Stir in vanilla.
4. Immediately pour tahini mixture over quinoa mixture, stirring with a spatula until quinoa mixture is coated.
5. Using your hands, a spatula or a large piece of waxed paper, press quinoa mixture firmly into prepared pan. Refrigerate for 30 minutes or until firm. Using foil liner, lift mixture from pan and invert onto a cutting board. Peel off foil and cut into 12 bars.

Crispy Coated Veggie Snacks

These healthy crispy baked tidbits are an appealing alternative to deep-fried fare.

Makes 3 dozen pieces

Tips

Experiment with other vegetables, such as cauliflower, broccoli or white turnip.

Use any leftover savory bread, such as Seedy Brown Bread (page 182) or Old-Fashioned Cornbread (page 185) to make the bread crumbs.

Serve with salsa, GF sour cream or your favorite dipping sauce.

Nutrients per 3 pieces (1 each zucchini, sweet potato and mushroom)	
Calories	53
Fat	2 g
Sodium	46 mg
Carbohydrate	7 g
Fiber	0 g
Protein	2 g
Calcium	55 mg
Magnesium	5 mg
Potassium	80 mg

- **Preheat oven to 375°F (190°C)**
- **Baking sheet, lightly greased**

1	small zucchini	1
1	small sweet potato	1
12	small mushrooms	12
3 cups	dry GF bread crumbs	750 mL
1 cup	freshly grated Parmesan cheese	250 mL
1 tbsp	dried rosemary or thyme	15 mL
Pinch	cayenne pepper	Pinch
2 cups	plain yogurt	500 mL
	Honey Mustard Dipping Sauce (page 225) or Plum Dipping Sauce (page 224)	

1. Peel zucchini, cut in half crosswise and cut each half lengthwise into quarters.
2. Peel sweet potato, cut in half lengthwise and cut into slices 1/4 inch (0.5 cm) thick.
3. Remove stems from mushrooms.
4. In a shallow dish or pie plate, combine bread crumbs, Parmesan cheese, rosemary and cayenne pepper.
5. Working with a few pieces at a time, dip zucchini, sweet potato and mushroom caps into yogurt to generously coat. Then dip into crumb mixture, pressing to coat well.
6. Arrange on prepared baking sheet in a single layer. Bake in preheated oven for 20 to 25 minutes or until vegetables are tender and coating is golden.
7. Transfer to a serving plate and serve immediately with dipping sauce.

Health Tip

- If you have a GI condition that is aggravated by hot or spicy foods, omit the cayenne pepper and serve hot sauce at the table for others to season to taste.

Spicy, Crispy Roasted Chickpeas

Chickpeas sprinkled with cayenne and lemon, then roasted until crispy, are a habit-forming snack. They're also great tossed into salads.

Makes 8 servings

Variation

You can use any ground spice or dried herb in place of, or in addition to, the cayenne.

- **Preheat oven to 425°F (220°C)**
- **Large rimmed baking sheet, lined with parchment paper**

1	can (14 to 19 oz/398 to 540 mL) chickpeas, drained, rinsed and patted dry	1
3/4 tsp	fine sea salt	3 mL
1/8 tsp	cayenne pepper	0.5 mL
2 tsp	extra virgin olive oil	10 mL
1 tsp	freshly squeezed lemon juice	5 mL

1. In a large bowl, combine chickpeas, salt, cayenne, oil and lemon juice. Spread in a single layer on prepared baking sheet.
2. Bake in preheated oven for 32 to 38 minutes or until crisp and dry. Let cool completely in pan. Store in an airtight container at room temperature for up to 2 weeks.

Health Tip

- If you have a GI condition that is aggravated by hot or spicy foods, omit the cayenne pepper and serve hot sauce at the table for others to season to taste.

Nutrients per serving	
Calories	50
Fat	2 g
Sodium	373 mg
Carbohydrate	7 g
Fiber	2 g
Protein	1 g
Calcium	8 mg
Magnesium	0 mg
Potassium	1 mg

Salty Almonds with Thyme

When entertaining in winter, light a fire and place small bowls full of these tasty nibblers where they are easily accessible to guests.

Makes 2 cups (500 mL)

Tip

You can make these nuts in a larger (5-quart) slow cooker, but watch carefully and stir every 15 minutes, because the nuts will cook quite quickly (in just over an hour).

Nutrients per ¼ cup (60 mL)	
Calories	238
Fat	21 g
Sodium	1050 mg
Carbohydrate	8 g
Fiber	5 g
Protein	8 g
Calcium	97 mg
Magnesium	97 mg
Potassium	256 mg

- **Small to medium (1½- to 3½-quart) slow cooker**

2 cups	unblanched almonds	500 mL
½ tsp	ground white pepper	2 mL
1 tbsp	fine sea salt (or to taste)	15 mL
2 tbsp	extra virgin olive oil	30 mL
2 tbsp	fresh thyme	30 mL

1. In slow cooker stoneware, combine almonds and white pepper. Cover and cook on High for 1½ to 2 hours, stirring every 30 minutes, until nuts are nicely toasted.
2. In a mixing bowl, combine salt, olive oil and thyme. Add to hot almonds in stoneware and stir thoroughly to combine. Spoon mixture into a small serving bowl and serve hot or let cool.

Health Tips

- Fresh herbs increase the alkalizing effect of this dish, as does the slow-cooking method.
- Almonds are a high source of potassium.

Sesame Ginger Cashews

A hint of sesame adds a whole new dimension to these rich spicy nuts.

Makes 2 cups (500 mL)

Nutrients per ¼ cup (60 mL)	
Calories	213
Fat	18 g
Sodium	181 mg
Carbohydrate	11 g
Fiber	1 g
Protein	5 g
Calcium	16 mg
Magnesium	90 mg
Potassium	198 mg

- **Preheat oven to 375°F (190°C)**

1 tbsp	sesame oil	15 mL
1½ tsp	ground ginger	7 mL
½ tsp	kosher or sea salt	2 mL
2 cups	raw cashews	500 mL

1. In a large bowl, combine oil, ginger and salt and mix to a paste. Add cashews and toss to coat nuts in spicy paste. Spread nuts in a single layer on a baking sheet. Roast in preheated oven, stirring occasionally, until light golden and aromatic, 10 to 12 minutes.
2. Transfer toasted nuts to a bowl and toss gently while still warm to redistribute the flavors and oils.

Buttery Peanuts

Everyone loves these hot buttery peanuts. Use peanuts with skins on or buy them peeled, depending upon your preference. Both work well in this recipe.

Makes 2 cups (500 mL)

Tip

You can make these nuts in a larger (5-quart) slow cooker, but watch carefully and stir every 15 minutes, because the nuts will cook quite quickly (in just over an hour).

Nutrients per ¼ cup (60 mL)	
Calories	264
Fat	24 g
Sodium	703 mg
Carbohydrate	8 g
Fiber	3 g
Protein	9 g
Calcium	21 mg
Magnesium	64 mg
Potassium	242 mg

- **Small to medium (1½- to 3½-quart) slow cooker**

2 cups	raw peanuts	500 mL
¼ cup	melted butter or butter substitute	60 mL
2 tsp	fine sea salt	10 mL

1. In slow cooker stoneware, combine peanuts and butter. Cover and cook on High for 2 to 2½ hours, stirring occasionally, until peanuts are nicely roasted. Drain on paper towels.
2. Place in a bowl, sprinkle with salt and stir to combine.

Variation

Curried Buttery Peanuts: In a small bowl, combine sea salt with 2 tsp (10 mL) curry powder and a pinch of cayenne pepper. Substitute for plain salt.

Cinnamon Apple Chips

Eating some of these apple chips each day might keep the doctor away, but the cinnamon would share the credit: recent studies indicate that eating as little as ½ tsp (2 mL) of ground cinnamon per day can lower LDL ("bad") cholesterol levels, boost cognitive function and memory, and even have a regulatory effect on blood sugar levels.

Makes 8 servings

Tip

Be sure to transfer the chips from the parchment paper to a wire rack while still warm, or they will stick.

Variation

Pear Chips: Use 4 medium Bosc pears, halved and cored, in place of the apples.

- **Preheat oven to 325°F (160°C)**
- **2 rimmed baking sheets, lined with parchment paper**

4	large tart-sweet apples (such as Braeburn, Gala or Pippin), halved and cored	4
4 tsp	stevia powder	20 mL
½ tsp	ground cinnamon	2 mL
	Nonstick cooking spray (preferably olive oil)	

1. Using a very sharp knife or a mandoline, cut apples into ⅛-inch (3 mm) thick slices.
2. In a small bowl, combine stevia and cinnamon.
3. Arrange apple slices in a single layer on prepared baking sheets. Spray with cooking spray and sprinkle with stevia mixture.
4. Bake in preheated oven for 35 to 40 minutes or until edges are browned and slices are dry and crispy. Transfer chips to a wire rack and let cool completely (they will crisp more as they cool). Store in an airtight container at room temperature for up to 1 week.

Health Tip

- If you choose the pear variation, be aware that pears are high in fructose, which might contribute to diarrhea symptoms.

Nutrients per serving	
Calories	50
Fat	0 g
Sodium	1 mg
Carbohydrate	13 g
Fiber	2 g
Protein	0 g
Calcium	7 mg
Magnesium	5 mg
Potassium	98 mg

Crispy Multi-Seed Crackers

Whether being dipped in salsa or served with a bowl of hot soup, these crisp, lavosh-style crackers will add heart-healthy omega-3 fatty acids and fiber to your diet.

Makes about 40 crackers

Tips

Buy flax seeds already ground or grind your own in a clean coffee grinder.

For a thin crisp cracker, roll dough to an even thickness as thinly as possible. Don't worry if it breaks into pieces.

Pay close attention during the last few minutes of baking, as crackers can burn easily.

- **Preheat oven to 375°F (190°C)**
- **Food processor**
- **Baking sheets, ungreased**

1/2 cup	water	125 mL
2 tbsp	extra virgin olive oil	30 mL
1 tsp	cider vinegar	5 mL
1/2 cup	brown rice flour	125 mL
1/2 cup	sorghum flour	125 mL
1/4 cup	cornstarch	60 mL
1/3 cup	ground flax seeds (flaxseed meal)	75 mL
1 1/2 tsp	xanthan gum	7 mL
1/2 tsp	GF baking powder	2 mL
1 tsp	salt	5 mL
1/4 cup	freshly grated Parmesan cheese	60 mL
1/4 cup	sesame seeds	60 mL
3 tbsp	dried oregano	45 mL
2 tbsp	poppy seeds	30 mL

1. In a small bowl, combine water, olive oil and vinegar. Mix well and set aside.
2. In food processor, combine brown rice flour, sorghum flour, cornstarch, ground flax seeds, xanthan gum, baking powder, salt, Parmesan, sesame seeds, oregano and poppy seeds; pulse until mixed. With machine running, add liquid mixture through feed tube in a slow, steady stream. Process until dough forms a ball.
3. Divide dough into four pieces. Place each on plastic wrap and flatten into a disk; wrap well. Let dough rest in refrigerator for 10 minutes. Place one disk between two sheets of waxed or parchment paper. To prevent the paper from moving while you're rolling out the dough, place it on a lint-free towel. Using a heavy stroke with a rolling pin, roll out the dough as thinly as possible. Carefully remove the top sheet of paper. Invert the dough onto the baking sheet. Remove the remaining sheet of paper. Repeat with the remaining dough.

Nutrients per cracker	
Calories	38
Fat	2 g
Sodium	67 mg
Carbohydrate	4 g
Fiber	1 g
Protein	1 g
Calcium	29 mg
Magnesium	11 mg
Potassium	30 mg

Tips

If crackers become soft, re-crisp in a toaster oven or conventional oven at 350°F (180°C).

Just before baking, sprinkle with 1 tsp (5 mL) coarse salt or sesame seeds.

Substitute an equal amount of hempseed flour for the ground flax seeds.

4. Bake in preheated oven for 18 to 25 minutes or until browned and crisp. Remove to a cooling rack and cool completely. Break into pieces. Store at room temperature in an airtight container for up to 2 weeks or freeze for up to 3 months.

Health Tip

- This recipe contains several kinds of seeds and may not be suitable for those with some GI conditions.

Apple and Celery Flax Seed Crackers

These crackers are a great morning snack, full of heart-healthy flax seeds.

Makes 16 crackers

Tips

Brown flax seeds will produce a darker-colored cracker.

To soak the whole flax seeds for this recipe, place in a bowl with 4 cups (1 L) water. Cover and set aside for 30 minutes so the flax can absorb the liquid and swell. Drain, discarding soaking water. Rinse under cold running water until the water runs clear.

When spreading out raw breads or crackers on a dehydrator sheet, keep a small bowl of room-temperature water off to the side. Use this to wet your hands intermittently to prevent the dough from sticking to your hands.

Nutrients per cracker	
Calories	155
Fat	12 g
Sodium	100 mg
Carbohydrate	9 g
Fiber	8 g
Protein	5 g
Calcium	75 mg
Magnesium	111 mg
Potassium	250 mg

- **Food processor**
- **Electric food dehydrator**

1 cup	chopped peeled apple	250 mL
½ cup	chopped celery	125 mL
1 tsp	freshly squeezed lemon juice	5 mL
½ tsp	fine sea salt	2 mL
2 cups	whole flax seeds, soaked (see tips, at left)	500 mL
1 cup	ground flax seeds (flaxseed meal)	250 mL
1 cup	filtered water (approx.)	250 mL
¼ cup	chopped fresh parsley	60 mL

1. In food processor, combine apple, celery, lemon juice and salt; process until smooth.
2. In a large bowl, combine soaked whole flax seeds, ground flax seeds, water and parsley. Add apple mixture and mix well. The dough should be thick enough to spread but not so thick that it is difficult to stir. If needed, add up to ¼ cup (60 mL) additional water.
3. Transfer mixture to a nonstick dehydrator sheet and, using your hands, spread evenly in a thin layer, approximately ½ inch (1 cm) thick, across the entire area of the sheet. Using a small knife, cut into 16 equal portions. Dehydrate at 105°F (41°C) for 10 to 12 hours or until crispy. Allow to cool, then transfer to an airtight container. Store at room temperature for up to 2 weeks.

Health Tip

- Fresh herbs increase the alkalizing effect of this dish.

Swiss Chard Spring Rolls with Sesame Lime Dipping Sauce

Workaday Swiss chard leaves are transformed into elegant spring rolls stuffed with gorgeous ingredients from the garden. A tamari and lime dipping sauce makes an easy accompaniment.

Makes 8 rolls

Tip

Use the coarse side of a box grater to shred the carrots and beets. Or, to make quick work of the task, use the shredding disk on a food processor. To prevent the carrots from turning purple, shred them first, then measure them, then shred the beets.

Dipping Sauce

1/4 cup	reduced-sodium tamari or soy sauce (GF, if needed)	60 mL
2 tbsp	freshly squeezed lime juice	30 mL
2 tsp	toasted sesame oil	10 mL
2 tsp	brown rice syrup or liquid honey	10 mL
1/4 tsp	ground ginger	1 mL

Spring Rolls

8	Swiss chard leaves, tough stems trimmed off	8
3/4 cup	shredded carrots	175 mL
3/4 cup	shredded peeled beets	175 mL
3/4 cup	mung bean sprouts or sunflower sprouts	175 mL
1/2 cup	packed fresh basil leaves	125 mL

1. *Sauce:* In a small bowl, whisk together tamari, lime juice, oil, brown rice syrup and ginger.
2. *Spring Rolls:* Place Swiss chard leaves on a work surface. Fill each with an equal amount of carrots, beets, sprouts and basil. Roll leaves around filling, tucking in edges. Serve immediately, with sauce, or store loosely covered in the refrigerator for up to 4 hours.

Health Tip

- Tamari soy sauce is an alkalizing condiment.

Nutrients per roll	
Calories	41
Fat	1 g
Sodium	403 mg
Carbohydrate	6 g
Fiber	1 g
Protein	2 g
Calcium	20 mg
Magnesium	21 mg
Potassium	163 mg

Fresh Vegetable Spring Rolls with Filipino Garlic Sauce

*Most Southeast Asian countries have a version of fresh spring rolls. Filipinos have adapted the original Fukien unfried spring rolls (*lun bia*) to one of their national dishes, fresh lumpia. The Vietnamese are famous for a wide range of uncooked spring rolls wrapped in "rice paper" — thin, round sheets of cooked glutinous rice that merely have to be soaked in warm water and rolled up around a filling. Here, both traditions are combined.*

Makes 6 servings

Tips

Vary the amounts of the vegetables or change them according to personal taste and what is available.

Jicama is a large round tuber with a thick skin that must be peeled; the slightly sweet crunchy flesh is eaten raw. It's a bit like a cross between an apple and a potato. It is often available at grocery chains, as well as Asian and Central American grocers.

Nutrients per serving	
Calories	222
Fat	4 g
Sodium	418 mg
Carbohydrate	41 g
Fiber	2 g
Protein	6 g
Calcium	36 mg
Magnesium	26 mg
Potassium	245 mg

Garlic Sauce

1 tbsp	vegetable oil	15 mL
2 tbsp	minced garlic	30 mL
1 cup	ready-to-use vegetable or chicken broth	250 mL
1/2 cup	granulated sugar	125 mL
4 tsp	soy sauce (GF, if needed)	20 mL
1/4 tsp	freshly ground black pepper	1 mL
2 1/2 tbsp	rice vinegar (or 3 tbsp/45 mL lime juice)	37 mL
2 1/2 tsp	cornstarch, mixed with 1 tbsp (15 mL) water	12 mL

Spring Rolls

1/2	package (2 oz/50 g) bean threads (optional)	1/2
3 oz	string beans	90 g
3 oz	snow peas	90 g
3 oz	bean sprouts	90 g
2 oz	carrot, julienned	60 g
3 oz	jicama, julienned	90 g
1 oz	red bell pepper, julienned	30 g
12	sheets "rice paper" wrappers	12
6	leaf lettuce leaves, cut in half	6
1/4 cup	loosely packed Thai basil leaves (optional)	60 mL

1. *Sauce:* In a saucepan, heat oil over low heat; cook garlic 2 minutes without browning. Stir in broth, sugar, soy sauce and pepper; increase heat to simmer and cook 2 minutes. Stir in vinegar; cook 1 minute. Stir in cornstarch mixture; cook 30 seconds or until thickened. Transfer to a serving bowl; cool to room temperature.

Tip

Wrapping the spring rolls is an easily acquired skill; just don't be too frustrated if the first batch isn't perfect. Avoid trying to overstuff the wrappers; it is better to have extra filling to make more spring rolls than to struggle with overfilled rolls.

2. *Spring Rolls:* If using bean threads, soak them in cold water to cover until pliable. Bring a pot with 4 cups (1 L) water to a boil. Blanch bean threads for 20 seconds, string beans for 2 minutes, snow peas for 30 seconds, bean sprouts for 5 seconds and carrots for 30 seconds, rinsing them all in cold water immediately after blanching to stop further cooking; drain and dry vegetables. Cut beans and pea pods into juliennes by cutting lengthwise on a very oblique diagonal. Mix bean threads, string beans, snow peas, bean sprouts, carrots, jicama and red pepper.
3. Fill a large bowl with warm water and soak 1 wrapper until soft. Place wrapper on dry cloth, put a lettuce leaf half over it, make a line of 3 or 4 basil leaves and cover with vegetables; roll into a cylinder, tucking in the edges as you roll. Put on a tray and cover with a damp cloth. Repeat with the remaining wrappers and filling. Serve with garlic sauce on the side to be spooned over just before eating or, if serving the spring rolls as finger food, to be dunked into.

Variation

Strips of cold boiled, roasted or Chinese-style barbecued pork make a very nice addition to the spring rolls, as do cold poached shrimp.

Health Tips

- Sodium is a critical buffer that reduces acid in our bodies, but too much or the wrong kind can make things worse. Reducing sodium or using sea salt instead of table salt is a good way to improve your health — no matter what your condition is.
- Making your own broth or stock to replace a ready-made product will reduce sodium and increase the health benefits of this dish.

Mushroom Pinwheels

Use this versatile mushroom mixture to create many hot party snacks. Here, it's encased in puff pastry, but you can also use it as a filling for small phyllo pastry cups, mini vol-au-vent pastry shells, short-crust pastry shells, wonton wrappers, salad roll wrappers or gougères.

Makes 36 pinwheels

Tip

A soft-bristle pastry brush is a handy tool for gently brushing dirt from the cremini mushrooms.

- **Preheat oven to 400°F (200°C)**
- **Food processor**
- **2 baking sheets, lined with parchment paper**

2	packages (each ½ oz/14 g) dried porcini mushrooms	2
¼ cup	hot water	60 mL
8 oz	cremini mushrooms, quartered	250 g
1	shallot, roughly chopped	1
2	cloves garlic, roughly chopped	2
2 tbsp	olive oil	30 mL
1 tsp	finely chopped thyme	5 mL
½ tsp	finely chopped rosemary	2 mL
	Salt and freshly ground black pepper	
1 tbsp	sherry or Madeira	15 mL
1 lb	puff pastry	500 g
1	large egg, beaten	1

1. In a bowl, cover porcini mushrooms with hot water. Set aside to soak for 10 minutes. Remove mushrooms, squeeze out water and chop roughly. Strain soaking liquid to remove any grit and reserve ¼ cup (60 mL). Set aside.
2. In food processor, pulse porcini mushrooms, cremini mushrooms, shallot and garlic until finely chopped.
3. In a large skillet, heat oil over medium-high heat. Add mushroom mixture, thyme and rosemary and season lightly with salt and pepper. Sauté for 3 to 4 minutes. Deglaze pan with sherry, scraping up browned bits on bottom, and add porcini soaking liquid. Stir and cook until liquid is reduced and mushrooms are lightly browned, 2 to 3 minutes. Let cool.

Nutrients per pinwheel	
Calories	83
Fat	6 g
Sodium	37 mg
Carbohydrate	6 g
Fiber	0 g
Protein	2 g
Calcium	3 mg
Magnesium	3 mg
Potassium	31 mg

Variation

Mushroom Gruyère Crostini: Arrange crostini on a baking sheet. Spread with mushroom mixture and top with shaved Gruyère cheese. Bake in 350°F (180°C) oven until cheese is melted, about 5 minutes.

4. On a lightly floured surface, roll puff pastry to make a rectangle 18 by 9 inches (45 by 23 cm) and spread with a thin layer of mushroom mixture. Roll up pastry, jelly-roll style, to make a compact cylinder. Cut roll into $\frac{1}{2}$-inch (1 cm) slices. Arrange mushroom pinwheels on prepared baking sheet, about 2 inches (5 cm) apart. Pinwheels may be prepared ahead to this point. Cover and refrigerate for up to 4 hours.
5. Brush tops lightly with egg and bake in preheated oven until pastry is golden, 15 to 20 minutes. Serve warm.

Health Tip

- Save this snack for special occasions (as the acidifying part of a meal). It will make a great addition to any celebration!

Zucchini Fritters

Serve these fritters as part of an antipasti spread. They are great on their own or, if you like to gild the lily, even better with a bowl of tzatziki alongside.

Makes about 24 fritters

Tips

To expedite preparation, shred zucchini and set aside to sweat while you prepare the remaining ingredients.

For ease of preparation, use a food processor fitted with the shredding blade to shred the zucchini.

- **Preheat oven to 200°F (100°C)**

4 cups	shredded zucchini (about 3 medium)	1 L
1 tsp	coarse salt	5 mL
4 oz	feta cheese, crumbled	125 g
6	green onions (white part with a bit of green), minced	6
1/2 cup	finely chopped fresh dill fronds	125 mL
2	cloves garlic, minced	2
2	large eggs, beaten	2
1/2 cup	sorghum flour	125 mL
1 tbsp	cornstarch	15 mL
1/2 tsp	GF baking powder	2 mL
1/4 cup	vegetable oil (approx.)	60 mL

1. In a colander, placed over a sink, combine zucchini and salt. Toss well and set aside for 15 minutes to sweat. Using your hands, squeeze out as much water as possible. Spread on a clean tea towel and press to soak up as much liquid as possible, using a second tea towel, if necessary. (Zucchini should be as dry as possible; otherwise your fritters will be mushy.)
2. In a bowl, combine feta, green onions, dill and garlic. Add zucchini and eggs and mix well. Sprinkle sorghum flour, cornstarch and baking powder evenly over mixture and toss well.
3. In a large heavy skillet, heat oil over medium-high heat. Scoop out about 1 heaping tbsp (20 mL) of mixture at a time and drop into hot oil. Repeat until pan is full, leaving about 2 inches (5 cm) between fritters. Cook, turning once, until nicely golden, about 5 minutes per batch. Drain on paper towel–lined platter and keep warm in preheated oven while you complete the frying. Serve warm.

Health Tip

- Soft cheeses are less acidic than hard cheeses, such as Cheddar, but it is best to indulge in small servings of cheese on rare occasions, to balance your pH.

Nutrients per fritter	
Calories	55
Fat	4 g
Sodium	141 mg
Carbohydrate	3 g
Fiber	0 g
Protein	2 g
Calcium	35 mg
Magnesium	6 mg
Potassium	79 mg

Herbed Quinoa Deviled Eggs

Quinoa contributes a delicate sesame flavor and a toothsome texture to traditional deviled eggs. Replacing the mayonnaise with Greek yogurt lightens this into a healthy snack and adds another layer of flavor.

Makes 8 appetizers

Tip

To prepare ½ cup (125 mL) cooked quinoa, combine 2½ tbsp (37 mL) quinoa and ⅓ cup (75 mL) water in a medium saucepan. Bring to a boil over medium-high heat. Reduce heat to low, cover and simmer for 12 to 15 minutes or until water is just barely absorbed. Cover and let stand for 5 to 6 minutes. Fluff with a fork and let cool completely.

4	large eggs	4
	Cold water	
	Ice water	
½ cup	cooked quinoa (see tip, at left), cooled	125 mL
1½ tbsp	finely chopped fresh basil, parsley or dill	22 mL
3 tbsp	plain Greek yogurt	45 mL
1 tsp	Dijon mustard	5 mL
	Fine sea salt and freshly cracked black pepper	

1. Place eggs in a medium saucepan and add enough cold water to cover by 1 inch (2.5 cm). Bring to a boil over medium-high heat. Remove from heat, cover and let stand for 13 minutes. Drain and transfer eggs to a bowl of ice water. Let stand until cool.
2. Peel eggs and cut in half lengthwise. Transfer yolks to a medium bowl and mash with a fork until smooth. Stir in quinoa, basil, yogurt and mustard. Season to taste with salt and pepper.
3. Place egg whites, hollow side up, on a serving plate. Spoon yolk mixture into egg whites, dividing evenly. Cover and refrigerate for at least 15 minutes, until filling is set, or for up to 24 hours.

Variation

Southern Deviled Eggs: Omit the basil and add 1 tbsp (15 mL) sweet pickle relish to the egg yolk mixture. Garnish tops of eggs with ¼ tsp (1 mL) sweet paprika.

Nutrients per appetizer	
Calories	54
Fat	3 g
Sodium	53 mg
Carbohydrate	3 g
Fiber	0 g
Protein	4 g
Calcium	20 mg
Magnesium	11 mg
Potassium	56 mg

Health Tip

- Fresh herbs increase the alkalizing effect of this dish.

Mediterranean Pizza Squares

This vegetarian pizza, with an easy-to-prepare crust, is delicious served hot or at room temperature.

Makes 48 appetizers

Tips

To quickly roast a head of garlic, cut off top of head to expose clove tips. Drizzle with ¼ tsp (1 mL) olive oil and microwave on High for 70 seconds or until fork-tender. Or bake in a pie plate or baking dish at 375°F (190°C) for 15 to 20 minutes.

This is a very thin crust. There is enough dough to cover the bottom of the pan evenly with a thin layer. Take your time.

For fast, easy cutting, use a pizza wheel.

Nutrients per appetizer	
Calories	54
Fat	3 g
Sodium	115 mg
Carbohydrate	5 g
Fiber	1 g
Protein	2 g
Calcium	41 mg
Magnesium	2 mg
Potassium	52 mg

- **Preheat oven to 425°F (220°C)**
- **15- by 10-inch (40 by 25 cm) rimmed baking sheet, lightly greased and sprinkled with cornmeal**

1 cup	amaranth flour	250 mL
½ cup	quinoa flour	125 mL
¼ cup	cornstarch	60 mL
¼ cup	cornmeal	60 mL
1 tsp	xanthan gum	5 mL
1 tbsp	GF baking powder	15 mL
1 tsp	salt	5 mL
⅓ cup	vegetable shortening	75 mL
¾ cup	milk	175 mL
	Sweet rice flour	
3	plum (Roma) tomatoes, thinly sliced	3
4	cloves garlic, roasted (see tip, at left) and chopped	4
⅔ cup	sliced black olives	150 mL
¼ cup	snipped fresh basil	60 mL
¼ tsp	freshly ground black pepper	1 mL
1 cup	shredded Monterey Jack cheese	250 mL
1 cup	crumbled feta cheese	250 mL

Traditional Method

1. In a large bowl, stir together amaranth flour, quinoa flour, cornstarch, cornmeal, xanthan gum, baking powder and salt. Using a pastry blender or two knives, cut in shortening until mixture resembles coarse crumbs. Add milk, all at once, stirring with a fork to make a soft dough.

Food Processor Method

1. In a food processor fitted with a metal blade, pulse amaranth flour, quinoa flour, cornstarch, cornmeal, xanthan gum, baking powder and salt. Add shortening and pulse until mixture resembles small peas, about 5 to 10 seconds. With the machine running, pour milk through feed tube and process until dough just holds together.

Tips

You can also serve these pizza squares for lunch or as a snack, in which case they make 3 to 4 servings.

To make the pizza kid-friendly, top with their favorite fixings. Keep one in the freezer for when they are invited to a pizza party.

Variations

Substitute mozzarella, fontina or provolone cheese for the Monterey Jack.

Substitute an equal amount of chopped fresh rosemary for the basil.

For Both Methods

2. Transfer dough to prepared pan. Either cover with waxed paper and roll out with a rolling pin or gently pat out dough with fingers dusted with sweet rice flour to fill the pan evenly. Bake in the bottom third of preheated oven for 10 minutes or until slightly firm.

3. Arrange tomato slices over crust; sprinkle with garlic, olives, basil and pepper. Sprinkle with Monterey Jack and feta.

4. Bake for 20 to 25 minutes or until cheese is bubbly and crust is golden. Remove to a cutting board and cut into squares. Serve immediately. Transfer any extra squares to a cooling rack to prevent the crust from getting soggy.

Health Tips

- To achieve a healthy balance of acid and alkaline, you can include low-fat milk and small portions of cheese as the more acidic part of your meal. If you begin to use nut milks or other non-dairy milks, you may quickly find that you no longer prefer the flavor of regular milk. Including a leafy green salad or steamed greens as part of this meal (and in the next few) will help to rebalance your pH.
- Roma and cherry tomatoes are higher in fructose than other tomatoes. If you are at risk for diarrhea, substitute other tomatoes for this recipe.

Leek, Onion and Garlic Tart

This tart will support your immune system as well as tantalize your taste buds.

Makes 6 servings

Tips

A springform pan makes serving easier because the sides can be removed.

Serve hot or at room temperature. Slice in thin wedges for a first course or use larger servings for a vegetable side dish.

Variation

Substitute regular potatoes or ½ acorn or butternut squash for the sweet potatoes.

Nutrients per serving	
Calories	228
Fat	13 g
Sodium	145 mg
Carbohydrate	25 g
Fiber	4 g
Protein	4 g
Calcium	85 mg
Magnesium	29 mg
Potassium	483 mg

- **Preheat oven to 375°F (190°C)**
- **10-inch (25 cm) springform pan or round tart pan or shallow baking dish, buttered**

Base

3 cups	thinly sliced potatoes (unpeeled)	750 mL
1 cup	thinly sliced peeled sweet potatoes	250 mL
3 tbsp	honey mustard	45 mL
2 tbsp	olive oil	30 mL

Topping

¼ cup	sliced leek (white part only)	60 mL
4	cloves garlic, slivered	4
3 cups	sliced onions	750 mL
2 tbsp	olive oil	30 mL
3 tbsp	chopped fresh basil	45 mL
¼ cup	freshly grated Parmesan cheese	60 mL

1. *Base:* In a large bowl, toss potatoes with mustard and 2 tbsp (30 mL) oil. Spread in bottom of prepared pan. Press potatoes with the back of a spoon to compress. Season to taste with salt and pepper.
2. *Topping:* Spread leek and garlic evenly over potato base, then onions over top. If desired, season to taste with salt. Drizzle with oil. Bake in preheated oven for 40 minutes or until potatoes are tender and onions are golden. Sprinkle with basil and cheese; bake for another 5 minutes or until cheese has melted. Let stand for at least 10 minutes before serving.

Health Tip

- Vitamin-packed sweet potatoes are also high in fiber.

Dips and Sauces

Caramelized Onion Dip

This dip is one of life's guilty pleasures. Serve with potato chips or leaves of Belgian endive.

Makes about 1½ cups (375 mL)

Tip

The amount of salt you'll need to add depends upon the accompaniment. If you're serving this with salty potato chips, err on the side of caution.

Variation

For a more herbal flavor, add 2 tbsp (30 mL) chopped fresh thyme leaves along with the cream cheese.

- **Small (approx. 2-quart) slow cooker**
- **Food processor**

2	onions, thinly sliced on the vertical	2
4	cloves garlic, chopped	4
1 tbsp	melted butter	15 mL
4 oz	cream cheese, cubed and softened	125 g
½ cup	sour cream	125 mL
1 tbsp	dark miso (GF, if needed)	15 mL
	Salt (see tip, at left) and freshly ground black pepper	
	Finely snipped chives	

1. In slow cooker stoneware, combine onions, garlic and butter. Toss well to ensure onions are thoroughly coated. Place a clean tea towel, folded in half (so you will have two layers), over top of stoneware to absorb moisture. Cover and cook on High for 5 hours, stirring two or three times to ensure onions are browning evenly, replacing towel each time, until onions are nicely caramelized.
2. Transfer mixture to food processor. Add cream cheese, sour cream, miso and salt and pepper to taste. Process until well blended. Transfer to a serving dish and garnish with chives.

Health Tip

- Garlic, onions and chives counteract the acidic cheese in this recipe. Cooking in the slow cooker definitely helps reduce the acidifying impact. Save this mouthwatering treat for special occasions.

Nutrients per 1 tbsp (15 mL)	
Calories	24
Fat	2 g
Sodium	51 mg
Carbohydrate	2 g
Fiber	0 g
Protein	1 g
Calcium	24 mg
Magnesium	2 mg
Potassium	22 mg

Pumpkin Pepita Hummus

You'll love the contrasts at play in this dish, from its earthy and sweet flavors to its velvety and crisp textures. It proves that pumpkin is far more than pie filling.

Makes about 2 cups (500 mL)

Tips

If you use homemade pumpkin purée instead of canned, you'll need about 1¾ cups (425 mL).

Look for roasted green pumpkin seeds that are lightly seasoned with sea salt.

This spread can be stored in an airtight container in the refrigerator for up to 3 days.

- **Food processor**

2	cloves garlic, coarsely chopped	2
1	can (15 oz/425 mL) pumpkin purée (not pie filling)	1
2 tsp	ground cumin	10 mL
¾ tsp	fine sea salt	3 mL
⅛ tsp	cayenne pepper	0.5 mL
3 tbsp	tahini	45 mL
2 tbsp	freshly squeezed lemon juice	30 mL
2 tbsp	lightly salted roasted green pumpkin seeds (pepitas), chopped	30 mL
1 tbsp	chopped fresh flat-leaf (Italian) parsley	15 mL

1. In food processor, combine garlic, pumpkin, cumin, salt, cayenne, tahini and lemon juice; process until smooth.
2. Transfer to a serving dish and sprinkle with pumpkin seeds and parsley.

Health Tip

- This tasty alkalizing dip pairs well with raw veggies for a great snack.

Nutrients per 2 tbsp (30 mL)	
Calories	36
Fat	2 g
Sodium	74 mg
Carbohydrate	3 g
Fiber	1 g
Protein	1 g
Calcium	11 mg
Magnesium	10 mg
Potassium	82 mg

Green Pesto

Pesto can be used as a dip for fresh vegetables, a spread on a sandwich, a sauce for a main dish or a flavoring for a soup or sauce. In a few simple steps, you can make pesto at home in no time.

Makes 2 cups (500 mL)

Variations

Omit the walnuts and increase the parsley to 6 cups (1.5 L) and the olive oil to ¾ cup (175 mL).

Substitute an equal amount of fresh cilantro for the parsley or an equal amount of raw shelled hemp seeds for the walnuts.

- **Food processor**

4 cups	roughly chopped fresh flat-leaf (Italian) parsley leaves	1 L
½ cup	extra virgin olive oil	125 mL
½ cup	raw walnut halves	125 mL
¼ cup	freshly squeezed lemon juice	60 mL
½ tsp	fine sea salt	2 mL
3	cloves garlic	3

1. In food processor, combine parsley, olive oil, walnuts, lemon juice, salt and garlic; process until smooth, stopping motor and scraping down sides of work bowl as necessary.
2. Transfer to a bowl. Serve immediately or cover and refrigerate for up to 5 days.

Health Tip

- Although the fresh herbs increase the alkalizing effect of this dish, the acidifying walnuts bring the pH balance toward the acidifying. Serve with steamed beets or dark leafy greens to offset the acidity.

Nutrients per 1 tbsp (15 mL)	
Calories	42
Fat	4 g
Sodium	47 mg
Carbohydrate	1 g
Fiber	0 g
Protein	0 g
Calcium	12 mg
Magnesium	6 mg
Potassium	51 mg

Cashew Scallion Cream Cheese

This take on traditional cream cheese is rich and spreadable. Use it virtually anytime you want a spread, as a replacement for hummus or as a dip for carrot sticks and broccoli florets.

Makes about 2½ cups (625 mL)

Tip

This recipe was tested in a high-powered blender, but if you do not have one, you can use a food processor.

Variations

This recipe can be enhanced with a variety of herbs and spices or seasonings. For instance, try substituting parsley leaves for half of the green onion and adding a clove of garlic.

For a Thai-inspired version, in step 1, add 1 tbsp (15 mL) raw agave nectar, 1 tsp (5 mL) ground coriander, 1 tsp (5 mL) finely chopped gingerroot and ½ tsp (2 mL) apple cider vinegar.

Nutrients per 1 tbsp (15 mL)	
Calories	38
Fat	3 g
Sodium	69 mg
Carbohydrate	2 g
Fiber	0 g
Protein	1 g
Calcium	5 mg
Magnesium	17 mg
Potassium	44 mg

- **High-powered blender (see tip, at left)**

1 cup	chopped green onions (white and green parts), divided	250 mL
¼ cup	filtered water	60 mL
1 tbsp	freshly squeezed lemon juice	15 mL
1 tsp	fine sea salt	5 mL
2 cups	raw cashews, soaked (see box, below)	500 mL

1. In blender, combine ½ cup (125 mL) green onions, water, lemon juice and salt; blend on high speed until smooth. Add soaked cashews and blend on high speed until smooth, stopping the motor once and stirring the mixture with a rubber spatula.
2. Transfer to a serving bowl and stir in the remaining green onions. Serve immediately or cover and refrigerate for up to 3 days.

How to Soak Raw Cashews

To soak 2 cups (500 mL) raw cashews, place in a bowl and cover with 4 cups (1 L) water. Cover and set aside for 30 minutes. Drain, discarding soaking water, and rinse under cold running water until the water runs clear.

You can keep cashews soaking in the refrigerator for up to 3 days, submerged in water and covered. You will need to change the water once or twice daily to prevent the cashews from becoming sour or fermenting.

Herbed Cashew Cheese

This "cheese" is as creamy and filling as traditional cheese. Use it as a dip with fresh veggies or as a spread on crisp romaine lettuce leaves.

Makes 1½ cups (375 mL)

Tips

Substitute an equal quantity of pine nuts or macadamia nuts for the cashews. If using macadamia nuts, increase the water by 2 tbsp (30 mL).

Nutritional yeast flakes can be found in well-stocked supermarkets and natural foods stores. Nutritional yeast is fortified with vitamin B_{12}. It helps to produce umami, the savory flavor that is sometimes lacking in vegetarian cuisine.

Substitute an equal amount of chopped fresh rosemary for the thyme.

- **Food processor**

2 cups	raw cashews (see tip, at left)	500 mL
½ cup	filtered water	125 mL
¼ cup	freshly squeezed lemon juice	60 mL
¼ cup	nutritional yeast (see tip, at left)	60 mL
4 tsp	chopped fresh thyme leaves (see tip, at left)	20 mL
1 tsp	fine sea salt	5 mL

1. In food processor, combine cashews, water, lemon juice, nutritional yeast, thyme and salt; process until smooth, stopping motor to scrape down sides of work bowl as necessary.
2. Transfer to a bowl. Serve immediately or cover and refrigerate for up to 4 days.

Nutrients per 1 tbsp (15 mL)	
Calories	68
Fat	5 g
Sodium	114 mg
Carbohydrate	4 g
Fiber	1 g
Protein	2 g
Calcium	6 mg
Magnesium	29 mg
Potassium	91 mg

Simple Veggie Marinade

Toss cherry tomatoes, zucchini, green or red bell pepper chunks, eggplant, mushrooms and onions with this classic marinade. Or brush it on vegetables grilling on the barbecue.

Makes about ⅓ cup (75 mL)

¼ cup	freshly squeezed lemon juice	60 mL
3 tbsp	canola oil	45 mL
2	cloves garlic, minced	2
2 tbsp	chopped fresh oregano leaves (or 2 tsp/10 mL dried)	30 mL
	Salt and freshly ground black pepper	

1. In a tightly covered container, combine lemon juice, oil, garlic, oregano, salt and pepper. Shake until well blended.
2. Store in the refrigerator until needed for up to 1 week.

Health Tip

- Fresh herbs increase the alkalizing effect of this marinade.

Nutrients per 1 tbsp (15 mL)	
Calories	82
Fat	9 g
Sodium	1 mg
Carbohydrate	2 g
Fiber	1 g
Protein	0 g
Calcium	22 mg
Magnesium	4 mg
Potassium	33 mg

Chunky Tomato Sauce

If you plan to make only one homemade sauce, this is the one. It can be used in dozens of ways and tastes 100% better than any commercial variety. Seek out good-quality canned plum tomatoes or, best of all, use field-ripened fresh plum tomatoes in season.

Makes about 5 cups (1.25 L)

Tip

If you don't have fresh herbs on hand, use 1 tsp (5 mL) each dried basil and oregano. Add them with the garlic in step 1.

2 tbsp	extra virgin olive oil	30 mL
2	onions, chopped	2
2	stalks celery, chopped	2
2	cloves garlic, finely chopped	2
1/4 cup	tomato paste	60 mL
2	cans (each 28 oz/796 mL) diced tomatoes, with juice	2
1 tbsp	chopped fresh basil, divided	15 mL
1 tbsp	chopped fresh oregano, divided	15 mL
	Salt and freshly ground black pepper	
Pinch	granulated sugar (optional)	Pinch

1. In a large saucepan, heat oil over medium heat. Add onions and celery and sauté until softened but not browned, 5 to 6 minutes. Add garlic and sauté for 1 to 2 minutes. Add tomato paste and cook, stirring, for 1 minute. Add tomatoes and bring to a simmer.
2. Reduce heat and stir in 1 tsp (5 mL) basil, 1 tsp (5 mL) oregano, 1/2 tsp (2 mL) salt and 1/4 tsp (1 mL) pepper. Simmer, stirring occasionally and breaking up tomatoes with a wooden spoon as they soften, until sauce is smooth and nicely thickened, about 45 minutes. Add the remaining basil and oregano and taste and adjust seasoning. Add sugar, if needed.

Health Tip

- Although tomato sauce is slightly acidifying, serving it with fresh herbs, onions and garlic helps balance the pH of the dish. Enjoy!

Nutrients per 1/4 cup (60 mL)	
Calories	39
Fat	1 g
Sodium	184 mg
Carbohydrate	6 g
Fiber	1 g
Protein	1 g
Calcium	19 mg
Magnesium	3 mg
Potassium	62 mg

Roasted Red Pepper Pasta Sauce

Keep a jar of roasted red peppers on hand to make this gorgeous sauce. Better yet, roast your own when they are in season and freeze them.

Makes 1 cup (250 mL)

Tip

There are many different-size jars of roasted red peppers available. No matter which size you buy, use about 1 cup (250 mL) drained peppers to make this sauce.

- **Food processor**

1	jar (10½ oz/313 mL) roasted red bell peppers, drained (see tip, at left)	1
1 tbsp	olive oil	15 mL
2	cloves garlic, minced	2
1 tsp	dried oregano (or 1 tbsp/15 mL chopped fresh)	5 mL
	Salt and freshly ground black pepper	

1. In food processor, purée roasted peppers. Set aside.
2. Heat oil in a nonstick skillet over medium heat. Add garlic and oregano. Cook, stirring, for 30 seconds.
3. Add red pepper purée. Reduce heat and cook slowly for 2 minutes. Season to taste with salt and pepper. Store in refrigerator for 1 week or freeze for longer storage.
4. Serve the sauce over cooked pasta. As a final touch, you can sprinkle the cooked sauce and pasta with some grated Parmigiano-Reggiano cheese at serving time.

Nutrients per ¼ cup (60 mL)	
Calories	57
Fat	4 g
Sodium	271 mg
Carbohydrate	5 g
Fiber	1 g
Protein	1 g
Calcium	15 mg
Magnesium	1 mg
Potassium	9 mg

Cashew Alfredo Sauce

The deep, rich flavor and texture of this creamy sauce pair perfectly with gluten-free noodles topped with Parmesan cheese. It's also wonderful as a spread on crisp stalks of celery or fresh romaine lettuce leaves.

Makes 3 cups (750 mL)

Tip

If you have a high-powered blender, use it to make this sauce. It will be smoother and creamier than when made in a regular blender.

Variation

Instead of the cashews, substitute 1 cup (250 mL) macadamia nuts soaked in 2 cups (500 mL) water for 30 minutes, drained and rinsed, and an additional 1⁄4 cup (60 mL) olive or flaxseed oil.

Nutrients per 1⁄4 cup (60 mL)	
Calories	161
Fat	13 g
Sodium	292 mg
Carbohydrate	9 g
Fiber	1 g
Protein	5 g
Calcium	12 mg
Magnesium	60 mg
Potassium	174 mg

- **Blender**

2 cups	raw cashews, soaked (see box, page 217)	500 mL
3⁄4 cup	filtered water	175 mL
3 tbsp	nutritional yeast	45 mL
2 tbsp	extra virgin olive oil or flaxseed oil	30 mL
1 tbsp	brown rice miso	15 mL
1 tbsp	freshly squeezed lemon juice	15 mL
1	clove garlic	1
1 tsp	fine sea salt	5 mL

1. In blender, combine soaked cashews, water, nutritional yeast, olive oil, miso, lemon juice, garlic and salt. Blend on high speed until smooth.
2. Transfer to a bowl and serve immediately or cover and refrigerate for up to 3 days.

Health Tip

- Brown rice miso is highly alkalizing, which makes this a better choice than barbecue or a dish with cheese.

Yellow Coconut Curry Sauce

This raw curry sauce is delicious served with fresh zucchini noodles, marinated spinach or some raw cashews.

Makes 1 cup (250 mL)

Tips

Coconut oil is solid at room temperature but has a melting point of 76°F (24°C), so it is easy to liquefy. To melt it, place in a shallow glass bowl over a pot of simmering water.

Depending on the curry powder you use, this recipe can pack a punch. Add 2 tsp (10 mL) curry powder and then try a taste, adding more if you prefer.

Nutrients per ¼ cup (60 mL)	
Calories	189
Fat	18 g
Sodium	354 mg
Carbohydrate	6 g
Fiber	1 g
Protein	3 g
Calcium	11 mg
Magnesium	47 mg
Potassium	111 mg

- **Blender**

½ cup	raw cashews	125 mL
½ cup	filtered water	125 mL
3 tbsp	melted coconut oil (see tip, at left)	45 mL
2 to 3 tsp	mild curry powder (see tip, at left)	10 to 15 mL
1 tbsp	freshly squeezed lemon juice	15 mL
1 tsp	chopped gingerroot	5 mL
½ tsp	fine sea salt	2 mL

1. In blender, combine cashews, water, coconut oil, curry powder, lemon juice, ginger and salt. Blend on high speed until smooth.
2. Transfer to a bowl. Serve immediately or cover and refrigerate for up to 5 days.

Variation

For a spicier flavor, add ¼ tsp (1 mL) cayenne pepper, or more if you prefer.

Plum Dipping Sauce

Try this quick, easy and rich plum-colored sauce with Crispy Pecan Chicken Fingers (page 296).

Makes 1 cup (250 mL)

Tips

Sauce can be stored, covered, in the refrigerator for up to 2 weeks.

To prevent cross-contamination, set out individual bowls for dipping sauces for each person.

Serve sauce warm or cold — it's delicious either way!

- **Blender**

1	can (14 oz/398 mL) prune plums	1
1/3 cup	granulated sugar	75 mL
3 tbsp	white vinegar	45 mL

1. Drain plums, reserving 2 tbsp (30 mL) liquid. Remove pits from plums. In blender, purée plums and reserved liquid.
2. In a small saucepan, combine plum purée, sugar and vinegar. Heat over medium heat until mixture comes to a gentle boil. Remove from heat and let cool before serving.

Variations

In season, 8 fresh plums can be substituted for the canned plums. For an even quicker sauce, substitute one 7.5-oz (213 mL) jar of GF baby food strained plums.

To add tomato flavor, add 1 tbsp (15 mL) GF ketchup or GF barbecue sauce to the dipping sauce.

Nutrients per 1 tbsp (15 mL)	
Calories	25
Fat	0 g
Sodium	0 mg
Carbohydrate	7 g
Fiber	0 g
Protein	0 g
Calcium	2 mg
Magnesium	1 mg
Potassium	30 mg

Honey Mustard Dipping Sauce

Here is a perfect dip for when you're looking for that addictive bite of mustard.

Makes ½ cup (125 mL)

Nutrients per 1 tbsp (15 mL)	
Calories	34
Fat	0 g
Sodium	45 mg
Carbohydrate	9 g
Fiber	0 g
Protein	0 g
Calcium	1 mg
Magnesium	0 mg
Potassium	5 mg

¼ cup	Dijon mustard	60 mL
¼ cup	liquid honey	60 mL

1. In a small bowl, combine Dijon mustard and honey. Serve at room temperature. (If the honey becomes too thick to pour, microwave, uncovered, on Medium for a few seconds until it pours easily.)

Variation

Substitute prepared or grainy mustard for the Dijon.

Thai Dipping Sauce

This sauce turns plain chicken wings and shrimp into Thai delights.

Makes ½ cup (125 mL)

3 tbsp	finely minced shallots	45 mL
3 tbsp	freshly squeezed lime juice	45 mL
2 tbsp	reduced-sodium soy sauce (GF, if needed)	30 mL
2 tbsp	Bold Chili Sauce (page 226) or store-bought chili sauce	30 mL
1 tbsp	chopped fresh cilantro	15 mL
1 tbsp	lightly packed brown sugar	15 mL
½ tsp	Chinese five-spice powder	2 mL
	Freshly ground black pepper	

1. In a bowl, combine shallots, lime juice, soy sauce, chili sauce, cilantro, brown sugar and five-spice powder. Season to taste with pepper. Serve cold or hot. To reheat, place in the microwave for 30 seconds.

Health Tip

- If you have a GI condition that is aggravated by hot or spicy foods, choose a milder chili sauce for this dish.

Nutrients per 1 tbsp (15 mL)	
Calories	17
Fat	0 g
Sodium	191 mg
Carbohydrate	4 g
Fiber	0 g
Protein	0 g
Calcium	5 mg
Magnesium	3 mg
Potassium	45 mg

Bold Chili Sauce

This bold and spicy sauce is all you need on hot dogs or steak burgers.

Makes 3 cups (750 mL)

Tip

This sauce keeps well, covered and refrigerated, for up to 1 week.

- **Preheat oven to 400°F (200°C)**
- **Baking sheet, lined with parchment paper**
- **Food processor or blender**

16	dried guajillo chiles	16
2 tbsp	canola oil	30 mL
6	cloves garlic	6
1½ tbsp	extra virgin olive oil	22 mL
1½ tsp	granulated sugar	7 mL
1 tsp	dried oregano	5 mL
1 tsp	sea salt	5 mL
¼ tsp	freshly ground black pepper	1 mL
⅛ tsp	ground cumin	0.5 mL
3 cups	ready-to-use beef broth (GF, if needed)	750 mL

1. Place chiles on prepared baking sheet. Brush with canola oil. Roast in preheated oven until soft, about 15 minutes. Split the chiles and discard the seeds. Place in a bowl with enough hot water to cover and let soak for 10 minutes.
2. Drain chiles, transfer to food processor and process until smooth. Add garlic, olive oil, sugar, oregano, salt, pepper and cumin; process for 15 seconds.
3. Transfer mixture to a medium saucepan over medium heat. Add broth and simmer, stirring occasionally, until thickened, for 30 minutes. Let cool.

Health Tip

- If you have a GI condition that is aggravated by hot or spicy foods, omit the dried guajillo chiles and serve hot sauce at the table for others to season to taste.

Nutrients per 1 tbsp (15 mL)	
Calories	15
Fat	1 g
Sodium	61 mg
Carbohydrate	1 g
Fiber	0 g
Protein	0 g
Calcium	3 mg
Magnesium	0 mg
Potassium	14 mg

No-Sugar Ketchup

Use this ketchup when you want to cut calories — most store-bought ketchups are packed with sugar.

Makes 2 cups (500 mL)

Tip

This ketchup keeps well, tightly covered and refrigerated, for up to 1 week.

3 cups	tomato juice	750 mL
1/4 cup	cider vinegar	60 mL
1/4 cup	sugar substitute (such as Splenda)	60 mL
1 1/2 tsp	dried green pepper flakes	7 mL
1/2 tsp	dried onion flakes	2 mL
1/4 tsp	freshly ground black pepper	1 mL
1/8 tsp	dried rosemary	0.5 mL
1/8 tsp	dried thyme	0.5 mL
1/8 tsp	dried basil	0.5 mL
1/8 tsp	dried parsley	0.5 mL

1. In a large saucepan, combine tomato juice, vinegar, sugar substitute, green pepper flakes, onion flakes, black pepper, rosemary, thyme, basil and parsley. Bring to a boil over medium heat. Reduce heat and simmer, stirring occasionally, until thickened, about 1 hour. Let cool.

Health Tip

- To increase the alkalinity of this ketchup recipe, use dried organic sugarcane in place of the sugar substitute.

Nutrients per 1 tbsp (15 mL)	
Calories	5
Fat	0 g
Sodium	16 mg
Carbohydrate	3 g
Fiber	0 g
Protein	0 g
Calcium	3 mg
Magnesium	3 mg
Potassium	45 mg

Avocado Mayonnaise

Here's a no-egg mayonnaise that you can also use as a spread.

Makes 1 cup (250 mL)

Nutrients per 1 tbsp (15 mL)	
Calories	34
Fat	3 g
Sodium	42 mg
Carbohydrate	1 g
Fiber	1 g
Protein	0 g
Calcium	2 mg
Magnesium	4 mg
Potassium	60 mg

- **Food processor**

1	ripe avocado, cut into quarters	1
2 tbsp	freshly squeezed lime juice	30 mL
2 tbsp	fresh cilantro	30 mL
1/4 tsp	sea salt	1 mL
1/4 tsp	freshly ground black pepper	1 mL
2 tbsp	extra virgin olive oil	30 mL

1. In food processor, combine avocado, lime juice, cilantro, salt and pepper; process until smooth.
2. With the motor running, slowly drizzle oil through the small hole in the feed tube until it has been incorporated into mayonnaise. Use within a few hours.

Health Tip

- This is an excellent alkalizing mayonnaise for the everyday.

Big-Batch Marrakech Rub for Chicken, Pork or Lamb

Mix up a batch of this zesty rub and keep it for days when you want to make Roast Lamb with Marrakech Rub (page 279). It's also great for seasoning vegetables for roasting or meats for grilling.

Makes 3/4 cup (175 mL)

Nutrients per 1 tsp (5 mL)	
Calories	6
Fat	0 g
Sodium	2 mg
Carbohydrate	1 g
Fiber	1 g
Protein	0 g
Calcium	11 mg
Magnesium	2 mg
Potassium	26 mg

1/4 cup	paprika	60 mL
2 tbsp	ground coriander	30 mL
2 tbsp	ground cumin	30 mL
2 tbsp	ground cinnamon	30 mL
1 tbsp	cayenne pepper	15 mL
1 tbsp	ground allspice	15 mL
1 tsp	ground ginger	5 mL
1 tsp	ground cloves	5 mL

1. In a small bowl, combine paprika, coriander, cumin, cinnamon, cayenne, allspice, ginger and cloves.
2. Transfer to an airtight container and store in a cool, dark place for up to 6 months.

Soups

Chicken Stock

Homemade stock adds extra goodness to soups, stews and sauces without excess salt or chemical flavor enhancers and preservatives often found in store-bought options.

Makes 8 cups (2 L)

Tip

Add a small amount of salt to help bring out flavors of other ingredients during cooking, but do not add more salt to finished stock since it will be used in many applications and seasoned again later. Here is the opportunity to make a salt-free stock if health concerns dictate.

Variation

Turkey Stock: Replace chicken pieces with turkey and include any giblets (neck, heart, gizzard) that you have saved in the freezer. The liver makes stock bitter. Discard it or save separately for later use.

- **8-quart (8 L) stockpot**
- **Fine sieve, lined with cheesecloth**

2 lbs	whole chicken or chicken pieces	1 kg
2	onions, quartered	2
1	carrot, quartered	1
1	stalk celery, quartered	1
1	leek (white and light green parts only), halved	1
1	tomato, quartered	1
4 quarts	cold water	4 L
1	bay leaf	1
2	sprigs fresh thyme	2
2	sprigs fresh parsley	2
1	sprig fresh rosemary	1
1 tsp	whole black peppercorns	5 mL
1 tsp	kosher salt	5 mL

1. Rinse chicken in cold water. Place in stockpot. Add onions, carrot, celery, leek, tomato and water. Tie bay leaf, thyme, parsley and rosemary in a bundle with kitchen string and add to the pot with peppercorns and salt.
2. Bring to a boil over medium heat. Reduce heat to low and simmer until liquid is flavorful, 3 to 4 hours. Regularly skim off and discard foam and impurities that come to the surface.
3. Remove pot from heat and lift out chicken and vegetables with a slotted spoon. Pour stock into a large bowl through prepared sieve. Discard solids. Let cool.
4. Refrigerate, covered, until cold. Remove fat that congeals on top. Simmer stock to reduce and intensify flavor, if needed. Keep in refrigerator in a covered container for up to 4 days or freeze for up to 3 months.

Health Tip

- This stock — with all of its alkalizing fresh herbs — is a healthier option than ready-made chicken stock.

Nutrients per ½ cup (125 mL)	
Calories	81
Fat	2 g
Sodium	172 mg
Carbohydrate	3 g
Fiber	1 g
Protein	13 g
Calcium	21 mg
Magnesium	17 mg
Potassium	188 mg

Korean Cold Cucumber Soup

Cucumber soup is refreshing on a sultry summer day and helps to stimulate the appetite.

Makes 4 servings

Tip

Toast sesame seeds in a dry pan over medium heat for 3 to 4 minutes until fragrant; remove from pan and let cool.

Variations

For a vegetarian version of this soup, replace fish sauce with a 2-inch (5 cm) square piece of dried kelp.

A few slices of apple or pear can be added to the soup; place them over the radish.

Health Tip

- Use organic dried sugarcane rather than granulated sugar to increase the alkalizing effect of this recipe.

Nutrients per serving	
Calories	45
Fat	1 g
Sodium	2344 mg
Carbohydrate	9 g
Fiber	2 g
Protein	2 g
Calcium	21 mg
Magnesium	24 mg
Potassium	160 mg

5 cups	water	1.25 L
5	slices gingerroot	5
3	sprigs watercress	3
3	green onions (bottom two-thirds only), sliced (or 1 small onion, sliced)	3
1	small apple, sliced	1
4 tsp	fish sauce (or 6 dried anchovies, heads removed)	20 mL
½ tsp	whole black peppercorns	2 mL
2 tsp	rice vinegar or cider vinegar	10 mL
1½ tsp	soy sauce (GF, if needed)	7 mL
¼ tsp	granulated sugar	1 mL
1½ cups	thinly sliced cucumbers	375 mL
1 tsp	salt	5 mL
⅔ cup	thinly sliced daikon radish or red or icicle radish	150 mL
2 tsp	salt	10 mL
¼ tsp	granulated sugar	1 mL
1 tsp	ground dried chile peppers (optional)	5 mL
1½ tbsp	thinly sliced green onions	22 mL
1 tsp	toasted sesame seeds	5 mL

1. In a large saucepan, combine water, ginger, watercress, green onions, apple, fish sauce and peppercorns. Bring to a boil; reduce heat and simmer 20 minutes. Add vinegar, soy sauce and sugar; cook 30 seconds. Strain stock into a large bowl; discard solids. Let stock cool to room temperature; refrigerate.
2. In a bowl, combine cucumbers and 1 tsp (5 mL) salt. In another bowl, combine radish and 2 tsp (10 mL) salt. Set bowls aside for 30 minutes. In a sieve, quickly rinse cucumber under cold running water; drain, squeezing solids hard to remove extra moisture. Refrigerate. Repeat draining procedure with radish; transfer to a bowl and stir in sugar and chiles (if using). Refrigerate for at least 1 hour. Soak green onions in cold water.
3. Mound the cucumber slices in 4 individual soup bowls and top with radish. Carefully ladle stock into bowls without disturbing mounded vegetables; sprinkle with drained green onions and toasted sesame seeds.

Dairy-Free Cream of Celery Soup

The addition of millet is what makes this soup creamy without any cream. These small, golden round seeds are a very important staple to Africans because the millet plant is drought resistant and the grain is high in protein. Although millet is most commonly used in North America as birdseed, it can make a delicious and nutritious addition to soups, croquettes, muesli and puddings.

Makes 6 servings

Tip

Do not use vegetables from the *Brassica* family, such as broccoli or turnips, to make the stock; their flavor is too strong.

Nutrients per serving	
Calories	77
Fat	3 g
Sodium	60 mg
Carbohydrate	12 g
Fiber	2 g
Protein	2 g
Calcium	40 mg
Magnesium	25 mg
Potassium	224 mg

- **Food processor**

Vegetable Stock

	Vegetable trimmings such as parsley stems, carrot ends, celery leaves and leek "beards"	
1	6-inch (15 cm) piece of kombu seaweed	1
2	bay leaves (optional)	2
1	sprig thyme (optional)	1
2	cloves garlic, crushed (optional)	2
1	onion, quartered (optional)	1
10 to 12 cups	water	2.5 to 3 L

Celery Soup

3 cups	sliced celery, cut on a ½-inch (1 cm) bias	750 mL
¼ cup	millet (see tip, page 170)	60 mL
1 tbsp	extra virgin olive oil	15 mL
1 cup	finely chopped onions	250 mL
2 tsp	chopped garlic	10 mL
½ cup	julienned carrots	125 mL
	Salt	
	Chopped fresh parsley	

1. *Stock:* In a saucepan, combine vegetable trimmings, kombu and optional ingredients, if using. Add water or just enough to cover. Bring to a boil and cook for 15 minutes; strain stock through a sieve. (Stock may be used in stews, soups, sauces and vegetable casseroles.)
2. *Soup:* In a large pot with a lid, combine celery and millet with 4½ cups (1.125 L) stock. Cover and bring to a boil. Simmer 20 minutes or until both the celery and millet are cooked.

Variation

Blend in some chopped fresh herbs, such as thyme, to give the soup an additional fresh garden taste, or add a little grated lemon zest or juice.

3. In another pot, heat oil over medium heat; add onions and sauté until softened. Add garlic and carrots; cook until soft. Add about 2 cups (500 mL) more stock; bring to a boil. Reduce heat and simmer.

4. Transfer celery mixture to food processor and purée until very smooth. Pour over sautéed vegetables. Add salt to taste and more stock, if necessary, to achieve desired consistency. Serve garnished with parsley.

This recipe courtesy of Ron Farmer.

Health Tip

- This soup is especially alkalizing because of the kombu seaweed.

Cabbage Borscht

Served with dark rye bread, this hearty soup makes a soul-satisfying meal, particularly in the dark days of winter.

Makes 8 servings

Tip

If you prefer a smoother soup, do not purée the vegetables in step 2. Instead, wait until they have finished cooking, and purée the soup in the stoneware using an immersion blender before adding the vinegar and cabbage. Allow the soup time to reheat (cook on High for 10 or 15 minutes) before adding the cabbage to ensure that it cooks.

- **Blender or food processor**
- **Large (approx. 5-quart) slow cooker**

1 tbsp	olive oil	15 mL
2	onions, finely chopped	2
4	stalks celery, diced	4
2	carrots, diced	2
4	cloves garlic, minced	4
1 tsp	caraway seeds	5 mL
1 tsp	salt	5 mL
$\frac{1}{2}$ tsp	cracked black peppercorns	2 mL
1	can (28 oz/796 mL) tomatoes, with juice, coarsely chopped	1
1 tbsp	packed brown sugar	15 mL
3	beets, peeled and diced	3
1	potato, peeled and diced	1
4 cups	enhanced ready-to-use vegetable broth (see box, opposite)	1 L
1 tbsp	red wine vinegar	15 mL
4 cups	finely shredded cabbage	1 L
	Sour cream (optional)	
	Finely chopped fresh dill	

1. In a skillet, heat oil over medium heat. Add onions, celery and carrots and cook, stirring, until softened, about 7 minutes. Add garlic, caraway seeds, salt and peppercorns and cook, stirring, for 1 minute.
2. Transfer to blender (see tip, at left), add half the tomatoes and process until smooth. Transfer to slow cooker stoneware.
3. Add the remaining tomatoes, brown sugar, beets and potato to stoneware. Add vegetable broth.

Nutrients per serving	
Calories	118
Fat	2 g
Sodium	654 mg
Carbohydrate	23 g
Fiber	6 g
Protein	3 g
Calcium	93 mg
Magnesium	22 mg
Potassium	626 mg

Tip

To make ahead, complete steps 1 and 2. Cover and refrigerate for up to 2 days. When you're ready to cook, complete the recipe.

4. Cover and cook on Low for 6 hours or on High for 3 hours, until vegetables are tender. Add vinegar and cabbage, in batches, stirring until each is submerged. Cover and cook on High for 20 to 30 minutes, until cabbage is tender. To serve, ladle into bowls, add a dollop of sour cream (if using) and garnish with dill.

How to Enhance Prepared Vegetable Broth

To enhance prepared vegetable broth before use, combine it in a large saucepan with 1 carrot, peeled and coarsely chopped, 1 1/2 tsp (7 mL) tomato paste, 1/2 tsp (2 mL) celery seed, 1/2 tsp (2 mL) cracked black peppercorns, 1/4 tsp (1 mL) dried thyme, 2 fresh parsley sprigs, 1 bay leaf and 1/2 cup (125 mL) white wine. Bring to a boil over medium heat. Reduce heat to low, cover and simmer for 30 minutes, then strain and discard solids.

Health Tip

- This recipe contains caraway seeds and may not be suitable for those with some GI conditions.

Leafy Greens Soup

This delicious country-style soup is French in origin and based on the classic combination of leeks and potatoes, with the addition of healthful leafy greens.

Makes 8 servings

Tips

To clean leeks, fill a sink full of lukewarm water. Split the leeks in half lengthwise and submerge them in the water, swishing them around to remove all traces of dirt. Transfer to a colander and rinse thoroughly under cold water.

This soup can be partially prepared before it is cooked. Complete step 1, cover and refrigerate overnight or for up to 2 days. When you're ready to cook, continue with steps 2 and 3.

Health Tip

- The leafy greens in this recipe increase the alkalizing effect of the dish.

Nutrients per serving	
Calories	126
Fat	3 g
Sodium	508 mg
Carbohydrate	23 g
Fiber	3 g
Protein	3 g
Calcium	90 mg
Magnesium	38 mg
Potassium	212 mg

- **Large (approx. 5-quart) slow cooker**
- **Food processor, blender or immersion blender**

1 tbsp	butter or olive oil	15 mL
1 tbsp	olive oil	15 mL
6	small leeks (white and light green parts only), thinly sliced	6
4	cloves garlic, minced	4
1 tsp	sea salt	5 mL
1 tsp	dried tarragon	5 mL
½ tsp	cracked black peppercorns	2 mL
6 cups	ready-to-use vegetable or chicken broth (GF, if needed)	1.5 L
3	potatoes, peeled and cut into ½-inch (1 cm) cubes	3
4 cups	packed torn Swiss chard leaves (about 1 bunch)	1 L
1 cup	packed torn sorrel, arugula or parsley leaves	250 mL
	Heavy or whipping (35%) cream (optional)	
	Garlic-flavored croutons (optional)	

1. In a large skillet over medium heat, melt butter and olive oil. Add leeks and cook, stirring, until softened, about 5 minutes. Add garlic, salt, tarragon and peppercorns and cook, stirring, for 1 minute. Add broth and bring to a boil. Transfer to slow cooker stoneware.
2. Stir in potatoes. Cover and cook on Low for 8 hours or on High for 4 hours, until potatoes are tender. Add Swiss chard and sorrel, in batches, stirring after each to submerge the leaves in the liquid. Cover and cook on High for 20 minutes, until greens are tender.
3. Working in batches, purée soup in food processor. (You can also do this in the stoneware using an immersion blender.) Spoon into individual serving bowls and drizzle with cream and/or top with croutons, if desired.

Health Tip

- Use homemade chicken or vegetable stock instead of the ready-made version to increase the health benefits of this recipe.

Butternut Apple Soup with Swiss Cheese

Topped with melted cheese, this creamy and delicious soup makes a light main course, accompanied by a green salad. It can also be served as a starter to a more substantial meal.

Makes 6 to 8 servings

Tips

To save time, you can use precut squash (often available in the produce section) or frozen diced squash. You will need 2 lbs (1 kg) or 7 cups (1.75 L).

To make ahead, complete step 1. Cover and refrigerate for up to 2 days. When you're ready to cook, complete the recipe.

Health Tip

- Use homemade chicken stock to increase the health benefits of this recipe.

Nutrients per serving (1 of 8)	
Calories	174
Fat	6 g
Sodium	621 mg
Carbohydrate	29 g
Fiber	4 g
Protein	6 g
Calcium	187 mg
Magnesium	59 mg
Potassium	605 mg

- **Medium to large (3½- to 5-quart) slow cooker**
- **Immersion blender, food processor or blender**
- **6 to 8 ovenproof bowls**

1 tbsp	olive oil	15 mL
2	onions, chopped	2
4	cloves garlic, minced	4
2 tsp	dried rosemary, crumbled (or 1 tbsp/15 mL chopped fresh)	10 mL
½ tsp	cracked black peppercorns	2 mL
5 cups	ready-to-use vegetable broth (GF, if needed)	1.25 L
2	tart apples (such as Granny Smith), peeled and coarsely chopped	2
1	butternut squash (about 2½ lbs/1.25 kg), peeled and cut into 1-inch (2.5 cm) cubes	1
	Salt (optional)	
1 cup	shredded Swiss cheese	250 mL
½ cup	finely chopped walnuts (optional)	125 mL

1. In a skillet, heat oil over medium heat. Add onions and cook, stirring, until softened, about 3 minutes. Add garlic, rosemary and peppercorns and cook, stirring, for 1 minute. Transfer to slow cooker stoneware. Stir in broth.
2. Add apples and squash and stir well. Cover and cook on Low for 6 hours or on High for 3 hours, until squash is tender. Preheat broiler.
3. Purée soup using an immersion blender. (You can also do this in batches in a food processor or blender.) Season to taste with salt (if using).
4. Ladle into ovenproof bowls. Sprinkle with cheese and broil until cheese melts, about 2 minutes. (You can also do this in batches in a microwave oven on High, about 1 minute per batch.) Sprinkle with walnuts, if desired. Serve immediately.

Health Tip

- Fresh herbs and the slow-cooking preparation method increase the alkalizing effect of this dish.

Spicy Thai Pumpkin and Coconut Soup

This soup has been freely adapted from a traditional Thai soup made with calabaza (tropical pumpkin).

Makes 4 to 6 servings

Tips

Calabaza is also known as "Jamaican pumpkin" in the Caribbean and "calabash" in the southern U.S. It is usually sold cut into sections at West Indian stores and some grocery chains. Butternut or another type of orange-fleshed squash is also suitable.

Dried shrimp are available at any Chinese or Southeast Asian grocer. Store them in the refrigerator or freezer to maintain their color and freshness.

Nutrients per serving (1 of 6)	
Calories	219
Fat	18 g
Sodium	297 mg
Carbohydrate	14 g
Fiber	3 g
Protein	6 g
Calcium	45 mg
Magnesium	48 mg
Potassium	518 mg

- **Blender or food processor**

4 cups	ready-to-use chicken broth (GF, if needed)	1 L
1 tbsp	chopped fresh galangal (or 3 pieces dried galangal soaked in 1 cup/250 mL water until softened, or 2 tsp/10 mL chopped gingerroot)	15 mL
1 tbsp	vegetable oil	15 mL
2 tsp	dried shrimp, soaked in water to cover for 5 minutes, then drained	10 mL
½ cup	finely chopped red bell peppers	125 mL
2 tbsp	chopped shallots (or ¼ cup/60 mL chopped onions)	30 mL
1 to 4 tsp	chopped fresh red chile peppers	5 to 20 mL
1 tsp	minced garlic	5 mL
2	stalks fresh cilantro (including roots), finely chopped	2
1 tbsp	fish sauce (or 3 anchovies)	15 mL
1 tsp	light brown or granulated sugar	5 mL
½ tsp	freshly ground white pepper	2 mL
2 cups	cubed calabaza or squash (such as butternut)	500 mL
1½ cups	coconut milk	375 mL
1½ tsp	freshly squeezed lime juice	7 mL
	Fresh cilantro leaves	
	Chopped red chile pepper (optional)	

1. In a large saucepan, combine broth and dried galangal with its soaking liquid (if using dried). Bring to a boil; reduce heat to medium and cook until reduced to 3 cups (750 mL). Remove from heat; let cool. Remove galangal and discard.
2. In a nonstick skillet, heat oil over medium-high heat; cook shrimp for a few seconds. Stir in red peppers, shallots, chiles to taste, garlic, cilantro and fresh galangal or ginger (if using); cook until vegetables begin to wilt and color. Add fish sauce, sugar and white pepper; cook for another 30 seconds. Remove from heat; stir in 1 cup (250 mL) broth.

Tip

Adjust the amount of chiles to taste: 1 tsp (5 mL) for a mild soup or up to 4 tsp (20 mL) for a very spicy version. For a more authentic Thai flavor, use red bird's eye chiles — but not more than 2 tsp (10 mL), as they really pack a punch!

3. Transfer mixture to blender and purée until very smooth.
4. Add purée to the remaining broth (use some to rinse out the blender); bring to a boil. Reduce heat to low and add calabaza; simmer, stirring often, until the calabaza falls apart when stirred. Whisk the soup until smooth (or purée in blender). Increase heat to high. When the soup begins to boil, slowly add coconut milk, stirring continuously, until it reaches a full boil. Remove from heat and stir in the lime juice. Serve garnished with cilantro and a little chile pepper, if desired.

Variations

Replace the cilantro garnish with a few leaves of Thai basil and 1 or 2 red bird's eye chiles, quartered lengthwise. Or garnish with julienned Italian basil and a few threads of seeded red chile.

Reserve about one-third of the pumpkin or squash and cut it into attractive bite-size pieces. Cook these first in the chicken broth until tender but not falling apart. Remove them from the broth and put aside. Add them to the soup after the rest of the squash has been puréed; heat through before serving.

Health Tips

- Use homemade chicken stock to increase the health benefits of this recipe.
- Fresh herbs increase the alkalizing effect of this dish.

Fennel-Scented Tomato and Wild Rice Soup

If you get cravings for tomatoes, this soup is for you. The fennel brings intriguing licorice flavor, and the wild rice adds texture, to make this soup particularly enjoyable.

Makes 8 servings

Tip

Toasting fennel seeds intensifies their flavor. To toast, stir seeds in a dry skillet over medium heat until fragrant, about 3 minutes. Immediately transfer to a mortar or spice grinder and grind finely.

Nutrients per serving	
Calories	134
Fat	2 g
Sodium	222 mg
Carbohydrate	26 g
Fiber	5 g
Protein	5 g
Calcium	80 mg
Magnesium	59 mg
Potassium	527 mg

- **Immersion blender, food processor or blender**
- **Medium to large (3½- to 5-quart) slow cooker**

1 tbsp	vegetable oil	15 mL
2	leeks (white and light green parts only), sliced	2
1	bulb fennel, cored and thinly sliced on the vertical	1
3	cloves garlic, sliced	3
1 tsp	fennel seeds, toasted and ground (see tip, at left)	5 mL
½ tsp	salt (optional)	2 mL
½ tsp	freshly ground black pepper	2 mL
1	can (28 oz/796 mL) crushed tomatoes	1
4 cups	ready-to-use vegetable broth (GF, if needed), divided	1 L
¾ cup	wild rice, rinsed and drained	175 mL
	Heavy or whipping (35%) cream or non-dairy alternative (optional)	
	Finely chopped fresh fennel fronds or flat-leaf (Italian) parsley	

1. In a large skillet, heat oil over medium heat. Add leeks and fennel slices and cook, stirring, until softened, about 7 minutes. Add garlic, fennel seeds, salt (if using) and pepper and cook, stirring, for 1 minute. Stir in tomatoes and 2 cups (500 mL) broth. Remove from heat.
2. Purée using an immersion blender. (You can also do this in batches in a food processor or stand blender.) Transfer to slow cooker stoneware.

Tips

For a slightly different tomato flavor, substitute 2 cans (each 14 oz/398 mL) fire-roasted tomatoes, with juice, for the crushed tomatoes.

To make ahead, complete steps 1 and 2. Cover and refrigerate for up to 2 days. When you're ready to cook, complete the recipe.

3. Add the remaining broth and wild rice. Cover and cook on Low for 6 hours or on High for 3 hours, until rice is tender and grains have begun to split.

4. Ladle into bowls, drizzle with cream, if desired, and garnish with fennel fronds.

How to Prepare Bulb Fennel

Before removing the core, chop off the top shoots (which resemble celery) and discard. If desired, save the feathery green fronds to use as a garnish. If the outer sections of the bulb seem old and dry, peel them with a vegetable peeler before using.

Health Tips

- The slow-cooking preparation method increases the alkalizing effect of this dish.
- Choosing a non-dairy alternative will increase the health benefits of this recipe.

Sprouted Lentil and Spinach Soup

Perfectly sprouted lentils are the key to this flavorful soup. You will need to start sprouting them at least 2 days before you want to make the soup.

Makes 4 servings

Tip

To soak the sun-dried tomatoes for this recipe, place in a bowl and add 1 cup (250 mL) water. Cover and set aside for 30 minutes. Drain, discarding any remaining water.

- **Food processor**

½ cup	green lentils, sprouted (see box, opposite)	125 mL
¼ cup	dry-packed sun-dried tomatoes, soaked (see tip, at left)	60 mL
2 cups	baby spinach	500 mL
¼ cup	extra virgin olive oil, divided	60 mL
¼ cup	freshly squeezed lemon juice, divided	60 mL
1 tsp	fine sea salt	5 mL
2 cups	chopped tomatoes	500 mL
1 cup	filtered water	250 mL
1 tsp	wheat-free tamari (GF, if needed)	5 mL
1	clove garlic	1
½ tsp	dried oregano	2 mL
¼ tsp	dried basil	1 mL

1. In a bowl, toss together the spinach, 1 tbsp (15 mL) olive oil, 1 tbsp (15 mL) lemon juice and the salt. Set aside to marinate for 15 to 20 minutes.
2. In food processor, process chopped tomatoes, water, tamari, garlic, oregano, basil, sun-dried tomatoes and the remaining lemon juice and olive oil until smooth and no large pieces remain.
3. Add marinated spinach and sprouted lentils and process for 10 to 15 seconds or until the soup is slightly puréed but still retains some texture. Serve immediately or cover and refrigerate for up to 2 days.

Nutrients per serving	
Calories	230
Fat	14 g
Sodium	881 mg
Carbohydrate	22 g
Fiber	6 g
Protein	7 g
Calcium	37 mg
Magnesium	19 mg
Potassium	544 mg

Variations

You can replace the sprouted lentils with an equal quantity of any sprouted legume, such as chickpeas or mung beans. Follow the same instructions as for sprouting lentils.

If baby spinach is not available, substitute 1½ cups (375 mL) spinach leaves. Mature spinach will create a deeper flavor, which is why you need less. If using mature spinach, make sure to rinse it well, as it generally contains a large amount of grit.

How to Sprout Lentils

To sprout ½ cup (125 mL) green lentils, soak in 2 cups (500 mL) water at room temperature for 24 hours, changing the water every 3 hours. Transfer to a colander and rinse under cold running water. Place the colander over a bowl and set aside in a dry area of your kitchen. Rinse the lentils every 2 to 3 hours to keep them damp but not moist. Before going to bed, rinse the lentils and place a damp cloth overtop. In the morning, rinse again. Repeat this process for 2 days, until tails approximately ¼ inch (0.5 cm) long have sprouted from the lentils. Rinse and drain. The lentils are now ready for use in your recipe, or you can cover them and refrigerate for up to a week.

Health Tip

- If you are increasing the amount of fiber in your diet, begin gradually with small servings of lentils, chickpeas or mung beans.

Minestrone Soup

This recipe is proof that lettuces can be cooked. Savoy cabbage deliciously ups the green content. This makes a big batch — feed your friends or freeze the leftovers.

Makes 8 to 12 servings

Tips

The tender inner stalks of celery are called the celery heart.

Fire-roasted canned tomatoes are sold in well-stocked supermarkets and gourmet food shops. They add a delicious smoky flavor to the minestrone. If you can't find any, use regular canned diced tomatoes and, if desired, a dash of liquid smoke.

Nutrients per serving (1 of 12)	
Calories	141
Fat	5 g
Sodium	625 mg
Carbohydrate	20 g
Fiber	5 g
Protein	5 g
Calcium	64 mg
Magnesium	26 mg
Potassium	328 mg

1/4 cup	extra virgin olive oil	60 mL
1	large onion, diced	1
2	large cloves garlic, chopped	2
4	carrots (8 oz/250 g total), sliced	4
2	stalks celery heart with leaves (see tip, at left)	2
2 oz	savoy cabbage, finely shredded (about 2 cups/500 mL, loosely packed)	60 g
4 oz	green beans, halved (about 1 1/4 cups/300 mL)	125 g
3 oz	small cauliflower florets (about 1 cup/250 mL)	90 g
1/2 cup	thinly sliced fennel	125 mL
2 tsp	kosher salt or coarse sea salt	10 mL
6 cups	ready-to-use vegetable broth (GF, if needed)	1.5 L
4 cups	water	1 L
1	can (14 oz/398 mL) diced fire-roasted tomatoes (see tip, at left)	1
1	can (19 oz/540 mL) romano beans, rinsed and drained	1
1 cup	elbow pasta (GF, if needed)	250 mL
1	zucchini (6 oz/175 g), halved lengthwise and sliced	1
1/4 cup	chopped fresh parsley leaves	60 mL
1 tbsp	chopped fresh oregano leaves	15 mL
1 tbsp	chopped fresh basil leaves	15 mL
1/4 tsp	freshly ground black pepper	1 mL
3	leaves romaine, finely chopped (about 2 cups/500 mL, loosely packed)	3
	Freshly grated Parmesan cheese (optional)	

Tip

If you prefer a thinner soup, add extra vegetable broth, to taste, at the end.

1. In a large pot over medium heat, heat oil until shimmery. Add onion and garlic and cook, stirring often, for about 3 minutes, until softened. Add carrots, celery, cabbage, green beans, cauliflower, fennel and salt. Cook, stirring often, for about 5 minutes, until softened. Add broth, water and tomatoes. When mixture comes to a simmer, cover, reduce heat to low and simmer for 15 to 20 minutes, until vegetables are tender-crisp.
2. Stir in romano beans, pasta, zucchini, parsley, oregano, basil and pepper. Increase heat to medium and return to a simmer. Cover, reduce heat to low and cook for about 15 minutes or until pasta is al dente. Stir in romaine. Season to taste with salt. Ladle into serving bowls. Sprinkle with cheese, if desired. Serve hot.

Health Tip

- Fresh herbs increase the alkalizing effect of this dish.

Turkey and Black Bean Soup

This hearty soup is a meal in a bowl. Serve it with a simple green or shredded carrot salad and crusty whole-grain bread for a great weeknight meal.

Makes 8 servings

Tips

If you don't have ancho chile powder, you can substitute an equal quantity of New Mexico chile powder, your favorite chili powder blend or 1/4 tsp (1 mL) cayenne pepper.

This quantity of ancho chile powder, combined with a chipotle pepper, produces a zesty result. If you're heat-averse, reduce the quantity of chile powder and use a jalapeño instead of a chipotle pepper.

Nutrients per serving	
Calories	231
Fat	5 g
Sodium	364 mg
Carbohydrate	24 g
Fiber	8 g
Protein	25 g
Calcium	101 mg
Magnesium	75 mg
Potassium	983 mg

- **Large (minimum 6-quart) slow cooker**

1 tbsp	olive oil	15 mL
2	onions, finely chopped	2
2	carrots, diced	2
2	stalks celery, diced	2
4	cloves garlic, minced	4
1 tbsp	dried oregano, crumbled	15 mL
1 tsp	cracked black peppercorns	5 mL
1 tsp	finely grated lime zest	5 mL
2 tbsp	cumin seeds, toasted (see box, opposite)	30 mL
1/4 cup	tomato paste	60 mL
6 cups	Chicken or Turkey Stock (page 230) or ready-to-use chicken broth (GF, if needed)	1.5 L
2	cans (14 to 19 oz/398 to 540 mL) black beans, drained and rinsed	2
	Salt (optional)	
2 1/2 cups	cubed boneless skinless turkey breast	625 mL
2 tsp	ancho chile powder, dissolved in 2 tbsp (30 mL) freshly squeezed lime juice	10 mL
1	jalapeño pepper (or chipotle pepper in adobo sauce), minced	1
1	green bell pepper, finely chopped	1
1	red bell pepper, finely chopped	1

1. In a skillet, heat oil over medium heat for 30 seconds. Add onions, carrots and celery and cook, stirring, until softened, about 7 minutes. Add garlic, oregano, peppercorns, lime zest and toasted cumin and cook, stirring, for 1 minute. Add tomato paste and stir well. Transfer to slow cooker stoneware. Stir in stock and beans. Season to taste with salt (if using).

Tips

If you prefer a thicker, more integrated soup, purée the drained beans in a food processor or mash with a potato masher before adding to the stoneware.

You can also make this soup using cooked leftover turkey. Use 2½ cups (625 mL) of shredded turkey and add it along with the bell peppers.

This dish can be partially prepared before it is cooked. Complete step 1. Cover and refrigerate overnight or for up to 2 days. When you're ready to cook, continue with steps 2 and 3.

2. Add turkey and stir well. Cover and cook on Low for 6 hours or on High for 3 hours, until turkey is cooked and mixture is bubbly.
3. Add ancho solution and stir well. Add jalapeño and green and red bell peppers and stir well. Cover and cook on High for 20 minutes, until peppers are tender.

How to Toast Cumin Seeds

To toast cumin seeds, place seeds in a dry skillet over medium heat and cook, stirring, until fragrant and seeds just begin to brown, about 3 minutes. Immediately transfer to a mortar or a spice grinder and grind.

Health Tips

- Use homemade chicken stock to increase the health benefits of this recipe.
- If you have a GI condition that is aggravated by hot or spicy foods, reduce the amount of ancho chile powder in the recipe and serve hot sauce at the table for others to season to taste.

Chickpea Soup

This simple recipe is a great accompaniment to any meal.

Makes 6 to 8 servings

Tip

A 19-oz (540 mL) can of chickpeas will yield about 2 cups (500 mL) once the beans are drained and rinsed. If you have smaller or larger cans, you can use the volume called for or just add the amount from your can.

8	small potatoes, cut into bite-size pieces	8
4 cups	ready-to-use reduced-sodium vegetable or chicken broth (GF, if needed)	1 L
2 cups	rinsed drained canned chickpeas	500 mL
½ tsp	dried rosemary	2 mL

1. In a large pot, combine potatoes, broth, chickpeas, rosemary and 4 cups (1 L) water. Bring to a boil over medium-high heat. Cover, leaving lid ajar, reduce heat to low and simmer, stirring occasionally, for 30 minutes or until potatoes are tender (or for up to 1 hour if you prefer a very soft texture).

Health Tip

- Use homemade vegetable or chicken stock to increase the health benefits of this recipe.

Nutrients per serving (1 of 8)	
Calories	208
Fat	1 g
Sodium	442 mg
Carbohydrate	45 g
Fiber	6 g
Protein	6 g
Calcium	41 mg
Magnesium	57 mg
Potassium	820 mg

Salads

Dandelion Salad with Balsamic Pepper Strawberries

If you haven't tried strawberries with balsamic vinegar and pepper, now's the time. Check out the amazing combination in this simply dressed, bitter/sweet dandelion salad.

Makes 2 to 4 servings

Tips

Sweet onions are mild. The best-known variety is Vidalia. If desired, substitute red onion.

To toast almonds, cook them in a dry skillet over medium heat, stirring often, for 2 to 3 minutes, until golden and aromatic.

1	bunch dandelion greens (10 to 12 oz/ 300 to 375 g), trimmed and coarsely chopped (about 5 cups/1.25 L)	1
1 cup	thinly sliced sweet onion	250 mL
2 tsp	freshly squeezed lemon juice	10 mL
2 tbsp	extra virgin olive oil	30 mL
1/2 tsp	kosher salt or coarse sea salt	2 mL
	Freshly ground black pepper	
1 lb	ripe strawberries, quartered	500 g
1 tbsp	balsamic vinegar	15 mL
1 tsp	granulated sugar	5 mL
1/4 cup	slivered almonds, toasted (see tip, at left)	60 mL

1. In a large bowl, toss dandelion leaves and onion with lemon juice. Add oil and toss again to coat. Season to taste with salt and pepper. Divide greens equally among serving dishes.
2. In a small bowl, toss strawberries with vinegar, sugar, salt and pepper to taste. Spoon over greens. Scatter almonds overtop and serve immediately.

Variation

Dandelion Salad with Roasted Strawberries: Replace the fresh berries with roasted berries, which have a concentrated flavor and creamy texture. To roast them, halve the berries and transfer to a baking sheet. Add 2 tsp (10 mL) extra virgin olive oil, 1 tsp (5 mL) granulated sugar and salt and pepper to taste. Combine with a spatula. Arrange berries cut side down. Roast in a preheated 400°F (200°C) oven for 5 to 8 minutes, until caramelized but still holding their shape. Spoon over greens in step 2.

Health Tip

- Substitute the granulated sugar for dried organic sugarcane to increase the health benefits of this recipe.

Nutrients per serving (1 of 4)	
Calories	186
Fat	11 g
Sodium	407 mg
Carbohydrate	21 g
Fiber	6 g
Protein	4 g
Calcium	176 mg
Magnesium	62 mg
Potassium	552 mg

Nice 'n' Nutty Slaw

Used instead of the usual creamy coleslaw dressing, this oil-and-vinegar version allows you to marinate the slaw for several hours. It is a colorful addition to potlucks or picnics. Feel free to experiment with your own combination of shredded vegetables.

Makes 8 servings

Tips

Fennel is a slightly sweet licorice-flavored vegetable with the crunch of celery. If you have difficulty finding it in your local supermarket, look in an Italian fruit and vegetable store.

Experiment with other cabbages, such as napa and Chinese cabbage.

Salad can be prepared through step 2, covered and stored in the refrigerator for up to 1 day. Dressing can be stored in an airtight container in the refrigerator for up to 2 weeks.

Variation

Substitute an equal amount of bok choy for the fennel. It adds a wonderful crunch!

Nutrients per serving	
Calories	179
Fat	13 g
Sodium	175 mg
Carbohydrate	14 g
Fiber	4 g
Protein	4 g
Calcium	87 mg
Magnesium	37 mg
Potassium	270 mg

- **Preheat oven to 350°F (180°C)**
- **Baking sheet**

1/2 cup	sliced unblanched almonds	125 mL
1/4 cup	sesame seeds	60 mL
3	green onions, sliced	3
3 cups	shredded red cabbage	750 mL
3 cups	shredded green cabbage	750 mL
2 cups	alfalfa sprouts or sunflower sprouts	500 mL
1 cup	sliced fennel or celery	250 mL
1/2 cup	chopped fresh parsley	125 mL
1	apple, sliced	1

Poppy Seed Dressing

1/4 cup	white wine vinegar or freshly squeezed lemon juice	60 mL
2 tbsp	chopped onion	30 mL
2 tbsp	granulated sugar	30 mL
1 tbsp	poppy seeds	15 mL
1/2 tsp	salt	2 mL
1/4 tsp	freshly ground black pepper	1 mL
1/4 cup	vegetable oil	60 mL

1. Spread almonds and sesame seeds on baking sheet. Bake in preheated oven for 10 to 12 minutes or until golden brown. Let cool.
2. In a large bowl, combine onions, red and green cabbage, sprouts, fennel and parsley.
3. *Dressing:* In a small bowl, whisk together vinegar, onion, sugar, poppy seeds, salt and pepper. Whisk in oil.
4. Up to 4 hours before serving, toss almonds, sesame seeds and apples with cabbage mixture; toss with dressing until well mixed. (Longer marinating will cause apples to brown and almonds to become soggy.)

Health Tips

- Substitute the granulated sugar for dried organic sugarcane to increase the health benefits of this recipe.
- This recipe contains poppy and sesame seeds and may not be suitable for those with some GI conditions.

Sunny Lettuce and Avocado Salad

Butter lettuce is paired with avocado and a sun-dried tomato dressing in this pretty salad. Add crusty bread and you have a light meal.

Makes 2 to 4 servings

Tips

To dice avocados, slice each avocado in half lengthwise and discard pit. Using a paring knife, cut a crosshatch pattern in each half, all the way to the skin, then scoop out the pieces with a spoon.

Toast green pumpkin seeds in a dry skillet over medium heat for 2 to 3 minutes, stirring often, until they are turning golden and start to pop.

Variation

Don't waste the radish leaves. If desired, sprinkle some finely chopped leaves over the lettuce at the end of step 2.

Nutrients per serving (1 of 4)	
Calories	243
Fat	22 g
Sodium	171 mg
Carbohydrate	13 g
Fiber	7 g
Protein	3 g
Calcium	15 mg
Magnesium	50 mg
Potassium	526 mg

1	large head butter lettuce (6 oz/175 g), cored and leaves separated	1
2	small avocados, diced (see tip, at left)	2
½ cup	Sun-Dried Tomato Vinaigrette (page 268)	125 mL
2 tbsp	green pumpkin seeds (pepitas), toasted (see tip, at left)	30 mL
4	small red radishes, sliced	4

1. Line serving plates with lettuce leaves. Set aside.
2. In a bowl, gently toss avocado with vinaigrette to taste (you will have some left over). Spoon avocado onto lettuce, dividing equally. Scatter with pepitas. Arrange radishes in overlapping slices alongside avocado. Serve immediately.

Health Tip

- Pumpkin seeds (pepitas) increase the alkalizing effect of this recipe.

Warm Sweet-and-Sour Beet Salad

Beets are a super food with many health benefits. Enjoy this unusual salad!

Makes 4 to 6 servings

Tips

This salad can also be served cold the next day.

Remember to peel nonorganic fruits and vegetables.

Variation

Substitute 4 cups (1 L) washed torn spinach for the beet tops.

Nutrients per serving (1 of 6)	
Calories	131
Fat	5 g
Sodium	125 mg
Carbohydrate	23 g
Fiber	4 g
Protein	1 g
Calcium	22 mg
Magnesium	20 mg
Potassium	350 mg

4	beets, including greens	4
2 tbsp	olive oil	30 mL
1	red onion, quartered	1
½ cup	ready-to-use vegetable broth (GF, if needed)	125 mL
½ cup	apple juice or apple cider	125 mL
2	green apples, cored and quartered	2
10 to 12	dried apricots, quartered	10 to 12
2 tbsp	raspberry vinegar or red wine vinegar	30 mL

1. Cut greens off beets; wash thoroughly. Chop stems and shred tender leaves; set aside. Trim root and coarse skin off beets; cut into wedges.
2. In a Dutch oven or roasting pan with lid, heat oil over medium heat. Add onion and cook for 5 minutes or until tender. Add beets, broth and apple juice. Bring to a boil; cover, reduce heat and simmer for about 20 minutes.
3. Stir in apples, cover and cook, stirring occasionally, for 6 minutes or until beets are tender. Stir in apricots, vinegar and beet stems and tops. Increase heat to medium-high; cook, stirring, for 10 minutes or until liquid evaporates and vegetables are coated with sauce. Season to taste with salt and pepper, if desired. Serve warm.

Health Tips

- Beets are a great addition to any recipe because they increase the alkalizing effect — and in this salad, the healthy beet greens are included too. This salad makes a fantastic partner to a more acidifying recipe, to balance the pH.
- If you have a GI condition that is aggravated by insoluble fiber, peel the apple before adding it to the salad.

Salad of Warm Wild Mushrooms

In North America, the term "mesclun" is applied to any mixture of tender young lettuces, herbs and other greens. Some mesclun mixtures also include edible flowers.

Makes 4 servings

Tips

Use this dish as a dramatic first course at a dinner party or as a light lunch after foraging for wild greens. Either way, your taste buds will dance with pleasure.

Omit the nasturtium and chive flowers if not available.

Shiitake, maitake or button mushrooms can also be used in place of the wild mushrooms. Spinach or lettuce can be substituted for the mesclun.

Nutrients per serving	
Calories	254
Fat	20 g
Sodium	115 mg
Carbohydrate	12 g
Fiber	1 g
Protein	8 g
Calcium	211 mg
Magnesium	50 mg
Potassium	413 mg

- **Preheat oven to 375°F (190°C)**
- **Baking sheet, lightly oiled**

¼ cup	olive oil	60 mL
2 tbsp	chopped fresh chives	5 mL
1	large clove garlic, chopped	1
8 oz	wild mushrooms, such as chanterelles, cèpes or oyster mushrooms, sliced	250 g
4 oz	soft goat cheese, cut into 4 rounds	125 g
4 cups	mesclun or French sorrel	1 L
2 tbsp	chopped fresh hyssop or sage	30 mL
2 tbsp	fresh tarragon	30 mL
2 tbsp	fresh chervil	30 mL
½ cup	fresh nasturtium flowers	125 mL
2 tbsp	fresh chive flowers	30 mL
2 tbsp	balsamic vinegar	30 mL

1. In a skillet over medium heat, heat 2 tbsp (30 mL) oil. Add chives and garlic; cook for 1 to 2 minutes. Add mushrooms and sauté for 1 minute or until barely tender. Season to taste with salt and pepper. Using a slotted spoon, lift mushrooms out of pan onto prepared baking sheet, dividing into 4 portions. Place goat cheese in center of each portion. Bake in preheated oven for about 4 minutes, allowing cheese to melt but not brown.
2. Meanwhile, wash and dry mesclun, hyssop, tarragon and chervil. Place in a medium bowl and toss with nasturtium and chive flowers. Divide into 4 portions and arrange on plates.
3. Add the remaining oil to skillet over medium heat. Stir to collect pan juices and bits. Add vinegar; simmer until slightly reduced.
4. Spoon hot mushrooms and their juices over mesclun mixture; drizzle with hot oil and vinegar. Serve immediately.

Health Tip

- The mushroom and fresh herb combination makes this a great alkalizing salad.

Garden Pea, Butter Lettuce and Radish Salad

Shaved radishes and their greens add a bit of bite and a dash of color to this refined salad with a citrusy herb dressing.

Makes 2 to 4 servings

Tips

You'll need about 6 oz (175 g) green peas in the pod for 1 cup (250 mL) shelled. If the peas are not young and tender, cook them in a saucepan of boiling salted water for 3 to 4 minutes. Drain well and cool to room temperature before using. Fresh peas are seasonal, but you can turn this into a year-round salad by substituting thawed frozen peas. In a large, microwave-safe bowl, heat peas on High for about 1 minute, until warm and tender, then drain and cool to room temperature.

If you have one, use a mandoline to shave the radishes very thinly.

Nutrients per serving (1 of 4)	
Calories	130
Fat	11 g
Sodium	114 mg
Carbohydrate	6 g
Fiber	2 g
Protein	2 g
Calcium	15 mg
Magnesium	12 mg
Potassium	74 mg

1	medium-large head butter lettuce, cored and torn into bite-size pieces (about 6 cups/1.5 L, loosely packed)	1
½ cup	Lime Herb Dressing (page 269)	125 mL
1 cup	shelled tender green peas (see tip, at left)	250 mL
4	green onions (white and light green parts), cut diagonally into ½-inch (1 cm) pieces	4
2	red radishes, thinly sliced (see tip, at left)	2
¼ cup	loosely packed chopped radish greens	60 mL

1. In a bowl, toss lettuce with dressing to taste (you will have some left over).
2. Transfer prepared lettuce to a serving platter. Scatter peas, green onions, radishes and radish greens overtop. Serve immediately.

Salad of Fresh Spring Greens, New Potatoes and Asparagus

This beautiful salad is a true celebration of spring or summer.

Makes 6 servings

Tips

This salad is wonderful as a bed for grilled salmon. Sprinkle it with herbs and serve with lemon wedges.

For the best taste and freshness, choose asparagus with a bright green stalk and tightly closed, purple-tinged tips.

Choose fiddleheads that are tightly closed and bright green in color. Rinse them in several changes of water to remove any debris, then trim the root ends.

Instead of the field greens, try shredded kale, napa cabbage or Chinese cabbage.

12	small new potatoes, scrubbed	12
1 lb	asparagus, tough ends removed	500 g
8 oz	fiddleheads	125 g
16 cups	assorted field greens (beet greens, watercress, Boston, leaf, romaine, arugula)	4 L
2	large hothouse tomatoes, cut into wedges	2

Herbal Vinaigrette

1	clove garlic, minced	1
1/4 cup	white wine vinegar	60 mL
1/4 cup	water	60 mL
1/4 cup	vegetable oil	60 mL
1/4 cup	extra virgin olive oil	60 mL
2 tsp	chopped fresh tarragon, thyme or rosemary	10 mL
2 tsp	Dijon mustard	10 mL
1 tsp	salt	5 mL
1 tsp	granulated sugar	5 mL
1/4 tsp	freshly ground black pepper	1 mL

1. In a steamer over simmering water, steam potatoes until tender, about 15 minutes. Drain well.
2. Meanwhile, in a large pot of boiling water, cook asparagus and fiddleheads for 2 to 3 minutes or until tender-crisp. Drain and refresh under cold water. Cut asparagus into 2-inch (5 cm) pieces.
3. *Vinaigrette:* In a small bowl, whisk together garlic, vinegar, water, vegetable oil, olive oil, tarragon, mustard, salt, sugar and pepper until smooth.
4. In a large bowl, toss together greens, potatoes, asparagus and fiddleheads with enough dressing to coat. Arrange on a platter or individual plates. Garnish with tomato wedges.

Health Tip

- This super alkalizing salad will rebalance your pH after acid-heavy meals.

Nutrients per serving	
Calories	362
Fat	17 g
Sodium	507 mg
Carbohydrate	47 g
Fiber	6 g
Protein	9 g
Calcium	176 mg
Magnesium	81 mg
Potassium	1877 mg

Hot Sweet Potato Salad

Adding cloves and nutmeg to this healthy casserole will fill your home with a warm, welcoming fragrance.

Makes 4 to 6 servings

Variations

Substitute white potatoes for the sweet potatoes.

Add 1 cup (250 mL) cubed rutabaga with the sweet potatoes.

- **Preheat oven to 375°F (190°C)**
- **9-inch (23 cm) casserole dish, lightly oiled**

3	large sweet potatoes, cut into large chunks	3
3 tbsp	olive oil	45 mL
1	leek (white and light green parts only), sliced	1
1	onion, chopped	1
1 cup	ready-to-use vegetable broth (GF, if needed)	250 mL
$\frac{1}{4}$ tsp	ground cloves	1 mL
$\frac{1}{4}$ tsp	ground nutmeg	1 mL

1. In a large saucepan, cover sweet potatoes with water. Bring to a boil, reduce heat and simmer for 20 minutes or until just tender. Drain.
2. In a large skillet, heat oil over medium heat. Add leek and onion; sauté until soft. Stir in stock; bring to a boil and cook, stirring occasionally, for 1 minute or until stock is thick and slightly reduced.
3. In prepared casserole dish, toss potatoes with onion mixture, cloves and nutmeg. If desired, season to taste with salt and pepper. Cover and bake in preheated oven for 30 to 40 minutes.

Health Tip

- Use homemade stock rather than a ready-to-use version to increase the health benefits of this recipe.

Nutrients per serving (1 of 6)	
Calories	135
Fat	7 g
Sodium	63 mg
Carbohydrate	17 g
Fiber	3 g
Protein	1 g
Calcium	37 mg
Magnesium	23 mg
Potassium	274 mg

Sesame Noodle Salad

This is a great salad to serve a crowd, especially with food from the grill marinated in Asian flavors.

Makes 6 to 8 servings

Tip

To string edible-pod peas, use a sharp paring knife to cut across the stem end of the peas toward the inside edge and pull away the thin cellulose string that holds the two sides of the pod together.

7 oz	rice vermicelli noodles	210 g
1/2	red bell pepper	1/2
1/2	green bell pepper	1/2
2 oz	snow peas, trimmed (see tip, at left)	60 g
1	stalk celery	1
2	green onions	2
1 cup	bean sprouts	250 mL
1 to 1 1/4 cups	Sesame Ginger Dressing and Dip (see recipe, opposite)	250 to 300 mL

1. Blanch rice vermicelli in a large pot of boiling water for 1 minute, or prepare noodles according to package instructions. Drain and rinse under cold water. Set aside.
2. Cut red and green bell peppers into julienne. Cut snow peas, celery and green onions into fine slivers on the diagonal.
3. In a large bowl, combine noodles, bell peppers, snow peas, celery, green onions and beans sprouts and toss with dressing.

Nutrients per serving (1 of 8)	
Calories	215
Fat	9 g
Sodium	240 mg
Carbohydrate	30 g
Fiber	1 g
Protein	3 g
Calcium	31 mg
Magnesium	17 mg
Potassium	153 mg

Sesame Ginger Dressing and Dip

Mirin, a sweetened rice wine, adds kick to this chock-full-of-flavor dressing.

Makes 1¾ cups (425 mL)

Tips

If you don't have a food processor or blender, a mortar and pestle does a great job. Grind the chopped and dry ingredients (garlic, gingerroot, sugar, etc.) together first. Stir in the liquid flavoring ingredients, then whisk in the oil until sauce is smooth and the desired consistency.

Tahini, a creamy paste made from ground sesame seeds, is used in many Middle Eastern sauces and dressings to drizzle over legumes, vegetables and salads, and in popular dips such as hummus and baba ghanoush. It is readily available in jars at supermarkets.

Nutrients per 1 tbsp (15 mL)	
Calories	53
Fat	4 g
Sodium	109 mg
Carbohydrate	3 g
Fiber	0 g
Protein	1 g
Calcium	5 mg
Magnesium	3 mg
Potassium	22 mg

- **Food processor or blender**

⅓ cup	tahini	75 mL
¼ cup	soy sauce (GF, if needed)	60 mL
3 tbsp	sweet chili sauce	45 mL
3 tbsp	mirin	45 mL
2 tbsp	packed brown sugar or palm sugar	30 mL
1 tbsp	chopped gingerroot	15 mL
2 tsp	chopped garlic	10 mL
½ tsp	sambal oelek	2 mL
⅓ cup	vegetable oil	75 mL

1. In food processor, combine tahini, soy sauce, chili sauce, mirin, brown sugar, ginger, garlic and sambal oelek. With motor running, slowly drizzle in oil through the feed tube. Add about ¼ cup (60 mL) water. Add more water, 1 tbsp (15 mL) at a time, to make sauce a thick, creamy consistency.

Variation

Peanut Sauce: Replace tahini with natural unsweetened peanut butter to make an irresistible sauce to accompany salad rolls or anything that needs a peanut dip.

Health Tip

- Mirin is a type of Japanese rice wine. If you are sensitive to alcohol or allergic to fermented foods, omit it from the recipe.

Quinoa Salad

This simple, delicious salad packs a nutritional punch. Thanks to the quinoa, it even provides a complete protein, so it's a great choice for vegetarians. Whether it serves 2 or 4 depends on how much you're willing to share!

Makes 2 to 4 servings

Variation

If you're making this salad for non-vegetarians, you can substitute ready-to-use reduced-sodium chicken or turkey broth for the vegetable broth.

1¼ cups	ready-to-use reduced-sodium vegetable broth (GF, if needed)	300 mL
¾ cup	quinoa, rinsed	175 mL
½ cup	thawed frozen peas	125 mL
¼ cup	finely chopped orange bell pepper	60 mL
¼ cup	finely chopped yellow bell pepper	60 mL
1 tbsp	finely chopped red onion	15 mL
2 tbsp	extra virgin olive oil	30 mL
1 tbsp	chopped fresh parsley	15 mL
1 tsp	dried thyme	5 mL
1 tsp	freshly squeezed lemon juice	5 mL
	Salt and freshly ground black pepper	

1. In a saucepan, bring broth to a boil over high heat. Add quinoa, reduce heat to low, cover and simmer for 20 minutes or until quinoa is tender and liquid is almost absorbed. Remove from heat and let stand, covered, for 5 minutes or until liquid is absorbed.
2. In a large bowl, combine quinoa, peas, orange pepper, yellow pepper and red onion.
3. In a small bowl, whisk together oil, parsley, thyme and lemon juice. Drizzle over salad and toss to coat. Season to taste with salt and pepper. Serve warm or cover and refrigerate for 1 hour, until chilled, and serve cold.

Nutrients per serving (1 of 4)	
Calories	201
Fat	9 g
Sodium	315 mg
Carbohydrate	25 g
Fiber	4 g
Protein	6 g
Calcium	27 mg
Magnesium	71 mg
Potassium	256 mg

Fast Egg Salad

Dilweed adds extra flavor to this family standard. You can serve this salad on toasted bread or on a bed of greens.

Makes 4 servings

8	hard-cooked eggs, chopped	8
1/2	red onion, minced	1/2
1/4 cup	mayonnaise	60 mL
2 tbsp	Dijon mustard	30 mL
1 tsp	dried dillweed	5 mL
1 tsp	Hungarian paprika	5 mL
1/2 tsp	sea salt	2 mL
1/2 tsp	freshly ground black pepper	2 mL

1. In a bowl, using a fork, stir together eggs, onion, mayonnaise, mustard, dill, paprika, salt and pepper until blended. Use immediately or cover and refrigerate for up to 3 days.

Health Tip

- If you have a GI condition that is aggravated by hot or spicy foods, reduce the amount of paprika in this recipe.

Nutrients per serving	
Calories	220
Fat	16 g
Sodium	757 mg
Carbohydrate	6 g
Fiber	1 g
Protein	13 g
Calcium	61 mg
Magnesium	14 mg
Potassium	177 mg

Salmon and Wild Rice Salad

Try this salad throughout the seasons, varying the vegetables with the freshest ones available. When you accompany this with good bread and a green salad in spring or summer or a hearty soup in fall or winter, you have a satisfying meal.

Makes 6 servings

Tips

Canned salmon with the bones is an excellent source of calcium and vitamin D, essential for the absorption of calcium. Be sure to mash the bones and add them to the salad for added calcium.

Cover and store in the refrigerator for up to 1 day.

Nutrients per serving	
Calories	540
Fat	25 g
Sodium	1060 mg
Carbohydrate	54 g
Fiber	5 g
Protein	27 g
Calcium	235 mg
Magnesium	105 mg
Potassium	803 mg

1 cup	wild rice	250 mL
5 cups	water, divided	1.25 L
1½ tsp	salt, divided	7 mL
2	bay leaves	2
1 cup	long-grain parboiled rice	250 mL
1 lb	broccoli florets	500 g
2	cans (each 6 oz/170 g) sockeye salmon	2
8 oz	whole mushrooms	250 g
½ cup	chopped fresh parsley	125 mL
4	green onions, chopped	4
½	red bell pepper, chopped	½

Dressing

1	clove garlic, minced	1
½ cup	vegetable oil	125 mL
¼ cup	red wine vinegar	60 mL
1 tbsp	granulated sugar	15 mL
½ tsp	salt	2 mL
¼ tsp	freshly ground black pepper	1 mL

1. Rinse wild rice and cover with cold water. Let soak for 30 minutes. Drain.
2. In a large saucepan, combine 3 cups (750 mL) water, 1 tsp (5 mL) salt and 1 bay leaf; bring to a boil over high heat. Stir in wild rice; bring back to boil. Reduce heat to medium and cook, covered, until tender, about 25 minutes. Drain and let cool. Discard bay leaf.
3. In a medium saucepan, bring the remaining water, the remaining salt and the remaining bay leaf to a boil over high heat. Add parboiled rice; reduce heat to medium and simmer, covered, for 15 minutes. Remove from heat and let stand, covered, for 5 minutes or until all liquid is absorbed. Let cool. Discard bay leaf.

Variation

Peas, asparagus spears, green beans, fiddleheads or sliced zucchini may be substituted for the broccoli florets. To prepare asparagus, break off tough root end. Slice zucchini; leave green beans whole but cut off ends. Fiddleheads are the tightly coiled emerging fronds of the ostrich fern. They need to be rinsed in several changes of water to remove any debris. Trim root end. All green vegetables should be cooked uncovered to maintain their bright green color.

4. Meanwhile, in a large pot of rapidly boiling salted water, cook broccoli, uncovered, until tender-crisp, about 2 to 3 minutes. Drain and refresh under cold water.

5. Drain salmon; discard skin and mash bones. In a large bowl, combine cooled wild and parboiled rice, broccoli, salmon with mashed bones, mushrooms, parsley, green onions and red pepper.

6. *Dressing:* In a small bowl, whisk together garlic, oil, vinegar, sugar, salt and pepper. Pour over salad and toss gently.

Health Tips

- Replace the long-grain rice with brown rice to increase the alkalizing effect of this recipe.
- Wild rice is a highly alkalizing food.

Tuna Avocado Salad

A great lunchbox idea, this salad can be served on its own over a green salad or stuffed into a pita or tortilla for a delicious healthy sandwich.

Makes 4 servings

Tip

This recipe makes enough salad to serve as a side dish for 4 or as lunch for 2. For a stylish presentation for 2, reserve the hollowed-out avocado skins to use as serving dishes and top each serving with a sprig of fresh parsley.

1	can (6 oz/170 g) water-packed tuna, drained	1
1	avocado, cut into bite-size pieces	1
1	small tomato, diced	1
1/2	small red onion, finely chopped	1/2
1/4 cup	frozen corn kernels, thawed	60 mL
2 tbsp	chopped fresh parsley	30 mL
2 tbsp	olive oil	30 mL
1 tsp	freshly squeezed lemon juice	5 mL
	Freshly ground black pepper (optional)	
	Hot pepper sauce (optional)	

1. In a small bowl, combine tuna, avocado, tomato, red onion, corn, parsley, olive oil, lemon juice, pepper (if using) and hot pepper sauce (if using).

This recipe courtesy of Cindy McKenna.

How to Prepare an Avocado

First cut around the avocado lengthwise, cutting through to the pit. Twist one half to separate the avocado into two halves. To easily pop out the pit, use a sharp knife to pierce the pit; turn the knife and twist. Cut avocado flesh inside the skin in a crisscross pattern; remove avocado pieces with a large spoon. Avocados brown easily, so once cut, dip the pieces in lemon juice.

Health Tips

- If you have a GI condition that is aggravated by hot or spicy foods, omit the optional hot pepper sauce and serve it at the table for others to season to taste instead.
- Fresh herbs increase the alkalizing effect of this recipe.

Nutrients per serving	
Calories	220
Fat	15 g
Sodium	30 mg
Carbohydrate	8 g
Fiber	4 g
Protein	13 g
Calcium	19 mg
Magnesium	33 mg
Potassium	450 mg

Salad of Chicken and Peaches on Seedlings with Grilled Pepper Dressing

For an unequaled taste experience, try this satisfying chicken salad.

Makes 4 servings

Variation

The chicken and peaches can also be grilled. Place them on bamboo skewers (that have been soaked in water for 30 minutes) so they won't fall through the cracks.

Health Tip

- This recipe contains optional toasted pine nuts and may not be suitable for those with some GI conditions.

Nutrients per serving	
Calories	624
Fat	48 g
Sodium	171 mg
Carbohydrate	22 g
Fiber	5 g
Protein	29 g
Calcium	45 mg
Magnesium	73 mg
Potassium	955 mg

1 lb	boneless chicken, cut into 1-inch (2.5 cm) pieces	500 g
1/4 cup	chopped fresh lemon basil	60 mL
1/4 cup	julienned wild leeks	60 mL
1	small red onion, chopped	1
1 tbsp	black peppercorns, crushed	15 mL
1/2 cup	virgin olive oil	125 mL
2	firm peaches, pitted and cut into 1/4-inch (0.5 cm) thick slices (or 2 cups/500 mL frozen peach slices)	2
3	red bell peppers, grilled, peeled and seeded	3
2 tbsp	finely minced shallots	30 mL
2 tbsp	balsamic vinegar	30 mL
1 tsp	Dijon mustard	5 mL
3 tbsp	virgin olive oil	45 mL
	Salt and freshly ground white pepper	
2 oz	mixed seedlings (sunflower, radish or corn)	60 g
	Toasted pine nuts (optional)	

1. In a bowl, toss together the chicken, lemon basil, leeks, red onion, peppercorns and olive oil; marinate, covered, in refrigerator for at least 2 hours. Add peach slices and marinate another 30 minutes.
2. In food processor, purée red peppers with shallots, balsamic vinegar and mustard. Whisk in olive oil to emulsify. Season to taste with salt and pepper. Pour dressing on the bottom of a serving plate; top with seedlings.
3. Sauté chicken and peaches over high heat until chicken is lightly browned and just cooked. Place on top of seedlings and serve immediately. Garnish with pine nuts sprinkled around the salad, if desired.

This recipe courtesy of Kenneth Peace.

Chinese Chicken Salad

Serve this homemade version of takeout Chinese salad for lunch or dinner. The dressing also makes an easy marinade for pork or chicken.

Makes 4 servings

Tip

Make the dressing 2 to 3 days ahead to let the flavors develop, then cover and refrigerate it. So they don't get soggy, add the almonds just before serving the salad.

Variation

Try using fresh spinach leaves instead of salad greens for a heartier meal.

4 cups	salad greens	1 L
1 lb	cooked chicken pieces	500 g
1/4 cup	cider vinegar	60 mL
2 tbsp	freshly squeezed orange juice	30 mL
2 tbsp	granulated sugar	30 mL
1 tsp	Dijon mustard	5 mL
1 tsp	sea salt	5 mL
1/2 cup	canola oil	125 mL
2 tbsp	poppy seeds	30 mL
2 tbsp	sliced almonds, toasted	30 mL

1. Place 1 cup (250 mL) of greens on each plate. Top with chicken pieces. Set aside.
2. In a bowl, whisk together vinegar, orange juice, sugar, mustard and salt. While whisking, pour in oil in a thin, steady stream until emulsified. Stir in poppy seeds and almonds. Drizzle on salad.

Health Tips

- Some brands of Dijon mustard have sulfites, such as sodium metabisulfite, added as a preservative. If you are sensitive to sulfites, this could exacerbate some gastrointestinal conditions, so look for a brand that is sulfite-free.

Nutrients per serving	
Calories	516
Fat	35 g
Sodium	836 mg
Carbohydrate	12 g
Fiber	3 g
Protein	37 g
Calcium	87 mg
Magnesium	57 mg
Potassium	367 mg

Apple Cider Vinaigrette

This vinaigrette can be served warm. Simply microwave the dressing for 15 seconds and it's perfect for a wilted spinach salad.

Makes about 1 cup (250 mL)

Tip

You should take about 45 seconds to incorporate the oil to ensure it gets emulsified with the other ingredients. If you pour too fast, it will float on top.

2 tbsp	balsamic vinegar	30 mL
2 tbsp	apple cider vinegar	30 mL
1 tbsp	liquid honey	15 mL
1/2 tsp	sea salt	2 mL
3/4 cup	vegetable or peanut oil	175 mL

1. In a bowl, whisk together balsamic and cider vinegars, honey and salt.
2. While whisking, pour in oil in a thin, steady stream until emulsified.

Nutrients per 1 tbsp (15 mL)	
Calories	93
Fat	10 g
Sodium	83 mg
Carbohydrate	1 g
Fiber	0 g
Protein	0 g
Calcium	1 mg
Magnesium	0 mg
Potassium	3 mg

Sun-Dried Tomato Vinaigrette

Sun-dried tomatoes give this dressing added oomph. It's great with assertive greens.

Makes about ½ cup (125 mL)

Tips

For the finest minced garlic, push it through a press.

Kosher salt tastes better than iodized table salt and (ideally) contains no additives.

You can whisk vinaigrettes in a small bowl, but a medium bowl is a better choice. It gives you more room to whisk vigorously without accidental spatter.

2 tbsp	white wine vinegar, divided	30 mL
2	oil-packed sun-dried tomatoes, drained and finely chopped	2
1	large clove garlic, minced	1
½ tsp	granulated sugar	2 mL
1 tsp	kosher or coarse sea salt	5 mL
⅛ tsp	freshly ground black pepper	0.5 mL
¼ cup	extra virgin olive oil	60 mL

1. In a bowl, whisk together 1½ tbsp (22 mL) vinegar, tomatoes, garlic, sugar, salt and pepper. Gradually whisk in oil. Add some or all of the remaining vinegar, if desired.
2. Transfer to an airtight container and refrigerate for up to 2 weeks.

Variation

Replace some of the olive oil with the oil from the sun-dried tomatoes.

Health Tip

- Sun-dried tomatoes tend to be highly salted, so be cautious about your overall sodium intake on the day you enjoy this dressing. You may want to avoid adding salt to your food that day.

Nutrients per 1 tbsp (15 mL)	
Calories	63
Fat	7 g
Sodium	251 mg
Carbohydrate	1 g
Fiber	0 g
Protein	0 g
Calcium	1 mg
Magnesium	1 mg
Potassium	19 mg

Lime Herb Dressing

Bursting with tart lime and fresh herbs, this dressing gives all kinds of salads a wonderful lift.

Makes about ½ cup (125 mL)

Tip

Kosher salt tastes better than iodized table salt and (ideally) contains no additives.

Variation

Neon Lime Herb Dressing: Increase the amount of each herb to 1 tbsp (15 mL), chopped coarsely rather than finely. Add the ingredients to a mini blender and purée.

2 tbsp	freshly squeezed lime juice	30 mL
2 tsp	finely chopped fresh parsley leaves	10 mL
2 tsp	finely chopped fresh tarragon leaves	10 mL
2 tsp	finely chopped fresh chives	10 mL
1 tbsp	granulated sugar	15 mL
¼ tsp	Dijon mustard	1 mL
¼ tsp	kosher salt or coarse sea salt	1 mL
⅛ tsp	freshly ground black pepper	0.5 mL
⅓ cup	extra virgin olive oil	75 mL

1. In a bowl, whisk together lime juice, parsley, tarragon, chives, sugar, mustard, salt and pepper. Gradually whisk in oil.
2. Transfer to an airtight container and refrigerate for up to 1 week.

Health Tip

- Fresh herbs increase the alkalizing effect of this recipe.

Nutrients per 1 tbsp (15 mL)	
Calories	87
Fat	9 g
Sodium	64 mg
Carbohydrate	2 g
Fiber	0 g
Protein	0 g
Calcium	2 mg
Magnesium	1 mg
Potassium	10 mg

Asian Citrus Salad Dressing

In addition to salads, this dressing adds wonderful flavor served over steamed fish.

Makes about ½ cup (125 mL)

Nutrients per 1 tbsp (15 mL)	
Calories	40
Fat	3 g
Sodium	72 mg
Carbohydrate	2 g
Fiber	0 g
Protein	0 g
Calcium	7 mg
Magnesium	2 mg
Potassium	30 mg

1	orange	1
2 tbsp	sesame oil	30 mL
1 tbsp	soy sauce (GF, if needed)	15 mL
1 tbsp	rice vinegar	15 mL
	Salt and freshly ground black pepper	

1. Grate 1 tsp (5 mL) zest from orange and squeeze out juice to make ¼ cup (60 mL), reserve any extra for another use. Place zest and juice in a container with a tight-fitting lid. Add oil, soy sauce and vinegar. Shake well to combine. Season to taste with salt and pepper.
2. Refrigerate for several days or up to 1 week.

Health Tip

- Replace the soy sauce with reduced-sodium soy sauce to reduce the sodium load in this recipe.

Light Creamy Dill Dressing

Here is an easy, quick recipe that delivers lots of zing.

Makes about 1 cup (250 mL)

Tip

Use in a seafood salad, or serve as a tartar sauce with grilled fish.

Nutrients per 1 tbsp (15 mL)	
Calories	11
Fat	1 g
Sodium	36 mg
Carbohydrate	1 g
Fiber	0 g
Protein	0 g
Calcium	3 mg
Magnesium	0 mg
Potassium	5 mg

½ cup	2% yogurt	125 mL
2 tbsp	light mayonnaise	30 mL
3 tbsp	chopped fresh parsley	45 mL
¼ cup	chopped fresh dill (or 1½ tsp/7 mL dried dillweed)	60 mL
1 tsp	Dijon mustard	5 mL
¾ tsp	crushed garlic	3 mL
	Salt and freshly ground black pepper	

1. In bowl, combine yogurt, mayonnaise, parsley, dill, mustard and garlic. Season to taste with salt and pepper.

Health Tip

- Fresh herbs increase the alkalizing effect of this recipe.

Meaty Mains

Texas-Style Barbecue

In Texas and points south, "barbecue" has a distinct definition — beef or sometimes pork, slow-smoked over indirect heat to tender perfection. You can buy a small electric or charcoal home smoker to approximate true slow barbecue.

Makes 6 to 8 servings

1	beef brisket (about 4 lbs/2 kg)	1
1 tsp	freshly ground black pepper	5 mL
1 tbsp	olive oil	15 mL
1 tbsp	dry mustard	15 mL
2 tsp	dried oregano	10 mL
1 tsp	ground dried sage	5 mL
½ tsp	cayenne pepper	2 mL
5	cloves garlic, minced	5
1	1-inch (2.5 cm) piece gingerroot, minced	1
½ cup	ketchup	125 mL
¼ cup	light (fancy) molasses	60 mL
¼ cup	red wine vinegar	60 mL
¼ cup	tomato paste	60 mL

1. In a shallow glass baking dish, rub brisket with pepper; set aside.
2. In a saucepan, heat oil over medium heat. Add mustard, oregano, sage, cayenne pepper, garlic and ginger; cook for 4 minutes, stirring constantly. Stir in 1 cup (250 mL) of water, ketchup, molasses, wine vinegar and tomato paste. Bring to a boil, reduce heat to medium-low and cook for 15 minutes. Cool. Pour marinade over roast, cover and refrigerate for 1 to 2 days, turning meat occasionally.
3. If using a gas barbecue, light one burner only and place meat on unlit side with drip pan below grill and under roast; lower lid. In a conventional smoker, cook with beer or wine in the drip pan. For a covered charcoal barbecue, heat coals, then move them around the outside edges of grill with drip pan and meat in the middle. Maintain an even heat of 200°F (100°C), adding preheated coals throughout smoking period.
4. Cook 5 to 6 hours or until meat thermometer reads 150°F (65°C), turning occasionally and basting meat with marinade as it cooks. Add more coals as necessary to smoker or charcoal grill, and toss in some damp wood chips occasionally for smoke. Let stand 10 minutes before slicing. Serve with homemade or commercial barbecue sauce.

Nutrients per serving (1 of 8)	
Calories	557
Fat	20 g
Sodium	356 mg
Carbohydrate	14 g
Fiber	1 g
Protein	75 g
Calcium	80 mg
Magnesium	59 mg
Potassium	918 mg

Slow-Cooked Chili Flank Steak or Brisket

This is an ideal meal for entertaining because it can be prepared ahead of time and placed in the slow cooker earlier in the day to be ready for your company at night.

Makes 8 servings

Health Tips

- Replace the ready-to-use beef broth with a homemade version to reduce the sodium in this recipe.
- If you have a GI condition that is aggravated by hot or spicy foods, omit the chili powder and serve hot sauce at the table for others to season to taste.
- Slow cooking has more of an alkalizing effect than deep-frying or barbecuing.

Nutrients per serving	
Calories	208
Fat	8 g
Sodium	248 mg
Carbohydrate	8 g
Fiber	2 g
Protein	26 g
Calcium	66 mg
Magnesium	39 mg
Potassium	658 mg

- **Large (minimum 6-quart) slow cooker**

2 lbs	flank steak or beef brisket	1 kg
1/2 tsp	freshly ground black pepper	2 mL
1 tbsp	vegetable oil	15 mL
3	stalks celery, with leaves, cut into chunks and leaves chopped	3
2	cloves garlic, minced	2
1	onion, cut into chunks	1
1 cup	ready-to-use reduced-sodium beef broth (GF, if needed)	250 mL
1	can (19 oz/540 mL) chili-flavored or regular stewed tomatoes, with juice (about 2 1/3 cups/575 mL)	1
1	large carrot, cut into chunks	1
1	bay leaf	1
1/2 tsp	dried thyme	2 mL
2 tsp	chili powder	10 mL

1. Cut beef into large pieces that will comfortably fit in your slow cooker. Season with pepper.
2. In a large skillet, heat oil over medium-high heat. Cook beef for 3 to 4 minutes per side or until browned on all sides. Transfer beef to slow cooker.
3. In the fat remaining in the skillet, sauté celery (including leaves), garlic and onion until lightly browned, about 5 minutes. Add to slow cooker.
4. Add broth to skillet and scrape up any brown bits from the bottom. Pour liquid into slow cooker.
5. To the slow cooker, add tomatoes and juice, carrot, bay leaf, thyme and chili powder; stir to combine. Cover and cook on Low for 6 to 8 hours or until beef is fork-tender. Discard bay leaf.
6. Slice beef across the grain and arrange on a platter. Skim fat from sauce, pour sauce over meat and serve.

This recipe courtesy of Eileen Campbell.

Beef Tenderloin with Four-Peppercorn Crust

This is one of those show-stopper beef dishes for special dinners. Serve with garlic mashed potatoes or stuffed baked potatoes, and sautéed wild mushrooms.

Makes 12 to 14 servings

- **Preheat oven to 425°F (220°C)**
- **Shallow roasting pan with a rack**

2 tbsp	whole black peppercorns	30 mL
2 tbsp	whole white peppercorns	30 mL
2 tbsp	whole green peppercorns	30 mL
2 tbsp	whole pink peppercorns	30 mL
1 tbsp	coarse sea salt	15 mL
1	whole beef tenderloin (3 to 4 lbs/ 1.5 to 2 kg), well trimmed	1
3 tbsp	extra virgin olive oil	45 mL
	Mixed peppercorns and fresh thyme	

1. Combine the peppercorns in a bag. Crush coarsely with a mallet or rolling pin. Combine crushed peppercorns with salt.
2. Rinse beef and pat dry with paper towels, then rub with peppercorn-salt mixture, pressing the mixture into the meat. Let stand for 30 minutes at room temperature. (Recipe can be prepared to this point up to 2 days in advance; wrap meat tightly with plastic wrap and refrigerate. Bring to room temperature before proceeding with recipe.)
3. In a large nonstick skillet, heat oil over high heat until smoking. Cook tenderloin, turning frequently, for 5 minutes or until well-browned on all sides. Place tenderloin on rack in roasting pan. Roast for 30 minutes for medium-rare.
4. Tent meat with foil and let stand 15 minutes. Slice crosswise into ½-inch (1 cm) slices and serve garnished with a sprinkle of mixed peppercorns and a sprig of thyme.

Nutrients per serving	
Calories	128
Fat	6 g
Sodium	647 mg
Carbohydrate	0 g
Fiber	0 g
Protein	19 g
Calcium	0 mg
Magnesium	0 mg
Potassium	0 mg

Slow-Cooked Beef Stew

Do all the preparation the night before and place this stew in the slow cooker before you go to work in the morning. When you come home on a cold winter evening, a delicious meal will be ready for you.

Makes 8 servings

Tips

If you prefer, you could cook this on High for 4 to 5 hours instead.

Serve with egg noodles and a green salad for a complete and satisfying meal.

- **Large (minimum 6-quart) slow cooker**

1½ cups	dry red wine	375 mL
3 tbsp	vegetable oil, divided	45 mL
1	bay leaf	1
2 tsp	dried parsley	10 mL
1 tsp	dried thyme	5 mL
¼ tsp	freshly ground black pepper	1 mL
2 lbs	lean stewing beef, cut into cubes	1 kg
⅓ cup	all-purpose flour	75 mL
1	large onion, chopped	1
2	cloves garlic, minced	2
2 cups	sliced mushrooms	500 mL
18	small white onions (thawed if frozen)	18
1 cup	ready-to-use beef broth	250 mL
1 tbsp	tomato paste	15 mL

1. In a large bowl, whisk together wine, 1 tbsp (15 mL) oil, bay leaf, parsley, thyme and pepper. Stir in beef, coating evenly. Cover and refrigerate for at least 4 hours or overnight.
2. Drain beef, reserving 1 cup (250 mL) marinade. Place beef in slow cooker, sprinkle with flour and toss to coat.
3. In a small skillet, heat 1 tbsp (15 mL) oil over medium heat. Sauté chopped onion until lightly browned, about 5 minutes. Add garlic and sauté for a few seconds. Using a slotted spoon, transfer onions and garlic to slow cooker.
4. Add the remaining oil to skillet. Sauté mushrooms for 5 minutes or until they release their liquid. Using a slotted spoon, transfer mushrooms to slow cooker.
5. Add reserved marinade, small onions, broth and tomato paste to slow cooker; stir well. Cover and cook on Low for 8 to 10 hours or until beef is fork-tender.

This recipe courtesy of Eileen Campbell.

Health Tip

- Dishes prepared in a slow cooker are more alkalizing than those cooked in a deep-fryer or on the barbecue.

Nutrients per serving	
Calories	347
Fat	12 g
Sodium	101 mg
Carbohydrate	24 g
Fiber	4 g
Protein	28 g
Calcium	69 mg
Magnesium	57 mg
Potassium	852 mg

Indian Beef with Cauliflower and Peppers

If you have a hankering for something that resembles a beef curry but is more nutritious, here's the recipe for you. Serve over brown basmati rice, with a cucumber salad on the side.

Makes 8 servings

Tips

This quantity of black peppercorns provides a nicely zesty result. If you prefer a less peppery dish, reduce the quantity by half.

Cook cauliflower in rapidly boiling salted water until it's tender to the bite, about 3 minutes after the water has returned to a boil. Drain and add to the slow cooker.

Nutrients per serving	
Calories	243
Fat	11 g
Sodium	140 mg
Carbohydrate	10 g
Fiber	3 g
Protein	28 g
Calcium	64 mg
Magnesium	61 mg
Potassium	789 mg

- **Medium to large (3½- to 6-quart) slow cooker**

1 tbsp	olive oil (approx.)	15 mL
2 lbs	trimmed stewing beef, cut into ½-inch (1 cm) cubes	1 kg
2	onions, finely chopped	2
1 tbsp	minced gingerroot	15 mL
2	cloves garlic, minced	2
1	2-inch (5 cm) cinnamon stick	1
1 tsp	cracked black peppercorns (see tip, at left)	5 mL
2	bay leaves	2
2 tbsp	cumin seeds, toasted (see box, page 247)	30 mL
1 tbsp	coriander seeds, toasted	15 mL
1 cup	ready-to-use beef broth (GF, if needed)	250 mL
2 tbsp	tomato paste	30 mL
	Salt (optional)	
1	red bell pepper, finely chopped	1
1 to 2	long green chile peppers, minced	1 to 2
4 cups	cooked cauliflower florets (see tip, at left)	1 L
	Plain yogurt	
¼ cup	toasted slivered almonds	60 mL
½ cup	finely chopped cilantro leaves	125 mL

1. In a skillet, heat oil over medium-high heat for 30 seconds. Add beef, in batches, and cook, stirring, adding additional oil if necessary, until browned, about 3 minutes per batch. Transfer to slow cooker stoneware.
2. Reduce heat to medium. Add additional oil to pan if necessary. Add onions to pan and cook, stirring, until softened, about 3 minutes. Add gingerroot, garlic, cinnamon stick, peppercorns, bay leaves and toasted cumin and coriander and cook, stirring, for 1 minute. Add broth and tomato paste and bring to a boil, scraping up brown bits in the pan. Season to taste with salt (if using). Transfer to slow cooker stoneware. Stir well.

Tip

This dish can be partially prepared before it is cooked. Heat oil and complete step 2. Cover and refrigerate overnight or for up to 2 days. When you're ready to cook, either brown the beef as outlined in step 1 or add it to the stoneware without browning. Stir well and continue with step 3.

Variation

Substitute 4 cups (1 L) broccoli florets for the cauliflower.

3. Cover and cook on Low for 6 to 8 hours or on High for 3 to 4 hours, until beef is tender. Discard bay leaves and cinnamon stick. Add red pepper and chile pepper and stir well. Stir in cooked cauliflower. Cover and cook on High for 20 minutes, until pepper is tender. To serve, garnish with a drizzle of yogurt, toasted almonds and cilantro.

Health Tips

- If you have a GI condition that is aggravated by hot or spicy foods, omit the chile peppers in this recipe and serve hot sauce at the table for others to season to taste.
- This recipe contains almonds and coriander seeds and may not be suitable for those with some GI conditions.
- Fresh herbs increase the alkalizing effect of this dish.

Italian Meatballs with Chunky Tomato Sauce

This recipe is easily multiplied and is a favorite dish when families get together. Serve over spaghetti with extra grated Parmesan to sprinkle on top, and a dish of hot pepper flakes on the table for those who like to spice it up a little.

Makes 4 to 6 servings

Tip

Multiply this recipe to serve a large party or to make ahead and store in the freezer. For large quantities, instead of browning in a skillet, arrange the meatballs in single layers on large baking sheets and roast in a preheated 350°F (180°C) oven for about 20 minutes, shaking the pan occasionally so that the meatballs brown evenly on all sides. Heat Chunky Tomato Sauce in a large pot and combine browned meatballs with sauce and continue with step 3.

1½ lbs	lean ground beef	750 g
8 oz	ground pork	250 g
1	small onion, finely chopped	1
2	cloves garlic, finely chopped	2
¼ cup	fresh bread crumbs	60 mL
¼ cup	chopped fresh flat-leaf (Italian) parsley	60 mL
2 tbsp	freshly grated Parmesan cheese	30 mL
1 tbsp	chopped fresh basil (or 1 tsp/5 mL dried)	15 mL
1 tbsp	chopped fresh oregano (or 1 tsp/5 mL dried)	15 mL
1½ tsp	kosher or sea salt	7 mL
½ tsp	freshly ground black pepper	2 mL
1	large egg, lightly beaten	1
2 tbsp	olive oil	30 mL
	Chunky Tomato Sauce (page 220)	

1. In a large bowl, using a fork, combine beef and pork with onion, garlic, bread crumbs, parsley, Parmesan, basil, oregano, salt, pepper and egg. Scoop ¼ cup (60 mL) of the mixture and shape into a ball. Repeat with the remaining mixture.
2. In a large skillet, heat oil over medium-high heat. Add meatballs, in batches, and brown lightly on all sides. Do not crowd the pan. Set aside.
3. In a large pot, heat Chunky Tomato Sauce over medium heat until bubbling. Reduce heat to medium-low and add meatballs to the sauce. Use a wooden spoon to make room in the pot for all the meatballs and to ensure that they are all immersed in the sauce. Partially cover the pot and simmer until meatballs are no longer pink inside, 20 to 30 minutes.

Health Tips

- Fresh herbs increase the alkalizing effect of this recipe.
- If you are sensitive to gluten, choose GF bread crumbs.

Nutrients per serving (1 of 6)	
Calories	302
Fat	18 g
Sodium	835 mg
Carbohydrate	3 g
Fiber	0 g
Protein	31 g
Calcium	44 mg
Magnesium	13 mg
Potassium	166 mg

Roast Lamb with Marrakech Rub

This simple roast with the flavors of Morocco is easy to prepare if you have a batch of Marrakech Rub (page 228) on hand. It's great served hot, but would also be good served cold, with a hearty salad on the side.

Makes 8 servings

- **Roasting pan with rack, lightly sprayed with vegetable cooking spray**

3 lb	boneless leg of lamb, trimmed	1.5 kg
2 tbsp	Big-Batch Marrakech Rub for Chicken, Pork or Lamb (page 228)	30 mL
2 cups	ready-to-use reduced-sodium chicken broth (GF, if needed)	500 mL
1 cup	sliced dried apricots	250 mL

1. Place lamb in a large container and rub with Marrakech Rub. Cover and refrigerate for at least 1 hour or overnight. Preheat oven to 375°F (190°C).
2. Place lamb on prepared rack in roasting pan and roast for 25 minutes. Add 1 cup (250 mL) broth and the apricots to the drippings in the pan. Roast, adding more broth as the liquid evaporates, for 20 to 35 minutes or until lamb has reached an internal temperature of 150°F (65°C) for medium-rare, or until desired doneness. Transfer to a plate and cover with foil. Let rest for 15 minutes before carving.

This recipe courtesy of Eileen Campbell.

Nutrients per serving	
Calories	243
Fat	8 g
Sodium	125 mg
Carbohydrate	5 g
Fiber	2 g
Protein	37 g
Calcium	34 mg
Magnesium	53 mg
Potassium	644 mg

Veal Goulash

This version of goulash, a luscious Hungarian stew seasoned with paprika, is lighter than the traditional one made with beef.

Makes 8 servings

Tips

There is a hint of caraway flavor in this version. If you prefer a stronger caraway flavor, increase the quantity of caraway seeds to as much as 2 tsp (10 mL).

If you can't find whole small cremini mushrooms, white mushrooms or larger cremini mushrooms, quartered or sliced, depending upon their size, work well too.

Nutrients per serving	
Calories	216
Fat	7 g
Sodium	227 mg
Carbohydrate	11 g
Fiber	3 g
Protein	27 g
Calcium	55 mg
Magnesium	42 mg
Potassium	800 mg

- **Medium to large (3½- to 6-quart) slow cooker**

2 tbsp	olive oil, divided	30 mL
2 lbs	trimmed stewing veal, cut into 1-inch (2.5 cm) pieces	1 kg
2	onions, finely chopped	2
4	cloves garlic, minced	4
1 tsp	caraway seeds (see tip, at left)	5 mL
½ tsp	cracked black peppercorns	2 mL
1 lb	whole small cremini mushrooms	500 g
2 tbsp	all-purpose flour	30 mL
1	can (14 oz/398 mL) diced tomatoes, with juice	1
1 cup	ready-to-use chicken broth	250 mL
1 tbsp	sweet Hungarian paprika, dissolved in 2 tbsp (30 mL) water or chicken broth	15 mL
2	red bell peppers, finely chopped	2
½ cup	finely chopped fresh dill	125 mL
	Sour cream (optional)	

1. In a skillet, heat 1 tbsp (15 mL) oil over medium-high heat for 30 seconds. Add veal, in batches, and cook, stirring, adding more oil as necessary, until browned, about 5 minutes per batch. Using a slotted spoon, transfer to slow cooker stoneware.
2. Reduce heat to medium. Add onions to pan and cook, stirring, until softened, about 3 minutes. Add garlic, caraway seeds and peppercorns and cook, stirring, for 1 minute. Add mushrooms and toss to coat. Add flour and cook, stirring, for 1 minute. Add tomatoes and broth; bring to a boil. Transfer to slow cooker stoneware. Stir well.
3. Cover and cook on Low for 8 hours or on High for 4 hours, until veal is tender.
4. Add paprika solution to slow cooker stoneware and stir well. Add red peppers and stir well. Cover and cook on High for 30 minutes, until peppers are tender. To serve, ladle into bowls and top each serving with 1 tbsp (15 mL) dill and, if desired, a dollop of sour cream.

Tip

This dish can be partially prepared before it is cooked. Heat 1 tbsp (15 mL) oil and complete step 2. Cover and refrigerate overnight or for up to 1 day. When you're ready to cook, either brown the veal as outlined in step 1 or add it to the stoneware without browning. Stir well and continue with steps 3 and 4.

Health Tips

- If you have a GI condition that is aggravated by hot or spicy foods, omit the Hungarian paprika from this recipe. Set the hot sauce on the table for others to season to taste.
- This recipe contains caraway seeds and may not be suitable for those with some GI conditions.
- Replace the ready-to-use chicken stock with a homemade version to reduce the sodium in this recipe.

Dijon Ham Steaks

This simple ham steak can be served at a dinner party, dressed up with a fruity salsa.

Makes 4 servings

- **Preheat broiler**
- **Baking pan, lined with foil**

4	ham steaks (each 6 oz/175 g) or thick slices of ham	4
2 tbsp	Dijon mustard	30 mL
2 tbsp	packed brown sugar	30 mL
2 tbsp	pineapple or orange juice	30 mL

1. Place ham on prepared pan. Score edges to prevent curling during broiling.
2. In a small bowl, stir together mustard, sugar and juice. Spread over meat.
3. Broil in preheated broiler for 5 minutes or until golden brown and glazed. Serve immediately.

Nutrients per serving	
Calories	245
Fat	7 g
Sodium	2341 mg
Carbohydrate	9 g
Fiber	0 g
Protein	33 g
Calcium	14 mg
Magnesium	33 mg
Potassium	572 mg

Baked Pork Chops with Vegetable Rice

This savory one-dish meal can be prepared in advance and popped in the oven when you get home at night.

Makes 6 servings

Health Tips

- Replace the ready-to-use chicken broth with a homemade version to reduce the sodium in this recipe.
- Increase the alkalizing effect of this recipe by replacing the white rice with brown rice.

Nutrients per serving	
Calories	337
Fat	11 g
Sodium	554 mg
Carbohydrate	32 g
Fiber	2 g
Protein	25 g
Calcium	59 mg
Magnesium	75 mg
Potassium	1099 mg

- **Preheat oven to 350°F (180°C)**
- **13- by 9-inch (33 by 23 cm) baking dish with lid**

2 tsp	vegetable oil	10 mL
6	boneless pork loin chops, trimmed	6
1	onion, chopped	1
1	clove garlic, minced	1
1 cup	long-grain white rice	250 mL
1 tsp	curry powder	5 mL
1 tsp	ground cumin	5 mL
1 tsp	dried oregano	5 mL
2 cups	diced or sliced zucchini	500 mL
2 cups	ready-to-use chicken broth (GF, if needed)	500 mL
1½ cups	chopped plum (Roma) tomatoes	375 mL
1 cup	diced red or yellow bell pepper	250 mL
½ tsp	salt	2 mL
¼ tsp	freshly ground black pepper	1 mL
1	bay leaf	1

1. In a large skillet, heat oil over medium-high heat. Brown chops on both sides, about 4 minutes per side. Transfer to a plate.
2. Add onion and garlic to skillet and sauté for about 5 minutes or until softened. Add rice, curry powder, cumin and oregano; stir to coat rice. Add zucchini, broth, tomatoes, bell pepper, salt, pepper and bay leaf; bring to a boil. Reduce heat, cover and simmer for 10 minutes. Transfer to baking dish.
3. Nestle pork chops into rice mixture in baking dish and pour any juices from meat over top.
4. Cover and bake in preheated oven for 30 to 35 minutes or until rice is tender, liquid is absorbed and just a hint of pink remains in pork and it has reached an internal temperature of 160°F (71°C). Discard bay leaf.

This recipe courtesy of dietitian Patti Thomson.

Baked Ham with Citrus Glaze

A ham is a taste treat that is part of many a joyful gathering.

Makes 12 to 14 servings

Tip

Most commercially raised pigs today are bred and fed to grow and put on weight quickly. They produce very lean meat from large lean muscles with only a thin layer of fat. Today's pork tends to dry out very quickly during cooking and hams have to be given all kinds of flavor boosts to have any taste at all! Cook over medium heat and do not overcook. Seek out butchers who provide pork from local farmers who raise pigs on a smaller scale. Such prized breeds as Berkshire produce pork with a fine-grain marbling of fat, so the meat stays moist, juicy and flavorful. Every mouthful is succulent and tasty. You will be amazed and delighted.

Nutrients per serving (1 of 14)	
Calories	74
Fat	0 g
Sodium	282 mg
Carbohydrate	19 g
Fiber	0 g
Protein	0 g
Calcium	18 mg
Magnesium	4 mg
Potassium	69 mg

- **Preheat oven to 325°F (160°C)**
- **Large roasting pan**

1	bone-in cooked ham (about 12 lbs/5 kg)	1
15	whole cloves (approx.)	15
Citrus Glaze		
1 tbsp	minced gingerroot	15 mL
1 tbsp	grated orange zest	15 mL
2 tsp	grated lemon zest	10 mL
2 tsp	grated lime zest	10 mL
1 tbsp	minced shallots	15 mL
	Juice of 3 oranges (about 3⁄4 cup/175 mL)	
	Juice of 2 lemons (about 1⁄2 cup/125 mL)	
	Juice of 2 limes (about 1⁄4 cup/60 mL)	
1 cup	packed brown sugar	250 mL
3 tbsp	grainy Dijon mustard	45 mL
1 tsp	kosher or sea salt	5 mL
1⁄2 tsp	freshly ground black pepper	2 mL
2 tbsp	bourbon or rum (optional)	30 mL

1. If the ham has a rough, leathery skin on the surface, shave it off using a sharp knife until the layer of white fat is exposed. Score the fat to within about 1⁄2 inch (1 cm) of the flesh, making even strokes all in one direction in lines about 3⁄4 inch (2 cm) apart. Repeat making strokes perpendicular to the first cuts to form a pattern of squares. Press a whole clove into the fat in the center of each square.
2. Place ham in a large roasting pan and add 2 cups (500 mL) water. Bake in preheated oven for 2 hours, rotating the roasting pan occasionally to ensure even coloring.
3. *Glaze:* Meanwhile, in a small saucepan over medium-high heat, combine ginger, orange, lemon and lime zests, shallots and orange, lemon and lime juices. Bring to a boil. Reduce heat and simmer until juices are reduced by one-third, about 1 cup (250 mL). Stir in brown sugar, mustard, salt and pepper. Heat briefly to dissolve sugar. Stir in bourbon (if using).
4. Baste ham with glaze and continue baking, basting and rotating pan every 15 minutes, for about 1 hour or until an instant-read thermometer inserted in the center registers 140°F (60°C). Let stand for 10 minutes before carving.

Ribs with Hominy and Kale

This hearty stew is great on an early spring day when there is still a chill in the air but fresh radishes are appearing in the markets.

Makes 8 servings

Tips

Prepared hominy is available in well-stocked supermarkets or Latin American grocery stores. If you can't find it, chickpeas make an acceptable substitute.

If you are using small Hass avocados, use two in this recipe. Don't peel and dice avocados until you are ready to use them. Otherwise they will discolor.

Nutrients per serving	
Calories	343
Fat	17 g
Sodium	528 mg
Carbohydrate	28 g
Fiber	5 g
Protein	21 g
Calcium	159 mg
Magnesium	90 mg
Potassium	984 mg

- **Large (minimum 6-quart) slow cooker**

1 tbsp	olive oil	15 mL
2½ lbs	sliced country-style or side pork ribs, trimmed of fat	1.25 kg
2	onions, finely chopped	2
6	cloves garlic, minced	6
2 tsp	dried oregano (preferably Mexican), crumbled	10 mL
½ tsp	cracked black peppercorns	2 mL
1 tbsp	cumin seeds, toasted (see box, page 247)	15 mL
2 cups	ready-to-use chicken or vegetable broth (GF, if needed)	500 mL
2 tbsp	tomato paste	30 mL
3	cans (each 15 oz/425 g) hominy, drained and rinsed (see tip, at left)	3
1 tbsp	ancho chile powder, dissolved in 2 tbsp (30 mL) lime juice	15 mL
1	jalapeño pepper (or chipotle pepper in adobo sauce), minced	1
8 cups	chopped stemmed kale (about 1 large bunch)	2 L
½ cup	finely chopped red or green onion	125 mL
½ cup	finely chopped fresh cilantro	125 mL
1	avocado, peeled and diced (optional; see tip, at left)	1
	Sliced radishes (optional)	
	Lime wedges	

1. In a skillet, heat oil over medium-high heat for 30 seconds. Add ribs, in batches, and brown on both sides, about 5 minutes per batch. Transfer to slow cooker stoneware.
2. In same skillet, reduce heat to medium and add onions and cook, stirring, until softened, about 5 minutes. Add garlic, oregano, peppercorns and toasted cumin and cook, stirring, for 1 minute. Add broth and tomato paste; bring to a boil. Transfer to slow cooker stoneware.

Tip

This dish can be partially prepared before it is cooked. Heat 1 tbsp (15 mL) oil and complete step 2. Cover and refrigerate overnight or for up to 2 days. When you're ready to cook, brown the ribs as outlined in step 1 and add to stoneware. Stir well and continue with steps 3 and 4.

3. Add hominy and stir well. Cover and cook on Low for 8 hours or on High for 4 hours, until ribs are tender and falling off the bone.
4. Add chile powder solution and jalapeño pepper and stir well. Add kale, in batches, completely submerging each batch in the liquid before adding another. Cover and cook on High for 20 to 30 minutes, until kale is tender. To serve, ladle into bowls and garnish with onion and cilantro and, if desired, avocado and/or radishes. Pass lime wedges at the table.

Health Tips

- Replace the ready-to-use chicken or vegetable stock with a homemade version to reduce the sodium in this recipe.
- If you have a GI condition that is aggravated by hot or spicy foods, omit the jalapeño pepper and ancho chile powder from this recipe. Serve hot pepper sauce at the table for others to season to taste.
- Dishes prepared in a slow cooker are less acidifying than deep-fried or barbecued foods.

Vegetable Cobbler with Millet Crust

Not only is this tasty cobbler loaded with flavor, the distinctive millet crust makes it a delightfully different treat. Add a sliced tomato salad, in season, or a tossed green salad topped with shredded carrots to add color and nutrients.

Makes 8 servings

Tips

Be sure to rinse canned beans thoroughly under cold running water to remove as much sodium as possible. Alternatively, use 1 cup (250 mL) dried white beans, soaked, cooked and drained.

You can substitute 1 tbsp (15 mL) dried rosemary leaves, crumbled, for the fresh.

The small bit of pancetta (Italian-style cured pork) in this recipe adds so much flavor that it's worth including in keeping with "limited" consumption.

Nutrients per serving	
Calories	285
Fat	10 g
Sodium	507 mg
Carbohydrate	40 g
Fiber	9 g
Protein	11 g
Calcium	195 mg
Magnesium	157 mg
Potassium	1539 mg

- **Large (minimum 6-quart) slow cooker**

Topping

1 cup	millet (see tip, page 170)	250 mL
3 cups	water	750 mL
	Salt and freshly ground black pepper	
½ cup	freshly grated Parmesan cheese (optional)	125 mL

Cobbler

1 tbsp	olive oil	15 mL
1	chunk (3 oz/90 g) pancetta, diced	1
2	onions, finely chopped	2
4	carrots, peeled and diced	4
4	stalks celery, diced	4
2 tbsp	fresh rosemary leaves, finely chopped	30 mL
4	cloves garlic, minced	4
½ tsp	cracked black peppercorns	2 mL
1	can (28 oz/796 mL) tomatoes, with juice, coarsely chopped	1
	Salt (optional)	
1	can (14 to 19 oz/398 to 540 mL) white beans, drained and rinsed (see tip, at left)	1
12 oz	frozen sliced green beans (about 2 cups/500 mL)	375 g

1. *Topping:* In a saucepan over medium heat, toast millet, stirring constantly, until it crackles and releases its aroma, about 5 minutes. Add water, and salt and black pepper to taste, and bring to a boil. Reduce heat to low, cover and cook until millet is tender and all the water is absorbed, about 20 minutes. Stir in Parmesan (if using) and set aside.

Tip

This dish can be partially prepared before it is cooked. Complete step 2. Cover and refrigerate overnight or for up to 2 days. When you're ready to cook, continue with steps 1 and 3.

2. *Cobbler:* Meanwhile, in a large skillet, heat oil over medium heat for 30 seconds. Add pancetta and cook, stirring, until crispy, about 3 minutes. Add onions, carrots and celery and cook, stirring, until vegetables are softened, about 7 minutes. Add rosemary, garlic and peppercorns and cook, stirring, for 1 minute. Add tomatoes and bring to a boil. Add salt to taste (if using). Transfer to stoneware.
3. Add white beans and green beans and stir well. Spread millet evenly over the top. Cover and cook on Low for 8 to 10 hours or on High for 4 to 5 hours, until hot and bubbly.

Health Tip

- Fresh herbs increase the alkalizing effect of this dish.

Jambalaya

This is a great dish for a family dinner or a casual evening with friends. The robust flavors are delicious any time of the year, but particularly appreciated on a chilly night. All you need to add is warm whole-grain rolls, a big salad and, if you're feeling festive, some bold red wine.

Makes 6 servings

Tips

If you like heat, use hot Italian sausage and/or add the diced chile pepper.

Buy sausage from a butcher who makes it on-site and can tell you exactly what it contains.

Nutrients per serving	
Calories	378
Fat	10 g
Sodium	667 mg
Carbohydrate	29 g
Fiber	3 g
Protein	27 g
Calcium	124 mg
Magnesium	42 mg
Potassium	818 mg

3 cups	ready-to-use reduced-sodium chicken broth (GF, if needed)	750 mL
3/4 cup	Job's tears, soaked, rinsed and drained	175 mL
1 tbsp	olive oil	15 mL
8 oz	Italian sausage, removed from casings	250 g
1 lb	skinless boneless chicken thighs, cut into bite-size pieces	500 g
2	onions, finely chopped	2
2	stalks celery, diced	2
2	bell peppers (such as 1 green and 1 red), finely chopped	2
1	chile pepper, seeded and diced (optional)	1
4	cloves garlic, minced	4
2 tsp	Cajun seasoning	10 mL
1 tsp	dried thyme	5 mL
1	can (28 oz/796 mL) no-salt-added diced tomatoes, with juice	1
8 oz	medium shrimp, cooked, peeled and deveined (optional)	250 g

1. In a heavy saucepan with a tight-fitting lid, bring broth to a boil. Add Job's tears and return to a boil. Reduce heat to low. Cover and simmer for 30 minutes. (The Job's tears will not be fully cooked and liquid won't be completely absorbed.)
2. Meanwhile, in a Dutch oven, heat oil over medium heat for 30 seconds. Add sausage and cook, breaking up with a spoon, until no longer pink, about 4 minutes. Add chicken and cook, stirring, until very lightly browned, about 2 minutes. Transfer to a bowl. Drain off all but 1 tbsp (15 mL) fat from pan, if necessary.

Tips

Cajun seasoning should be simply a blend of spices, which are gluten-free, but some brands add wheat starch, so be sure to check the label if you are sensitive to gluten.

If you don't have Cajun seasoning, substitute 1 tsp (5 mL) paprika — sweet, hot or smoked, depending on your taste.

3. Add onions, celery, bell peppers and chile pepper (if using) and cook, stirring, until softened, about 5 minutes. Add garlic, Cajun seasoning and thyme and cook, stirring, for 1 minute. Add tomatoes and bring to a boil. Stir in partially cooked Job's tears with liquid and return sausage and chicken to pot. Stir well.

4. Reduce heat to low. Cover and simmer until Job's tears are tender and liquid is absorbed, about 30 minutes. Stir in shrimp (if using) and cook until heated through, about 10 minutes.

Health Tips

- If you have a GI condition that is aggravated by hot or spicy foods, omit the Cajun seasoning and serve hot sauce at the table for others to season to taste.
- Replace the ready-made chicken stock with a homemade version to reduce the sodium in this recipe.

Italian Sausage Patties

Serve these spicy meat patties over pasta, in a pesto sauce or with a mild tomato sauce. Make ahead and freeze for up to 3 months for a last-minute supper or snack.

Makes 12 patties

Tips

If you use an indoor contact grill, there is no need to turn the patties. Cooking time will be much shorter; check the manufacturer's instructions.

For a stronger flavor, substitute caraway or anise seeds for the fennel.

Variations

Substitute ground veal, pork, chicken or turkey for the ground beef.

Make into meatballs. Bake on a baking sheet at 400°F (200°C) for 15 to 20 minutes or until no longer pink in the center.

- **Barbecue, grill or broiler, preheated**

1 lb	lean ground beef	500 g
3	cloves garlic, minced	3
2 tsp	fennel seeds	10 mL
1 tsp	hot pepper flakes	5 mL
3/4 tsp	salt	3 mL
1/2 tsp	freshly ground black pepper	2 mL
1/4 tsp	cayenne pepper (optional)	1 mL

1. In a medium bowl, using a fork, gently combine beef, garlic, fennel seeds, hot pepper flakes, salt, pepper and cayenne pepper (if using). Form into 12 patties, 2 inches (5 cm) in diameter.
2. On preheated barbecue, grill patties for 2 to 3 minutes, turning only once, until meat thermometer registers 160°F (71°C) and patties are no longer pink inside.

Health Tip

- If you have a GI condition that is aggravated by hot or spicy foods, omit the hot pepper flakes and optional cayenne pepper. Instead, serve hot pepper flakes at the table for others to season to taste.

Nutrients per patty	
Calories	55
Fat	2 g
Sodium	171 mg
Carbohydrate	1 g
Fiber	0 g
Protein	8 g
Calcium	9 mg
Magnesium	10 mg
Potassium	142 mg

Poultry, Fish and Seafood Mains

Apple Harvest Chicken

Everyone will enjoy this fast and tasty chicken recipe. Serve with green beans and mashed potatoes for a simple weeknight dinner.

Makes 4 servings

- **Nonstick cooking spray**

4	boneless skinless chicken breasts	4
1/2 tsp	dried thyme	2 mL
	Salt and freshly ground black pepper	
2	medium apples, peeled and thickly sliced	2
1/4 cup	apple cider or apple juice	60 mL

1. Rinse and wipe chicken with paper towel. Sprinkle with thyme, salt and pepper.
2. In a large nonstick skillet lightly sprayed with cooking spray, sauté chicken on medium-high for 5 minutes on each side or until browned.
3. Add apples and cider. Cover, reduce heat to medium-low and cook gently for 10 minutes or until meat is no longer pink inside.

Health Tips

- Apples, apple cider and apple juice are all alkalizing foods. Increase your intake of alkalizing fruits and vegetables to balance foods that are highly acidifying, such as chicken, fish and beef.
- When cooking meats, choose a slower cooking method, such as steaming, slow-cooking or roasting. These methods have a reduced acidifying effect compared to deep-frying, frying or barbecuing.

Nutrients per serving	
Calories	249
Fat	3 g
Sodium	160 mg
Carbohydrate	29 g
Fiber	1 g
Protein	25 g
Calcium	122 mg
Magnesium	33 mg
Potassium	476 mg

Chicken Piccata

A light crispy coating keeps the skinless boneless chicken breast moist and flavorful. For extra piquancy, you could include 1 tbsp (15 mL) grated Parmesan cheese. Add a topping of tomato sauce and pile in a crusty bun for a delicious, if messy, hot sandwich.

Makes 6 servings

Variation

Pork or Veal Cutlets: Use the seasoned bread crumbs to coat thin cutlets of pork or veal. Bake in preheated oven as for Chicken Piccata, or sauté in a skillet over medium heat.

- **Preheat oven to 400°F (200°C)**
- **Baking sheet, lightly oiled**

6	boneless skinless chicken breasts	6
1 tsp	grated lemon zest	5 mL
1½ cups	fresh bread crumbs or panko	375 mL
2 tbsp	freshly squeezed lemon juice	30 mL
2 tbsp	finely chopped basil (or 2 tsp/10 mL dried)	30 mL
2 tbsp	finely chopped fresh flat-leaf (Italian) parsley	30 mL
2 tsp	finely chopped fresh rosemary (or ½ tsp/2 mL dried)	10 mL
½ tsp	kosher or sea salt	2 mL
½ tsp	freshly ground black pepper	2 mL
Pinch	cayenne pepper	Pinch
¼ cup	butter	60 mL
¼ cup	olive oil	60 mL

1. Pound chicken breasts between sheets of plastic wrap or parchment to an even thickness of about ½ inch (1 cm). Drizzle with lemon juice.
2. In a bowl, combine bread crumbs, lemon zest, basil, parsley, rosemary, salt, pepper and cayenne. Spread seasoned bread crumbs in a shallow dish.
3. In a small saucepan, melt butter and oil over low heat. Pat chicken dry. Dip chicken in melted butter and oil, one piece at a time, then coat in seasoned bread crumbs. Arrange in a single layer on prepared baking sheet. Discard any excess butter and bread crumb mixtures.
4. Bake in preheated oven until crust is crisp and golden and chicken is no longer pink inside, 12 to 15 minutes.

Health Tips

- If you are sensitive to gluten, choose GF bread crumbs.
- Fresh herbs increase the alkalizing effect of this recipe.

Nutrients per serving	
Calories	315
Fat	20 g
Sodium	430 mg
Carbohydrate	6 g
Fiber	0 g
Protein	26 g
Calcium	31 mg
Magnesium	36 mg
Potassium	470 mg

Chicken Pot Pie

Crave Grandma's country cooking? Take pleasure in the aroma of the chicken simmering when you're home during the weekend.

Makes 6 servings

Tips

For a more flavorful stock, use bone-in chicken. If available, add a couple of backs and necks.

If only boneless chicken pieces are available, purchase 2 lbs (1 kg) and add at least 2 to 3 tsp (10 to 15 mL) gluten-free chicken stock powder.

Freeze any leftover stock to use in other recipes.

Make stock in the slow cooker — just leave it on all day. Refrigerating the stock overnight makes it easier to remove any fat that has risen to the surface.

Variation

Make 4 to 6 individual pot pies, then freeze them. To serve, bake from frozen until hot and bubbly or a meat thermometer registers 170°F (77°C).

Nutrients per serving	
Calories	536
Fat	14 g
Sodium	675 mg
Carbohydrate	58 g
Fiber	5 g
Protein	46 g
Calcium	140 mg
Magnesium	58 mg
Potassium	1006 mg

- **8-cup (2 L) shallow casserole dish**

Stock

2½ lbs	whole chicken or bone-in chicken pieces	1.25 kg
1	carrot, coarsely chopped	1
1	onion, thickly sliced	1
8	whole black peppercorns	8
1	bay leaf	1
3 cups	water	750 mL

Stew

1 cup	green beans, cut into 1-inch (2.5 cm) pieces	250 mL
1 cup	baby carrots, cut in half	250 mL
2	potatoes, cut into ½-inch (1 cm) cubes	2
1	stalk celery, sliced	1
⅓ cup	cornstarch	75 mL
1 cup	milk	250 mL
2 tsp	dried thyme	10 mL
	Salt and freshly ground black pepper	
½	recipe Trendy Pastry (page 378)	½

1. *Stock:* In a large saucepan, combine chicken, carrot, onion, peppercorns, bay leaf and water. Bring to a boil. Then skim off froth. Reduce heat, cover and simmer for 60 minutes or until chicken is tender.
2. Strain, reserving 4 cups (1 L) stock. Discard carrot, onion, peppercorns and bay leaf. Cut chicken into large chunks. Skim fat off stock.
3. *Stew:* In a steamer or microwave, steam green beans, carrots, potatoes and celery just until tender. Set aside.
4. In a large saucepan, combine cornstarch, milk, thyme and reserved stock. Cook, stirring constantly, until mixture boils and thickens. Add chicken and vegetables. Spoon stew into the casserole dish.
5. Roll out pastry. Place on stew and cut steam vents. Bake in a 400°F (200°C) preheated oven for 25 to 35 minutes or until hot and bubbly.

Indian Chicken Kebabs

Curry and ginger provide a taste of India in this ever-so-easy-to-make entrée.

Makes 6 servings

- **Six skewers**

6	boneless skinless chicken breasts	6
1/2 cup	low-fat plain yogurt	125 mL
1 tbsp	grated gingerroot	15 mL
1 tbsp	curry paste	15 mL
	Salt and freshly ground black pepper	

1. Rinse and wipe chicken with paper towel. Cut into bite-size cubes.
2. In a bowl, whisk together yogurt, gingerroot, curry paste, and salt and pepper to taste. Add chicken and toss to coat. Cover and refrigerate for 1 hour.
3. Lightly grease barbecue and preheat to medium-high. Thread chicken loosely onto six skewers, discarding marinade. Place on prepared grill. Close lid and cook for 20 minutes, turning once or until meat is no longer pink inside.

Health Tips

- Curry, along with many other spices, is a highly alkalizing food. Increase your intake of alkalizing foods to balance those that are highly acidifying, such as chicken, fish and beef.
- When cooking meats, choose a slower cooking method, such as steaming, slow-cooking or roasting. These methods have a reduced acidifying effect compared to deep-frying, frying or barbecuing.

Nutrients per serving	
Calories	15
Fat	4 g
Sodium	152 mg
Carbohydrate	2 g
Fiber	0 g
Protein	26 g
Calcium	48 mg
Magnesium	37 mg
Potassium	504 mg

Crispy Pecan Chicken Fingers

Slender strips of succulent chicken inside a crunchy pecan coating — what a modern, healthier way to eat "fried" chicken! Serve with Plum Dipping Sauce (page 224) and Honey Mustard Dipping Sauce (page 225).

Makes 4 servings

Tips

Shake off excess egg and crumbs before baking.

Discard both leftover crumb mixture and the plastic bag — it is not safe to reuse either when raw chicken is involved.

Variations

Florentine Chicken Fingers: Top baked chicken fingers with grated Asiago cheese, 1 leaf of arugula and a strip of roasted red pepper and broil just until cheese is melted.

Pizza Chicken Fingers: Top baked chicken fingers with GF pizza sauce, grated mozzarella and, if desired, crumbled cooked bacon. Broil just until cheese melts.

Nutrients per serving	
Calories	450
Fat	20 g
Sodium	468 mg
Carbohydrate	35 g
Fiber	3 g
Protein	33 g
Calcium	52 mg
Magnesium	80 mg
Potassium	625 mg

- **Preheat oven to 425°F (220°C)**
- **Baking sheet, lightly greased**

4	boneless skinless chicken breasts (about 1 lb/500 g)	4
1⁄3 cup	brown rice flour	75 mL
2	large eggs, beaten	2
1 tbsp	water	15 mL
1 tbsp	Dijon mustard	15 mL
1 cup	fresh GF bread crumbs	250 mL
2⁄3 cup	pecans, coarsely chopped	150 mL
1⁄2 cup	cornmeal	125 mL
1⁄4 tsp	salt	1 mL
1⁄4 tsp	freshly ground black pepper	1 mL

1. Cut each breast into strips 3⁄4 inch (2 cm) wide. Pat dry.
2. Place the rice flour in a shallow dish or pie plate. In a second shallow dish or pie plate, whisk together eggs, water and Dijon mustard.
3. In a large plastic bag, combine bread crumbs, pecans, cornmeal, salt and pepper.
4. Coat chicken strips, a few at a time, first in rice flour, then in egg mixture. Shake in bread crumb mixture. Place in a single layer 1 inch (2.5 cm) apart on prepared baking sheet.
5. Bake in preheated oven for 20 to 25 minutes or until coating is golden brown and crispy and chicken is no longer pink inside.

Health Tips

- Use sea salt instead of iodized salt to increase your intake of trace minerals, which helps to buffer acids and balance pH.
- If you are experiencing flare-ups, brown or wild rice, both insoluble fiber foods, may worsen symptoms. Keep track of foods and symptoms in your health, life and diet diary to help identify troublesome foods.

Chicken, Hummus and Sautéed Veggie Wraps

This recipe is easy to prepare and full of flavor.

Makes 4 servings

Tip

This recipe can be fully prepared and refrigerated overnight for a great lunch, or its components can be stored separately in airtight containers for several days. Pop cold wraps in a toaster oven or microwave to heat through.

1 lb	small boneless skinless chicken breasts	500 g
	Salt and freshly ground black pepper	
	Nonstick cooking spray	
1 tbsp	olive oil	15 mL
2	cloves garlic, minced	2
1	green bell pepper, julienned	1
1	red bell pepper, julienned	1
1	yellow bell pepper, julienned	1
1	onion, cut into thin strips	1
2	carrots, julienned	2
½ cup	water	125 mL
2 to 3 tsp	chili powder	10 to 15 mL
½ cup	hummus	125 mL
4	10-inch (25 cm) whole wheat tortillas	4

1. Season chicken breasts with salt and pepper.
2. Heat a large skillet over medium heat. Spray with cooking spray. Cook chicken, turning once, for 5 minutes per side or until chicken is no longer pink inside and has reached an internal temperature of 170°F (77°C). Transfer to a clean plate and let cool. Cut into strips.
3. In the same skillet, heat olive oil over medium-high heat. Sauté garlic, green, red and yellow peppers, onion and carrots, stirring frequently, until beginning to brown, about 5 minutes. Add water and chili powder; season to taste with salt and pepper. Reduce heat to medium and cook until vegetables are tender-crisp and water has evaporated, about 5 minutes.
4. Spread 2 tbsp (30 mL) hummus up the middle of each tortilla. Top with chicken and vegetables. Roll up tortillas.

This recipe courtesy of Rena Hooey.

Health Tips

- If you have a GI condition that is aggravated by hot or spicy foods, omit the chili powder and serve hot sauce at the table for others to season to taste.
- If you are sensitive to gluten, choose GF tortillas.

Nutrients per serving	
Calories	392
Fat	13 g
Sodium	613 mg
Carbohydrate	38 g
Fiber	8 g
Protein	32 g
Calcium	49 mg
Magnesium	71 mg
Potassium	857 mg

Roast Turkey with Madeira Gravy

There is no need for stress when you're cooking for the holidays: make a list and prepare most of the meal ahead of time so that you can relax and enjoy the festivities. This turkey is roasted with aromatic vegetables and herbs in the central cavity and the stuffing baked on the side.

Makes 10 servings, plus leftovers

Tip

A large rectangular roasting pan made of heavy gauge aluminum for good heat distribution is indispensable in the kitchen for roasting turkeys and large cuts of meat. Select one that has a sturdy stand-up handle at each end; swinging handles that hang down are sometimes difficult to grab in a hot oven. Avoid nonstick coated ones because they often are not safe for use on the stovetop. A large V-shaped roasting rack keeps turkey suspended above the roasting fat and makes basting and handling easier.

Nutrients per serving (1 of 15)	
Calories	650
Fat	16 g
Sodium	374 mg
Carbohydrate	9 g
Fiber	1 g
Protein	107 g
Calcium	101 mg
Magnesium	127 mg
Potassium	1529 mg

- **Preheat oven to 325°F (160°C)**
- **Large stovetop-safe roasting pan**

1	turkey (16 lbs/8 kg)	1
1	lemon, quartered	1
	Salt and freshly ground black pepper	
1	onion, quartered	1
1	stalk celery, with leaves, roughly chopped	1
1	head garlic, loose skins removed, cut in half horizontally	1
3	sprigs fresh thyme	3
3	sprigs fresh flat-leaf (Italian) parsley	3
2	bay leaves	2
2 tbsp	melted butter or olive oil	30 mL
1 tbsp	dried sage	15 mL
1 tbsp	dried thyme	15 mL
	Apple Sage Stuffing (page 300)	

Madeira Gravy

1 cup	Madeira	250 mL
3½ cups	Turkey Stock (variation, page 230) or ready-to-use chicken broth (approx.)	875 mL
¼ cup	butter (optional)	60 mL
3	shallots, finely chopped	3
6 tbsp	all-purpose flour	90 mL
1 tsp	chopped thyme	5 mL
	Salt and freshly ground black pepper	

1. Remove giblets from turkey cavity; set aside for stock, if desired. Rinse turkey inside and out with cold water and pat dry thoroughly. Squeeze juice of one section of lemon into central cavity and season with salt and pepper. Add the remaining lemon quarters, onion, celery, garlic, thyme sprigs, parsley sprigs and bay leaves. Rub skin of bird with butter, dried sage, dried thyme, salt and pepper. To truss your turkey: Tuck the flap of skin at the neck and the wing tips under the bird. Loosely tie the drumsticks together.
2. Place turkey in a large roasting pan. Some cooks like to roast the turkey breast-side down for the first hour to keep the breast meat juicy; others prefer to baste with pan juices every 20 minutes or so. Roast turkey, basting occasionally

Tip

Lifting a heavy turkey from roasting pan to platter is often a two-man job. Make sure a large, warm platter is placed right beside the pan. Let turkey rest in the pan for 5 minutes. Stick the handle of a large wooden spoon into the cavity of the bird between the stuffing (if stuffed) and the breast bone and lift straight up and out of the pan. The helper is at hand to steady pan and platter and to guide the bird on both sides with hands protected by paper or tea towels. Cover loosely with foil and let rest while you complete the gravy.

with pan juices, until an instant-read thermometer inserted into the thickest part of the thigh registers 165°F (74°C) and when pierced the juices run clear, 3½ to 4 hours. It is important to turn the pan in the oven several times so that the bird cooks evenly and to cover the breast loosely with foil if it seems to be browning too quickly.

3. Remove pan from oven and let rest for 5 minutes. Lift turkey from pan, transfer to a warm platter and cover loosely with foil for about 30 minutes.
4. *Gravy:* Pour off fat and juices from roasting pan into a large measuring cup and place in the freezer for 2 to 3 minutes so that fat quickly rises to the surface. Transfer ¼ cup (60 mL) fat to a saucepan and skim off and discard the rest. Reserve the juices underneath.
5. Set roasting pan over medium-high heat. Carefully add Madeira and bring to a boil, scraping up browned bits on the bottom. Reduce heat and simmer for 5 minutes. Strain liquid and add to measuring cup. Add enough stock to make 4 cups (1 L).
6. In a saucepan, heat reserved turkey fat or butter over medium heat. Add shallots and sauté until soft and lightly browned, 4 to 5 minutes. Add flour and cook, stirring, until lightly browned, 3 to 4 minutes. Slowly whisk in Madeira mixture until smooth. Reduce heat. Add thyme and let sauce simmer, stirring occasionally, until desired flavor and consistency is reached, 5 to 10 minutes. Season to taste with salt and pepper.
7. Carve turkey and serve with Madeira Gravy and Apple Sage Stuffing.

Variation

Sage Butter Baste: A thin layer of flavored butter smoothed over the turkey breast under the skin adds moisture and flavor while the bird is cooking. Combine ⅓ cup (75 mL) soft butter with 2 tbsp (30 mL) chopped sage, 1 tsp (5 mL) grated lemon zest, ¼ tsp (1 mL) kosher salt and ¼ tsp (1 mL) freshly ground pepper. Use your hands to loosen the skin of the turkey from the breast meat and from the tops of the legs. Spread the herb butter over the meat and pat the skin to distribute the butter in an even layer.

Apple Sage Stuffing

This stuffing is moist and crunchy, with added zing from the fresh herbs.

Makes 10 servings or enough to stuff one 14- to 16-lb (7 to 8 kg) turkey

Tips

Use a country-style bread with good texture for stuffing — white, whole wheat or a mixture. It should be 1 to 2 days old and cut into ½-inch (1 cm) cubes or roughly torn.

Prepare stuffing and store separately in refrigerator up to 2 days ahead.

Nutrients per serving	
Calories	240
Fat	11 g
Sodium	242 mg
Carbohydrate	31 g
Fiber	3 g
Protein	4 g
Calcium	332 mg
Magnesium	12 mg
Potassium	183 mg

- **13- by 9-inch (33 by 23 cm) shallow baking dish, lightly buttered**

½ cup	butter, divided	125 mL
2 cups	chopped onions	500 mL
2 cups	chopped peeled firm tart apples	500 mL
1½ cups	chopped celery	375 mL
½ cup	chopped shallots	125 mL
¾ cup	chopped fresh flat-leaf (Italian) parsley	175 mL
1 tbsp	chopped fresh sage	15 mL
1 tbsp	chopped fresh thyme	15 mL
1 tsp	grated lemon zest	5 mL
¼ tsp	ground cloves	1 mL
	Salt and freshly ground black pepper	
1	large loaf country-style bread, cut into ½-inch (1 cm) cubes (10 to 12 cups/2.5 to 3 L)	1
½ to 1 cup	Turkey Stock (variation, page 230) or ready-to-use chicken broth	125 to 250 mL

1. In a large skillet, melt 2 tbsp (30 mL) butter over medium heat. Add onions and sauté until soft and lightly browned, 5 to 7 minutes. Scrape into a large bowl. Return skillet to heat and add the remaining butter. Add apples, celery and shallots and sauté until soft, 5 to 7 minutes. Add parsley, sage, thyme, lemon zest, cloves, 1 tsp (5 mL) salt and ¼ tsp (1 mL) pepper and sauté for 1 minute, then add to onions in bowl. Add bread cubes to bowl, moisten with enough stock until stuffing just holds together. Season to taste with salt and pepper.
2. Spread stuffing in prepared dish and cover with foil. About 30 minutes before the turkey is cooked, place dish in oven and bake for 30 minutes. Remove foil and bake until top is lightly browned, about 15 minutes more.

Health Tip

- Fresh herbs increase the alkalizing effect of this dish.

Turkey Meatloaf

Quick, easy and always popular, this meatloaf is great served with boiled new potatoes and fresh green beans.

Makes 6 servings

Tip

For a conventional meat loaf, top with Mustard Sauce, then bake in an ungreased 9- by 5-inch (23 by 12.5 cm) loaf pan in a 350°F (180°C) oven for 35 to 45 minutes.

- **Microwave-safe 9-inch (23 cm) ring mold, ungreased**

1½ lbs	extra-lean ground turkey	750 g
½ cup	tomato sauce	125 mL
⅓ cup	soft GF bread crumbs	75 mL
¼ cup	rice bran	60 mL
¼ cup	finely chopped onion	60 mL
1	large egg, lightly beaten	1
½ tsp	salt	2 mL
¼ tsp	freshly ground black pepper	1 mL
	Mustard Sauce (see recipe, below)	

1. In a bowl, gently mix together turkey, tomato sauce, bread crumbs, rice bran, onion, egg, salt and pepper.
2. Spoon into mold and cover with waxed paper. Microwave on High for 10 minutes or until partially set. Drain.
3. Spoon Mustard Sauce over meat loaf. Microwave on High for 2 to 3 minutes or until meat thermometer registers 170°F (77°C).
4. Let stand covered with foil for 5 minutes before serving.

Variation

Substitute extra-lean ground beef, veal, chicken or a combination for the turkey.

Nutrients per serving	
Calories	214
Fat	10 g
Sodium	391 mg
Carbohydrate	6 g
Fiber	1 g
Protein	25 g
Calcium	35 mg
Magnesium	78 mg
Potassium	361 mg

Mustard Sauce

This slightly tangy sauce complements meatballs, pork chops and veal.

Makes about ⅔ cup (150 mL)

½ cup	tomato sauce	125 mL
2 tbsp	packed brown sugar	30 mL
2 tbsp	freshly squeezed lemon juice	30 mL
1 tbsp	prepared mustard	15 mL

1. In a small bowl, combine tomato sauce, brown sugar, lemon juice and mustard.

Nutrients per 2 tbsp (30 mL)	
Calories	30
Fat	0 g
Sodium	164 mg
Carbohydrate	7 g
Fiber	0 g
Protein	1 g
Calcium	10 mg
Magnesium	6 mg
Potassium	99 mg

Brined Duck Breast

Some time in an aromatic brine adds moisture and flavor to duck and other poultry. Duck breasts cooked in this classic method are juicy and tender.

Makes 6 servings

Tips

Kosher salt tastes better than iodized table salt and (ideally) contains no additives.

Nutrients per serving	
Calories	170
Fat	4 g
Sodium	995 mg
Carbohydrate	13 g
Fiber	1 g
Protein	18 g
Calcium	59 mg
Magnesium	32 mg
Potassium	319 mg

Herbed Brine

8 cups	water	2 L
1/2 cup	kosher salt	125 mL
1/4 cup	packed brown sugar	60 mL
12	fresh sage leaves	12
6	sprigs fresh thyme	6
2	bay leaves	2
2	cloves garlic, coarsely chopped	2
1 tbsp	black peppercorns, crushed	15 mL
2 tsp	coriander seeds	10 mL
1 tsp	juniper berries	5 mL

Duck

6	duck breasts	6
2 tbsp	balsamic vinegar	30 mL
1 cup	Chicken Stock (page 230) or ready-to-use reduced-sodium chicken broth (GF, if needed)	250 mL
2 tbsp	port or Madeira	30 mL
	Freshly ground black pepper	
	Kosher or sea salt (optional)	

1. *Brine:* In a stockpot, combine water, salt, brown sugar, sage, thyme, bay leaves, garlic, peppercorns, coriander seeds and juniper berries over medium heat. Bring to a boil, stirring to dissolve salt and sugar. Reduce heat and simmer for 5 minutes. Pour into a large deep bowl and let cool. Refrigerate, covered, until cold.
2. *Duck:* Add duck breasts to cold brine, making sure that they are completely submerged; you may need to weight them down. (Insert a plate that fits into the pot, weighted down with a plastic container filled with water.) Cover and refrigerate for at least 6 hours or for up to 18 hours.

Health Tip

- If you are sensitive to alcohol or allergic to fermented foods, omit the port or Madeira from the recipe.

3. Drain duck and pat dry. Discard brine. Score the fat on the duck breast before cooking. Lay duck breast on a cutting board parallel to your body, take a sharp knife and run it through the fat at a slight angle all the way across the fat to within ¼ inch (0.5 cm) of the flesh; do not cut all the way through to the flesh. Turn the duck breast 180 degrees and cut lines perpendicular to the first set of cuts.
4. Heat a large heavy skillet over medium heat. Lay the duck breasts in pan, fat side down. You may have to cook duck in batches. Do not crowd the pan. Let duck breasts cook undisturbed for 5 minutes. Drain off fat regularly. Continue gentle cooking and rendering off fat until all but a scant ¼ inch (0.5 cm) of fat remains on the duck and the skin of the duck has browned to a rich, deep gold, 15 to 20 minutes. If the duck skin is getting too dark before enough fat has melted away, simply reduce the heat.
5. Turn duck breasts over and remove from heat. Let stand, loosely covered with foil, for 5 to 6 minutes. The duck will be cooked to a succulent rare to medium-rare.
6. Discard fat from skillet. Add vinegar and deglaze pan over high heat, scraping up browned bits on the bottom. Add stock and continue to cook until liquid is reduced to about ¾ cup (175 mL). Stir in port and season to taste with pepper. (Taste carefully before adding more salt: initial brining adds saltiness.) Spoon jus over duck breasts to serve.

Grilled Pheasant with Mustard Marinade

Grill the breasts on these simple but tasty kebabs to medium-rare perfection. If you can't find this tasty wild meat, substitute boneless skinless chicken breasts; grill until chicken is cooked through.

Makes 4 servings

- **Preheat barbecue**
- **8 bamboo skewers soaked in water or 8 metal skewers**

8	small red potatoes (about 1 lb/500 g)	8
3 tbsp	liquid honey	45 mL
2 tbsp	Dijon mustard	30 mL
1 tbsp	freshly squeezed lemon juice	15 mL
1/2 tsp	dried thyme	2 mL
1/4 tsp	freshly ground black pepper	1 mL
1 lb	boneless skinless pheasant breasts, cut into 16 strips	500 g
8	large mushrooms, stems removed, caps halved	8
16	cherry tomatoes	16

1. Cut potatoes in half. Put in saucepan with cold water to cover. Bring to a boil, reduce heat and simmer 10 minutes or until almost tender. Drain and set aside.
2. In a bowl, whisk together honey, mustard, lemon juice, thyme and pepper. Add the pheasant and mushrooms and toss to coat in marinade. Marinate 30 minutes at room temperature.
3. Alternately thread the pheasant, mushroom halves, tomatoes and potatoes on skewers, discarding the remaining marinade. Grill the kebabs on a covered grill for 8 minutes, turning occasionally, until pheasant is just cooked to medium-rare.

Health Tip

- Barbecuing meat increases the acidifying effect of the protein. To regain pH balance, increase your intake of alkalizing foods over the next few days.

Nutrients per serving	
Calories	468
Fat	4 g
Sodium	285 mg
Carbohydrate	73 g
Fiber	7 g
Protein	36 g
Calcium	50 mg
Magnesium	111 mg
Potassium	2144 mg

Fish Fillets with Chile Pepper Pesto

Here is an easy fish dish, full of the savory spices and feisty flavors of the West. Use boneless, skinless white fish fillets for this speedy but impressively flavored feast.

Makes 4 to 6 servings

Tip

Ancho or poblano peppers are about 4 inches (10 cm) long, cone-shaped, with a mild, almost raisin-like flavor. You can substitute the slightly hotter pasillas in this dish; they're also mild but are longer and narrower. You can find both dried anchos and pasillas in packages in the produce section of most major supermarkets.

Health Tip

- If you have a GI condition that is aggravated by seeds, omit the toasted pine nuts from this recipe.

Nutrients per serving (1 of 6)	
Calories	270
Fat	11 g
Sodium	296 mg
Carbohydrate	8 g
Fiber	3 g
Protein	33 g
Calcium	62 mg
Magnesium	77 mg
Potassium	947 mg

- **Preheat oven to 450°F (230°C)**
- **Food processor**
- **Large rimmed baking sheet, oiled**

3	dried ancho or pasilla chile peppers	3
2 tbsp	canola oil	30 mL
1	onion, chopped	1
1⁄4 cup	toasted pine nuts	60 mL
3	cloves garlic	3
1	large red bell pepper, chopped	1
2 tbsp	orange juice	30 mL
1 tsp	freshly squeezed lemon juice	5 mL
1⁄2 tsp	salt	2 mL
1 cup	fresh cilantro leaves	250 mL
2 lbs	fish fillets (such as snapper, halibut, perch or sole)	1 kg
	Lime wedges, chopped cilantro and Mexican-style rice	

1. Soak dried chiles in hot water for 30 minutes or until softened. Drain and discard seeds and stems. Set aside.
2. In a skillet, heat oil over medium-high heat. Cook onion for 8 minutes or until golden. Place in food processor with chiles, pine nuts, garlic, red pepper, orange juice, lemon juice and salt. Process to form a paste. Add cilantro and pulse until coarsely chopped.
3. Place fish fillets in a single layer on prepared baking sheet. Spread pesto over fish, smoothing it over the entire surface. Set aside for 10 minutes at room temperature to marinate.
4. Bake in preheated oven for 10 minutes per 1 inch (2.5 cm) of thickness, or until fish flakes easily when tested with a fork. Serve sprinkled with cilantro, with lime wedges and rice on the side.

Health Tip

- If you have a GI condition that is made worse by spicy ingredients, omit the dried chiles and set the hot sauce on the table for others to season to taste.

Simple Chinese Steamed Fish

This is an extremely simple way to cook fish, taking but minutes of preparation time. Whole or filleted fresh- and saltwater fish work well here, the best being those with a fairly delicate flavor and flesh, such as walleye (pickerel), whitefish, tilapia, flounder, halibut and small grouper.

Makes 4 servings

Tip

If you don't have a steamer (or have one that's too small to hold the fish plate or platter), a wok with a cover makes a great steamer, as does a large wide pot such as a Dutch oven. Simply rest the plate on a small rack or bowl inside the pot. Put a few fingers' depth of water in the pot and you have a steamer! Just make sure the bowl acting as a base for the plate also has some water in it (to avoid breakage).

1 to 2 lbs	whole fish or 1 lb (500 g) fish fillet or steak	500 g to 1 kg
1/4 to 1/2 tsp	salt	1 to 2 mL
1/4 tsp	freshly ground black or white pepper	1 mL
1 tsp	Chinese rice wine, sake or dry sherry (optional)	5 mL
2 tbsp	julienned gingerroot	30 mL
2 tsp	julienned finger chile pepper (optional)	10 mL
1 tbsp	soy sauce (GF, if needed)	15 mL
3 tbsp	julienned green onion	45 mL
2 tbsp	vegetable oil	30 mL
	Fresh cilantro sprigs	

1. If steaming whole fish, make a few cuts into the flesh on each side. Rub fish with salt, pepper and rice wine (if using). Put on a heatproof plate; cover with ginger and chile pepper (if using). Place in steamer over boiling water; cook, covered, over medium-high heat for 20 to 30 minutes or until cooked through (check the fish by making a small cut to the bone in the thickest area).
2. Remove plate from steamer and, if there is an excess, pour off some of the liquid that has accumulated on the plate. Pour soy sauce over fish and cover with green onion julienne. In a small saucepan, heat oil over high heat; when very hot, pour over fish, scalding the green onions (be careful: it may splatter a little). Garnish with coriander and serve immediately.

Nutrients per serving	
Calories	184
Fat	9 g
Sodium	363 mg
Carbohydrate	1 g
Fiber	0 g
Protein	24 g
Calcium	41 mg
Magnesium	39 mg
Potassium	501 mg

Health Tips

- Use reduced-sodium soy sauce to reduce the sodium level in this recipe.
- Steaming is one of the healthiest ways to cook fish, reducing the acidifying effect of the dish.

Variations

Mix 1 tbsp (15 mL) julienned Chinese or regular celery with the ginger.

A few drops of sesame oil can be drizzled over the fish before serving.

If you are on a low-fat diet, add soy sauce, two-thirds of the green onion and 1 tsp (5 mL) oil to fish before steaming. After fish is cooked, garnish with the remaining raw green onion and coriander sprigs. If desired, the juice can be poured off the fish and thickened with ½ tsp (2 mL) cornstarch dissolved in 1 tsp (5 mL) water.

Halibut with Beets and Beet Greens

Fresh halibut has a mild flavor of the sea, and fresh beets and their vibrant greens make a breathtaking accompaniment. A quick gremolata of orange zest, garlic and parsley simultaneously unites the dish's components and elevates the final result.

Makes 4 servings

Tip

Sea bass, cod or any other firm white fish fillets may be used in place of the halibut.

Nutrients per serving	
Calories	290
Fat	11 g
Sodium	157 mg
Carbohydrate	12 g
Fiber	3 g
Protein	36 g
Calcium	110 mg
Magnesium	64 mg
Potassium	762 mg

- **Preheat oven to 450°F (230°C)**
- **Large rimmed baking sheet, sprayed with nonstick cooking spray (preferably olive oil)**

Gremolata

1	clove garlic, minced	1
1/2 cup	packed fresh flat-leaf (Italian) parsley leaves, chopped	125 mL
1 tbsp	finely grated orange zest	15 mL

4	beets (about 2 inches/5 cm in diameter), with green tops attached	4
1/2 cup	thinly sliced shallots	125 mL
1/2 tsp	fine sea salt, divided	2 mL
6 tsp	extra virgin olive oil, divided	30 mL
4	skinless Pacific halibut fillets (each about 5 oz/150 g)	4

1. *Gremolata:* In a small bowl, combine garlic, parsley and orange zest. Set aside.
2. Trim leaves and stems from beets, reserving leaves and tender portion of stems, and scrub beets. Rinse and spin-dry beet greens and tender stems, then coarsely chop and set aside.
3. Place beets in a medium microwave-safe bowl and add enough water to cover halfway. Cover and microwave on High for 8 to 10 minutes or until just tender. Uncover, drain and let cool slightly. Peel beets and cut into 1/4-inch (0.5 cm) slices.
4. In the same bowl, combine sliced beets, shallots, half the salt, 1 tbsp (15 mL) gremolata and 2 tsp (10 mL) oil. Spread in a single layer on half of the prepared baking sheet.

Tip

The beets may be roasted instead of microwaved. Preheat oven to 400°F (200°C). Wrap each beet in foil. Place beets directly on oven rack and roast for 1½ hours or until fork-tender. Let cool slightly, then peel and slice beets.

5. Toss beet greens with 2 tsp (10 mL) oil. Mound on other side of baking sheet.
6. Sprinkle fish with the remaining salt and place on top of the beet greens. Brush fish with the remaining oil and sprinkle with 2 tbsp (30 mL) gremolata.
7. Roast in preheated oven for about 8 minutes or until fish is opaque and flakes easily when tested with a fork.
8. Divide fish, greens and beets among plates. Sprinkle with the remaining gremolata.

Poached Salmon

Salmon, with delicate pink flesh and mild flavor, is by far the most popular fish, especially in summer.

Makes 6 servings

Tip

If you would prefer to bake the salmon, pour the simmering Court Bouillon into a large ovenproof baking dish and arrange salmon in bouillon in a single layer. Bake in a preheated 350°F (180°C) oven for 10 to 15 minutes or until fish flakes easily when tested with the tip of a sharp knife.

Nutrients per serving	
Calories	240
Fat	8 g
Sodium	596 mg
Carbohydrate	2 g
Fiber	1 g
Protein	35 g
Calcium	23 mg
Magnesium	49 mg
Potassium	664 mg

7 to 8 cups	Court Bouillon (see recipe, opposite)	1.75 to 2 L
6	salmon fillets (each about 6 oz/175 g), skin removed	6
6	small sprigs fresh dill	6
1	lemon, thinly sliced	1

1. In a large skillet, heat Court Bouillon over medium heat until simmering.
2. Arrange salmon in bouillon in a single layer. Simmer until fish flakes easily when tested with the tip of a sharp knife, 10 to 15 minutes. Lift salmon fillets from poaching broth with a slotted spoon and transfer to a cooling rack to remove excess liquid. Serve warm or chilled and garnish with dill and lemon.

Variation

Poached Shrimp: Bring Court Bouillon to a simmer. Add 2 lbs (1 kg) shrimp in shell. Bring back to a simmer and cook until pink and just firm to the touch when pinched, 3 to 5 minutes for medium-size shrimp. When cool enough to handle, remove shell and devein.

Court Bouillon

Use this flavorful broth to poach fish, seafood or vegetables, such as mushrooms, leeks or shallots, that you plan to serve cold. Remove the cooked fish or vegetables from the broth and reduce to make a flavorful glaze, if you like.

Makes 7 to 8 cups (1.75 to 2 L)

8 cups	water	2 L
½ cup	dry white wine (or ¼ cup/60 mL Pernod)	125 mL
½	lemon, thinly sliced	½
2	shallots, sliced (or ½ onion, sliced)	2
1	bay leaf	1
4	sprigs fresh flat-leaf (Italian) parsley	4
8	whole black peppercorns	8
1 tsp	fennel seeds	5 mL
1 tsp	sea salt	5 mL

1. In a large pot over medium-high heat, combine water, wine, lemon, shallots, bay leaf, parsley, peppercorns, fennel seeds and salt. Bring to a boil. Reduce heat to low and simmer for 20 minutes. Strain and let cool.
2. Use at once or freeze for later use. Store in a covered container in the refrigerator and use within 2 days or freeze for up to 6 months.

Nutrients per 1 cup (250 mL)	
Calories	16
Fat	0 g
Sodium	351 mg
Carbohydrate	1 g
Fiber	0 g
Protein	0 g
Calcium	6 mg
Magnesium	2 mg
Potassium	20 mg

Salmon with Spinach

Salmon will remain moist using this cooking procedure. Layer spinach and mushrooms, then top with salmon. Bake on high heat for 10 minutes per inch (2.5 cm) thickness of the fish. Due to the extra thickness of fish and vegetables, you may need a few extra minutes of baking time.

Makes 4 servings

Tip

For ease of serving fish fillets, cut them into serving-size pieces before baking.

Variations

In place of the salmon, any white or firm-fleshed fish, such as turbot, swordfish, halibut or tuna, will work.

Sprinkle toasted sesame seeds over the fish before baking to give it a pleasing crunch.

Nutrients per serving	
Calories	427
Fat	14 g
Sodium	291 mg
Carbohydrate	3 g
Fiber	2 g
Protein	68 g
Calcium	114 mg
Magnesium	140 mg
Potassium	1431 mg

- **Preheat oven to 450°F (230°C)**
- **Shallow oblong baking pan, greased**

1	package (10 oz/300 g) frozen chopped spinach, thawed	1
1 tbsp	grated gingerroot	15 mL
2	large mushrooms, thickly sliced	2
	Salt and freshly ground black pepper	
4	salmon steaks or fillets	4

1. In a sieve, drain spinach, pressing with a spoon to remove excess liquid. Discard liquid. Spread spinach in bottom of prepared pan in a shape resembling the size of the fish. Arrange gingerroot and mushrooms evenly over spinach. Season lightly with salt and pepper. Add fish. Sprinkle lightly with salt and pepper.
2. Cover pan loosely with a tent of foil. Bake for 15 minutes or until fish is opaque and flakes easily when tested with a fork.

Health Tips

- Baking salmon is less acidifying than barbecuing it.
- If you have a GI condition that is aggravated by seeds, omit the toasted sesame seeds.

Rainbow Trout Baked on Cedar with Maple, Mustard and Dill

This recipe requires a cedar board between 1/4 and 1/2 inch (0.5 and 1 cm) thick. Some stores that sell barbecue accessories now stock different woods for smoking, or visit a store that carries wood. Check that the wood has not been soaked in any chemicals. Soak the board for at least 6 hours prior to using.

Makes 4 servings

Tip

In place of the cedar, try another hardwood. Different woods bring unique flavors to the dish: cedar and hickory are mild and smoky; cherrywood is sweet and fruity; apple wood is sharp and tangy; maple and alder are mildly sweet; oak is spicy. Don't use softwood, though — it contains too much resin.

Nutrients per serving	
Calories	273
Fat	7 g
Sodium	257 mg
Carbohydrate	29 g
Fiber	0 g
Protein	23 g
Calcium	71 mg
Magnesium	37 mg
Potassium	526 mg

- **Cedar plank**

4	rainbow trout fillets (about 4 oz/125 g each), all fine bones removed	4
2 tbsp	Dijon mustard	30 mL
1/2 cup	pure maple syrup	125 mL
2 tbsp	chopped fresh dill	30 mL
1 tsp	Worcestershire sauce (GF, if needed)	5 mL

1. Set up the barbecue, piling 10 coals on 2 sides away from the center of the barbecue. Light the barbecue and allow the coals to burn down. (If you are using a gas barbecue, ignite burner on one side, set to high and let it heat up; place board on unlit side of barbecue and reduce heat to medium-high; continue to cook as for a charcoal fire.) When you can hold your hand 8 inches (20 cm) above the coals for 5 seconds, you have a slow fire and are ready to proceed.
2. In a bowl, mix together mustard, maple syrup, dill and Worcestershire sauce.
3. Lay trout fillets onto cedar plank. Liberally brush or spoon mustard marinade over trout.
4. Place cedar plank in the center of barbecue (or unlit side of a gas barbecue). Cover with lid or make a tent foil over the barbecue. Let fish cook for 12 to 15 minutes or until opaque.
5. Serve with a drizzle of the remaining warmed marinade.

This recipe courtesy of Peter Ochitwa.

Health Tip

- Barbecuing increases the acidifying effect of a meal, so increase your intake of alkalizing foods for the next few days to regain your pH balance.

Grilled Tuna with Roasted Pepper Sauce

An exceptionally tasty main dish for special occasions.

Makes 4 servings

Tip

Choose tuna that is exceptionally fresh, as it cannot be cooked very long or the lean flesh dries out. Never grill tuna beyond medium-rare. It is better to cut into the tuna steak and check it rather than risking it being overcooked. The center should be red (for rare) to light pink (for medium-rare) — just like a steak. If the tuna is white throughout, then it is overdone.

Nutrients per serving	
Calories	570
Fat	13 g
Sodium	187 mg
Carbohydrate	14 g
Fiber	2 g
Protein	95 g
Calcium	184 mg
Magnesium	173 mg
Potassium	2122 mg

- **Preheat barbecue grill or broiler**
- **Blender or food processor**

2	red bell peppers (or 1 red and 1 yellow or green pepper), cut in half and seeded	2
4	shallots (or ½ red onion, cut into 2 or 3 thick slices)	4
1	head garlic (unpeeled)	1
4 to 6	red and/or green finger chile peppers	4 to 6
2	stalks fresh cilantro (including stems), finely chopped	2
4	anchovies	4
2 to 6	dried red chile peppers	2 to 6
1 tbsp	freshly squeezed lime juice	15 mL
½ tsp	granulated sugar	2 mL
2 tbsp	peanut or vegetable oil	30 mL
4	tuna or swordfish steaks	4
	Salt and freshly ground black pepper	
	Lime wedges and sprigs of fresh cilantro	

1. Put red peppers (skin side down), shallots, garlic head and finger chiles on hot grill or under broiler. Cook peppers until skin blackens; cool, then peel and cut into julienne strips. Cook shallots until browned and heated through. Cook garlic until all the cloves feel soft when pressed; cool, then squeeze out the flesh. Cook chiles until skins are half-blackened; cool, then remove seeds.
2. In blender, combine shallots, garlic, finger chiles, cilantro and anchovies; chop until a coarse paste forms.
3. In a skillet, over medium heat, toast dried red chiles until fragrant and slightly darkened; grind. Mix with garlic-chile paste.

Tips

The sauce can be prepared ahead of time; just make sure it is fully at room temperature before serving.

The finger chiles are necessary, but the dried chiles can be adjusted to taste or omitted altogether for a mild sauce.

4. In a small bowl, combine paste, red pepper strips, lime juice and sugar until well mixed. Taste; adjust balance of sweet-and-sour by adding extra lime juice or sugar. Stir in 1 tbsp (15 mL) oil; set aside.
5. Lightly salt and pepper the fish and brush with oil. Grill or broil on both sides until rare for tuna, or just cooked through for swordfish. Put a generous dollop of sauce on each steak and garnish with lime wedges and sprigs of cilantro.

Variation

Thai basil is very good in this sauce; add 12 to 15 finely julienned or chopped basil leaves to the sauce with oil and garnish the fish with the basil flowers (regular or purple basil would also be fine). Or 2 tbsp (30 mL) of chopped mint is a delicious addition to the sauce, accompanied with just a touch more lime juice and sugar.

Health Tips

- If you have a GI condition that is aggravated by hot or spicy foods, set aside the chile peppers and put the hot sauce on the table for others to season to taste.
- This is an acidifying meal, so increase your alkalizing foods for the next few days to balance your pH.

Clams Steamed with Sake and Lemon

This is a very simple and quick Japanese-style method of cooking clams. Use any type of clam that lends itself to steaming, such as Pacific Manila clams, Atlantic soft-shell or razor clams, or littlenecks. Mussels can also be cooked in this manner.

Makes 4 servings

Tip

The Japanese pepper called sansho is not absolutely necessary, but adds a little more dimension to the flavor of the sauce. It is available at Japanese and some Korean grocers and is used in a wide range of Japanese dishes.

3 lbs	clams	1.5 kg
6	thin slices lemon	6
1 tbsp	finely julienned gingerroot	15 mL
2⁄3 cup	sake	150 mL
1⁄2 tsp	Japanese (sansho) pepper (optional)	2 mL

1. Clean the clams by rinsing under cold water and wiping with a cloth.
2. Place the clams in a saucepan, cover with lemon slices and ginger. Pour in the sake; sprinkle with Japanese pepper (if using). Cover the pot and cook over high heat until the clams open; discard any that remain closed. Stir once and serve, providing a soup spoon for the flavorful broth.

Health Tip

- Lemon, ginger and Japanese (sansho) pepper are all alkalizing foods that help to balance your diet.

Nutrients per serving	
Calories	349
Fat	3 g
Sodium	2046 mg
Carbohydrate	15 g
Fiber	0 g
Protein	50 g
Calcium	138 mg
Magnesium	69 mg
Potassium	187 mg

Mini Crab Quinoa Cakes

Earthy quinoa is the perfect foil for lemony crab. This sophisticated starter is deceptively easy to make, and the layered flavors will impress your guests.

Makes 2 dozen cakes

Tip

To prepare 1 cup (250 mL) cooked quinoa, combine ⅓ cup (75 mL) quinoa and ⅔ cup (150 mL) water in a medium saucepan. Bring to a boil over medium-high heat. Reduce heat to low, cover and simmer for 12 to 15 minutes or until water is just barely absorbed. Cover and let stand for 5 to 6 minutes. Fluff with a fork and let cool completely.

Nutrients per cake	
Calories	41
Fat	1 g
Sodium	196 mg
Carbohydrate	3 g
Fiber	0 g
Protein	4 g
Calcium	22 mg
Magnesium	13 mg
Potassium	79 mg

½ tsp	fine sea salt	2 mL
¼ tsp	freshly cracked black pepper	1 mL
¼ cup	olive oil mayonnaise	60 mL
2 tbsp	Dijon mustard	30 mL
1 tsp	finely grated lemon zest	5 mL
1½ tbsp	freshly squeezed lemon juice	22 mL
1 cup	cooked quinoa (see tip, at left), cooled	250 mL
¾ cup	panko or dry bread crumbs (GF, if needed)	175 mL
½ cup	drained roasted red bell peppers, chopped	125 mL
¼ cup	finely chopped green onions	60 mL
2	large egg whites, lightly beaten	2
1 lb	cooked backfin (lump) crabmeat, drained	500 g
	Olive oil	

1. In a large bowl, whisk together salt, pepper, mayonnaise, mustard, lemon zest and lemon juice. Stir in quinoa, panko, roasted peppers, green onions and egg whites. Gently fold in crab, being careful not to break it up much.
2. Divide crab mixture into 24 equal portions. Form each portion into a ½-inch (1 cm) thick patty and place on a plate. Cover loosely and refrigerate for at least 30 minutes, until chilled, or for up to 4 hours.
3. In a large nonstick skillet, heat 2 tsp (10 mL) oil over medium heat. Add 6 patties and cook for 2 to 3 minutes per side or until golden. Transfer to a plate lined with paper towels. Repeat with the remaining patties, adding more oil and adjusting heat as necessary between batches. Serve warm.

Shrimp Cakes with Cilantro Yogurt Sauce

Here, a simple sauce made from yogurt, cilantro and jalapeño enhances Indian-spiced shrimp and quinoa cakes to great effect.

Makes 2 dozen cakes

Tip

To prepare 3 cups (750 mL) cooked quinoa, combine 1 cup (250 mL) quinoa and 2 cups (500 mL) water in a medium saucepan. Bring to a boil over medium-high heat. Reduce heat to low, cover and simmer for 12 to 15 minutes or until water is just barely absorbed. Cover and let stand for 5 to 6 minutes. Fluff with a fork and let cool completely. Reserve the leftover ½ cup (125 mL) cooked quinoa for another purpose.

Nutrients per cake	
Calories	44
Fat	1 g
Sodium	118 mg
Carbohydrate	5 g
Fiber	1 g
Protein	4 g
Calcium	35 mg
Magnesium	19 mg
Potassium	90 mg

- **Food processor**

Cilantro Yogurt Sauce

1 cup	packed fresh cilantro leaves, chopped	250 mL
2 tsp	minced seeded jalapeño pepper	10 mL
1 cup	plain yogurt	250 mL
	Fine sea salt and freshly ground black pepper	

Shrimp Cakes

1 lb	medium shrimp, peeled and deveined	500 g
2½ cups	cooked quinoa (see tip, at left), cooled	625 mL
1 cup	chopped green onions (about 1 bunch)	250 mL
2 tsp	garam masala	10 mL
	Vegetable oil	

1. *Sauce:* In a small bowl, whisk together cilantro, jalapeño and yogurt. Season to taste with salt and pepper. Cover and refrigerate until ready to serve.
2. *Cakes:* In food processor, combine shrimp, quinoa, green onions and garam masala; pulse until texture is coarse. Season with salt and pepper.
3. Divide shrimp mixture into 24 equal portions. Form each portion into a ½-inch (1 cm) thick patty.
4. In a large nonstick skillet, heat 2 tsp (10 mL) oil over medium heat. Add 6 patties and cook for 2 to 3 minutes per side or until golden. Transfer to a plate lined with paper towels. Repeat with the remaining patties, adding more oil and adjusting heat as necessary between batches. Serve warm, with yogurt sauce.

Vegetarian Mains

Spring Greens Pie

When there's arugula and spinach in the garden and young dandelions in the lawn, this tasty dish makes a great lunch or fast supper. Without the crust, it's also relatively low in fat.

Makes 6 servings

Health Tip

- If you are sensitive to gluten, replace the fresh bread crumbs with a GF variety.

- **Preheat oven to 375°F (190°C)**
- **9-inch (23 cm) pie plate**

2 tbsp	olive oil	30 mL
1	onion, minced	1
2	cloves garlic, minced	2
12 cups	chopped Swiss chard (about 1½ lbs/750 g)	3 L
5 cups	chopped arugula (about 8 oz/250 g)	1.25 L
4½ cups	chopped dandelion greens (about 12 oz/375 g)	1.125 L
2	small zucchini, grated	2
½	yellow bell pepper, chopped	½
½ cup	chopped fresh parsley	125 mL
⅓ cup	chopped fresh basil	75 mL
½ tsp	salt	2 mL
¼ tsp	freshly ground black pepper	1 mL
3	extra-large eggs, lightly beaten	3
¼ cup	freshly grated Parmesan cheese	60 mL
¼ cup	shredded Swiss cheese	60 mL
¼ cup	fresh bread crumbs	60 mL

1. In a large saucepan or stockpot, heat 1 tbsp (5 mL) oil over medium heat. Add onion and garlic; cook for 5 minutes or until tender. Stir in Swiss chard, arugula, dandelion greens, zucchini, yellow pepper, parsley, basil, salt and pepper; cover and cook, stirring occasionally, for 10 minutes or until tender.
2. Remove cover and cook, stirring often, for 20 minutes longer or until all liquid is evaporated. Transfer to a bowl and cool slightly.
3. Beat the eggs into the greens and pour into pie plate. Sprinkle with cheeses. Mix bread crumbs with the remaining oil, then sprinkle over pie.
4. Bake in preheated oven for 25 to 30 minutes. Let stand at least 10 minutes before serving.

Nutrients per serving	
Calories	172
Fat	10 g
Sodium	499 mg
Carbohydrate	13 g
Fiber	4 g
Protein	10 g
Calcium	256 mg
Magnesium	102 mg
Potassium	739 mg

Zucchini Boats Filled with Ratatouille and Herbs

This wonderful vegetable dish includes a great selection of fresh herbs.

Makes 4 servings

Health Tip

- Fresh herbs increase the alkalizing effect of this recipe.

5	zucchini, 4 cut in half lengthways, 1 diced	5
4 tbsp	olive oil	60 mL
1	onion, chopped	1
2 tbsp	minced garlic	30 mL
1	large eggplant, diced	1
1	red bell pepper, finely chopped	1
1	green bell pepper, finely chopped	1
3	tomatoes, diced	3
1 tbsp	chopped fresh rosemary	15 mL
1 tbsp	chopped fresh thyme	15 mL
1 tbsp	chopped fresh oregano	15 mL
1 tbsp	chopped fresh basil	15 mL
1 tbsp	chopped fresh parsley	15 mL
2 tbsp	balsamic vinegar	30 mL
	Salt and freshly ground black pepper	
8	sprigs fresh marjoram	8

1. With a vegetable peeler or sharp knife, carefully shave the rounded side of the 4 halved zucchinis so that they will rest flat. With a melon baller, scoop out the flesh. Reserve scooped flesh for the ratatouille.
2. In a large skillet, heat 3 tbsp (45 mL) oil over medium heat. Add onion and garlic; cook until softened, about 5 minutes. Add eggplant; cook about 10 minutes. Add diced zucchini, scooped zucchini flesh, peppers and tomatoes; cook 5 minutes or until softened. Add rosemary, thyme, oregano, basil, parsley and vinegar. Season to taste with salt and pepper. Reduce heat and simmer for about 15 minutes.
3. Meanwhile, in another skillet, heat the remaining oil over medium heat. Add zucchini boats and cook until softened (or grill for about 5 minutes on each side).
4. Spoon the hot ratatouille into the zucchini boats and garnish with marjoram.

This recipe courtesy of Anthony Nuth and Mark Howatt.

Nutrients per serving	
Calories	257
Fat	16 g
Sodium	27 mg
Carbohydrate	26 g
Fiber	10 g
Protein	5 g
Calcium	127 mg
Magnesium	79 mg
Potassium	1133 mg

Chinatown Takeout Curry

This vegetarian recipe is an introduction to the wide world of Chinese curry sauces. It tastes of nostalgia.

Makes 4 to 6 servings

Tips

This recipe makes about 4 cups (1 L) curry sauce. That's enough to accommodate the addition of 1 lb (500 g) of protein, such as cubed tofu. Alternatively, you can pour any leftovers over sautéed vegetables or use the sauce as you would a gravy.

For the liveliest flavor, make sure your curry powder is fresh. The aroma should be pleasantly pungent, not faded. Its shelf life is 2 to 4 months; check the label for a best-before date.

Nutrients per serving (1 of 6)	
Calories	224
Fat	13 g
Sodium	691 mg
Carbohydrate	23 g
Fiber	4 g
Protein	3 g
Calcium	99 mg
Magnesium	17 mg
Potassium	240 mg

- **Wok**

Sauce

4	large cloves garlic, minced	4
2 tbsp	curry powder	30 mL
2 tbsp	soy sauce (GF, if needed)	30 mL
2 tsp	tomato paste	10 mL
2 tsp	puréed gingerroot	10 mL
2 tsp	granulated sugar	10 mL
1 tsp	Chinese five-spice powder	5 mL
½ tsp	cayenne pepper	2 mL
¼ cup	cornstarch	60 mL
4¼ cups	ready-to-use vegetable broth (GF, if needed), divided	1.05 L
¼ cup	vegetable oil	60 mL
1	large shallot, finely chopped	1
	Kosher or coarse sea salt	

Curry

1 tbsp	vegetable oil	15 mL
3½ cups	trimmed and chopped Chinese celery (4 oz/125 g)	875 mL
1	onion, cut into 1-inch (2.5 cm) chunks	1
1	green bell pepper, cut into 1-inch (2.5 cm) chunks	1
2	carrots (4 oz/125 g total), cut diagonally into ¼-inch (0.5 cm) thick slices and blanched (see tip, opposite)	2
½ tsp	kosher salt or coarse sea salt	2 mL
1	can (14 oz/398 mL) baby corn, drained, rinsed and cut into 1-inch (2.5 cm) pieces	1

1. *Sauce:* In a small bowl, combine garlic, curry powder, soy sauce, tomato paste, ginger, sugar, five-spice powder and cayenne. Set aside.
2. In another small bowl, combine cornstarch and ¼ cup (60 mL) broth. Set aside.

Tips

To blanch carrot slices, cook them in a pot of boiling water for 1 minute, then drain and immediately rinse with cold water to stop the cooking.

Make the sauce just before you plan to use it, and do not cover it once it is done. It will thin as it sits. To rethicken leftover sauce, combine equal amounts of cornstarch and water (about 1 tsp/5 mL each) and stir into the sauce while warming it over medium heat. Bring it to a boil to activate the thickening power of the cornstarch.

3. In a medium saucepan over medium heat, heat oil until shimmery. Add shallot and cook, stirring often, for 1 to 2 minutes, until softened. Add prepared spice paste and stir in for 30 to 60 seconds. Add the remaining broth and stir, scraping up brown bits from bottom of pan. When mixture comes to a simmer, reduce heat to medium-low and cook for about 15 minutes, until shallot is very tender. Stir cornstarch mixture to loosen, then gradually add to the pan, stirring well to combine. Simmer for about 2 minutes, until sauce is thick and bubbly. Remove pan from heat but do not cover it (see tip, at left). Season to taste with salt. Set aside.

4. *Curry:* Heat wok over medium-high heat for 1 minute. Add oil, swirling to coat bottom of pan. Add Chinese celery, onion, green pepper, carrots and salt. Stir-fry for about 5 minutes, until vegetables are tender-crisp. Stir in baby corn for 1 minute, until heated through. Remove from heat and pour sauce, to taste, over vegetables (you may have some left over). Serve immediately.

Variation

Try adding about 1 cup (250 mL) mushrooms or snow peas — or any other vegetable you fancy — to the curry in step 4.

Health Tips

- Replace the ready-made vegetable stock with a homemade version to reduce the sodium in this recipe.
- If you have a GI condition that is aggravated by hot or spicy foods, omit the cayenne pepper and serve hot sauce at the table for others to season to taste.

Chard-Studded Stew with Cornmeal Dumplings

In terms of old-fashioned goodness, it doesn't get much better than this lusciously rich and flavorful comfort food.

Makes 6 servings

Tips

If you are halving this recipe, be sure to use a small (1½ to 2 quart) slow cooker.

Like spinach, Swiss chard can be very gritty, so swish it around in a basin of lukewarm water before rinsing under cold running water to ensure all grit is removed. Unless your chard is very young, you'll need to remove the thick vein running up the center of the leaf before chopping.

Nutrients per serving	
Calories	217
Fat	8 g
Sodium	1072 mg
Carbohydrate	33 g
Fiber	4 g
Protein	6 g
Calcium	185 mg
Magnesium	46 mg
Potassium	561 mg

- **Medium to large (3½- to 5-quart) slow cooker**

1 tbsp	vegetable oil	15 mL
2	onions, finely chopped	2
4	carrots, diced	4
4	stalks celery, diced	4
4	cloves garlic, minced	4
1 tsp	dried thyme	5 mL
1 tsp	salt	5 mL
½ tsp	cracked black peppercorns	2 mL
2 cups	ready-to-use vegetable broth	500 mL
¼ cup	white miso	60 mL
4 cups	packed chopped Swiss chard leaves (see tip, at left)	1 L

Cornmeal Dumplings

¾ cup	all-purpose flour	175 mL
¼ cup	fine cornmeal	60 mL
1½ tsp	baking powder	7 mL
¼ tsp	salt	1 mL
½ cup	warm milk	125 mL
2 tbsp	melted butter	30 mL

1. In a skillet, heat oil over medium heat. Add onions, carrots and celery and cook, stirring, until softened, about 7 minutes. Add garlic, thyme, salt and peppercorns and cook, stirring, for 1 minute. Stir in broth. Transfer to slow cooker stoneware.
2. Cover and cook on Low for 5 hours or on High for 2½ hours. Turn heat to High, if necessary. Add miso and stir until it dissolves. Add chard, in batches, stirring after each addition to submerge the leaves in the liquid. Cover and cook for 20 minutes, until mixture returns to a simmer.

Tip

To make ahead, complete step 1. Cover and refrigerate for up to 2 days. When you're ready to cook, complete the recipe.

3. *Dumplings:* Meanwhile, in a bowl, combine flour, cornmeal, baking powder and salt. Make a well in the center. Pour in milk and butter and mix with a fork, just until mixture comes together. Drop dough by spoonfuls onto vegetables. Cover and cook on High for 30 minutes, until dumplings are cooked through.

Health Tip

- Replace the ready-made vegetable stock with a homemade version to reduce the sodium in this recipe.

Fennel-Spiked Lentil Cobbler with Red Pepper and Goat Cheese

The mild licorice flavor of the fennel combines beautifully with the hint of heat from the black peppercorns and the nicely acidic balsamic vinegar in this delicious casserole. The crisp crumbs provide texture and the goat cheese adds a pleasant bit of tang. Add a simple green salad to complete the meal.

Makes 6 servings

Tips

If you plan to serve this in the stoneware, make sure to use a large oval slow cooker. If you prefer a more elegant presentation, transfer the mixture to an ovenproof serving dish before adding the topping.

This amount of peppercorns adds a nice bite to the lentils. If you prefer a milder result, reduce the quantity.

To make ahead, complete step 1. Cover and refrigerate for up to 2 days. When you're ready to cook, complete the recipe.

Nutrients per serving	
Calories	267
Fat	8 g
Sodium	436 mg
Carbohydrate	37 g
Fiber	7 g
Protein	14 g
Calcium	109 mg
Magnesium	43 mg
Potassium	474 mg

- **Medium to large (4- to 5-quart) slow cooker**

1 tbsp	olive oil	15 mL
2	onions, diced	2
1	large fennel bulb, trimmed, cored and diced	1
4	cloves garlic, minced	4
1 tsp	dried thyme	5 mL
1 tsp	cracked black peppercorns (see tip, at left)	5 mL
1/2 tsp	salt	2 mL
1 cup	dried brown or green lentils, rinsed	250 mL
1 tbsp	balsamic vinegar	15 mL
3 cups	ready-to-use vegetable broth (GF, if needed)	750 mL
1	red bell pepper, finely chopped	1
2 cups	fresh bread crumbs (GF, if needed)	500 mL
4 oz	soft goat cheese, crumbled	125 g

1. In a skillet, heat oil over medium heat. Add onions and fennel and cook, stirring, until softened, about 5 minutes. Add garlic, thyme, peppercorns and salt and cook, stirring, for 1 minute. Add lentils and toss until well coated. Stir in vinegar and broth and bring to a boil. Transfer to slow cooker stoneware.
2. Cover and cook on Low for 6 hours or on High for 3 hours, until lentils are tender. Stir in bell pepper. Cover and cook on High for 15 minutes, until pepper is tender.
3. Meanwhile, preheat broiler. In a bowl, combine bread crumbs and goat cheese. Stir until combined. Spread as best you can over lentil mixture and broil until crumbs and cheese begin to brown. Serve immediately.

Black Bean Chili

Chickpeas and black beans add wholesome flavor and fiber to this twist on classic chili.

Makes 4 to 6 servings

Tip

Serve this robust chili over baked sweet or regular potatoes for a main dish or with whole-grain nachos for an appetizer or party dish.

Variation

Substitute 2 cups (500 mL) of any cooked beans for the black beans.

2 tbsp	olive oil	30 mL
1 cup	chopped onions	250 mL
3	cloves garlic, minced	3
1½ cups	chopped red bell peppers	375 mL
2	whole chile peppers, crushed	2
2 tsp	ground cumin	10 mL
1	can (28 oz/796 mL) diced tomatoes, with juice	1
1	can (19 oz/540 mL) black beans, drained and rinsed	1
1	can (19 oz/540 mL) chickpeas, drained and rinsed	1
2 tbsp	dried thyme	30 mL
1 tbsp	dried savory	15 mL
2 tbsp	chopped fresh parsley	30 mL

1. In a large skillet, heat oil over medium heat. Add onions, garlic, peppers and chiles; cook for 5 minutes or until soft.
2. Stir in cumin, tomatoes, black beans, chickpeas, thyme and savory. Bring to a boil; simmer for 5 minutes. Stir in parsley and serve.

Health Tips

- If you have a GI condition that is aggravated by hot or spicy foods, omit the whole chile peppers and serve hot sauce at the table for others to season to taste.
- Fresh herbs increase the alkalizing effect of this recipe.

Nutrients per serving (1 of 6)	
Calories	300
Fat	6 g
Sodium	926 mg
Carbohydrate	50 g
Fiber	15 g
Protein	12 g
Calcium	159 mg
Magnesium	74 mg
Potassium	888 mg

Lentil Sloppy Joes

This makes a great dinner for those busy nights when everyone is coming and going at different times. Leave the slow cooker on Low or Warm, the buns on the counter and salad fixings in the fridge, and let everyone help themselves.

Makes 4 servings

Tip

To make ahead, complete step 1. Cover and refrigerate for up to 2 days. When you're ready to cook, complete the recipe.

Nutrients per serving	
Calories	441
Fat	6 g
Sodium	758 mg
Carbohydrate	75 g
Fiber	12 g
Protein	26 g
Calcium	78 mg
Magnesium	85 mg
Potassium	840 mg

- **Small to medium (1½- to 4-quart) slow cooker**

1 tbsp	vegetable oil	15 mL
1	onion, finely chopped	1
4	stalks celery, diced	4
4	cloves garlic, minced	4
½ tsp	dried oregano	2 mL
½ tsp	salt	2 mL
	Freshly ground black pepper	
½ cup	ketchup	125 mL
¼ cup	water	60 mL
1 tbsp	balsamic vinegar	15 mL
1 tbsp	packed brown sugar	15 mL
1 tbsp	Dijon mustard	15 mL
1	can (14 to 19 oz/398 to 540 mL) green or brown lentils, drained and rinsed	1
	Hot pepper sauce (optional)	
	Toasted hamburger buns (GF, if needed)	

1. In a skillet, heat oil over medium heat. Add onion and celery and cook, stirring, until softened, about 5 minutes. Add garlic, oregano, salt, and pepper, to taste, and cook, stirring, for 1 minute. Stir in ketchup, water, balsamic vinegar, brown sugar and mustard. Transfer to slow cooker stoneware. Add lentils and stir well.
2. Cover and cook on Low for 6 hours or on High for 3 hours, until hot and bubbly. Add hot pepper sauce to taste, if desired. Ladle over hot toasted buns and serve immediately.

Chickpea Herb Burgers

A tasty vegetarian take on the standard burger, this seed and veggie combo will make your mouth water!

Makes 6 burgers

Tip

Whether grilled on the barbecue or baked in the oven, these burgers are great with all the trimmings.

- **Preheat oven to 375°F (190°C) or barbecue grill to high**
- **Food processor or blender**
- **Parchment-lined baking sheet or greased grill**

1 tbsp	vegetable oil	15 mL
1	can (19 oz/540 mL) chickpeas, drained	1
1/2 cup	grated onions	125 mL
2	cloves garlic, minced	2
3 cups	shredded carrots	750 mL
1/2 cup	spelt flakes	125 mL
1/4 cup	unblanched almonds	60 mL
1/4 cup	sunflower seeds	60 mL
2 tbsp	flax seeds	30 mL
2 tbsp	chopped fresh parsley	30 mL
2 tbsp	fresh basil leaves	30 mL
1 tbsp	fresh thyme leaves	15 mL
1	large egg	1
	Salt and freshly ground black pepper (optional)	

1. In food processor, process oil, chickpeas, onion, garlic and carrots until well combined.
2. Add spelt flakes, almonds, sunflower seeds, flax seeds, parsley, basil, thyme and egg. Process until finely chopped and holding together. Season to taste with salt and pepper, if desired.
3. Form mixture into 6 patties. Arrange patties on prepared baking sheet or grill. Bake in preheated oven or grill for 3 minutes per side, being careful to turn burgers gently.

Health Tips

- If you have a GI condition that is aggravated by seeds, this recipe may not be for you!
- The fresh herbs in this recipe add to the alkalizing effect of the veggies and help balance the acidifying impact of the barbecue.

Nutrients per burger	
Calories	275
Fat	12 g
Sodium	321 mg
Carbohydrate	36 g
Fiber	9 g
Protein	10 g
Calcium	90 mg
Magnesium	74 mg
Potassium	493 mg

Wild Rice Cakes

These make a nice light dinner accompanied by a salad. The red pepper coulis is delicious, but chili sauce, tomato sauce or even a dab of pesto also work quite well.

Makes 4 servings

Tips

If you are using pre-shredded cheese, check the label to make sure the manufacturer has not added a product containing gluten to prevent sticking.

Plain yogurt should be gluten-free, but you should check the label before purchasing. Manufacturers often add gluten to flavored varieties and formulas frequently change.

Nutrients per serving	
Calories	386
Fat	15 g
Sodium	547 mg
Carbohydrate	42 g
Fiber	4 g
Protein	21 g
Calcium	408 mg
Magnesium	106 mg
Potassium	491 mg

- **Preheat oven to 400°F (200°C)**
- **Large rimmed baking sheet, lightly greased**
- **Food processor**

2½ cups	water	625 mL
1 cup	wild and brown rice mixture, rinsed and drained	250 mL
½ tsp	salt	2 mL
1½ cups	shredded reduced-fat Swiss cheese	375 mL
½ cup	plain yogurt (preferably full fat)	125 mL
¼ cup	chopped red or green onion	60 mL
¼ cup	finely chopped fresh parsley	60 mL
2	large eggs, beaten	2
	Freshly ground black pepper	

Red Pepper Coulis

2	roasted red bell peppers	2
3	drained oil-packed sun-dried tomatoes, chopped	3
2 tbsp	extra virgin olive oil	30 mL
1 tbsp	balsamic vinegar	15 mL
10	fresh basil leaves (optional)	10

1. In a large saucepan, bring water to a rolling boil. Add rice and salt. Return to a boil. Reduce heat, cover and simmer until rice is tender and about half of the wild rice grains have split, about 1 hour. Set aside until cool enough to handle, about 20 minutes.
2. In a bowl, combine rice, Swiss cheese, yogurt, red onion, parsley, eggs and pepper to taste. Mix well. Using a large spoon, drop mixture in 8 batches onto prepared baking sheet. Flatten lightly with a spatula or large spoon.

Tips

The basil adds a nice note to the coulis, but if you can't get fresh leaves, omit it — the coulis will be quite tasty, anyway.

Be careful when turning the cakes, as they have a tendency to fall apart until they are thoroughly cooked.

These could also serve 8 as a substantial side dish.

3. Bake in preheated oven for 15 minutes, then flip and cook until lightly browned and heated through, about 5 minutes. Let cool on pan for 5 minutes before serving. Top with Red Pepper Coulis.

4. *Red Pepper Coulis:* In food processor, combine roasted peppers, sun-dried tomatoes, oil, balsamic vinegar and basil (if using); process until smooth.

Health Tips

- The wild rice makes this recipe highly alkalizing and helps balance your pH.
- If you are experiencing flare-ups related to a GI condition, brown or wild rice, both insoluble fiber foods, may worsen symptoms. Keep track of foods and symptoms in your health, life and diet diary to help identify troublesome foods.

Roasted Vegetable Pizza

Like lots of topping with every bite of pizza? Try this simplified version — thin, edgeless and filled to the brim!

Makes one 12-inch (30 cm) pizza, or 6 slices

Tips

You'll need about 10 oz (300 g) portobello mushrooms for 3 cups (750 mL) sliced.

Sprinkling some of the cheese on the crust before topping helps the vegetables remain on the pizza.

Variation

For a stronger cheese combination, try Asiago and Romano.

- **Preheat oven to 425°F (220°C)**
- **Roasting pan**

1 tbsp	extra virgin olive oil	15 mL
2	small Italian eggplants, cut into ½-inch (1 cm) cubes	2
1	large red bell pepper, cut into ½-inch (1 cm) slices	1
1	large yellow bell pepper, cut into ½-inch (1 cm) slices	1
3 cups	sliced portobello mushrooms (½-inch/1 cm thick slices)	750 mL
4	small zucchini, cut into ½-inch (1 cm) slices	4
6	cloves garlic, minced	6
⅔ cup	shredded mozzarella cheese	150 mL
½ cup	freshly grated Parmesan cheese	125 mL
1	Thin Pizza Crust (page 186), prepared through step 4	1

1. Pour oil into roasting pan. Add vegetables and garlic. Toss to coat. Roast in preheated oven, turning once, for 10 to 15 minutes or until tender. Do not overcook. Set aside to cool.
2. Sprinkle half the mozzarella cheese over the partially baked pizza crust. Top with roasted vegetables, the remaining mozzarella and Parmesan. Reduce oven temperature to 400°F (200°C) and bake for 12 to 15 minutes or until the topping is bubbly and cheese is melted, lightly browned and heated through. Serve immediately.

Nutrients per slice	
Calories	308
Fat	11 g
Sodium	467 mg
Carbohydrate	45 g
Fiber	9 g
Protein	13 g
Calcium	331 mg
Magnesium	50 mg
Potassium	925 mg

Macaroni and Cheese

This classic comfort food has been updated with a mixture of cheeses.

Makes 6 to 8 servings

Tips

Rinsing the cooked pasta well prevents the macaroni and cheese from becoming too thick.

Be sure to use orange-colored Cheddar cheese for a more attractive dish.

Wild rice elbow pasta works particularly well in this recipe.

Variation

To turn this into a casserole, add canned tuna, peas and chopped onion or celery, transfer to a greased baking dish and bake in preheated 350°F (180°C) oven until hot.

1 cup	shredded old Cheddar cheese	250 mL
1⁄2 cup	shredded Swiss cheese	125 mL
1⁄4 cup	freshly grated Parmesan cheese	60 mL
1 tbsp	sorghum flour	15 mL
1⁄2 tsp	dry mustard	2 mL
1⁄2 tsp	salt	2 mL
1⁄4 tsp	freshly ground white pepper	1 mL
Pinch	cayenne pepper	Pinch
2 cups	GF elbow pasta	500 mL
1	can (14 oz/385 mL) 2% evaporated milk	1
1⁄4 tsp	GF Worcestershire sauce	1 mL

1. In a small bowl, combine Cheddar, Swiss, Parmesan, sorghum flour, dry mustard, salt, white pepper and cayenne pepper. Set aside.
2. In a large saucepan, cook pasta in boiling water according to package instructions, until just tender. Rinse well under cold running water and drain well.
3. Return the pasta to the saucepan. Stir in milk, Worcestershire sauce and cheese mixture. Simmer, stirring gently, over low heat until mixture boils and thickens.

Health Tips

- If you have a GI condition that is aggravated by hot or spicy foods, omit the cayenne pepper and serve hot sauce at the table for others to season to taste.
- This dish is an excellent choice for the percentage of acidifying foods you need to balance your pH.

Nutrients per serving (1 of 8)	
Calories	210
Fat	9 g
Sodium	374 mg
Carbohydrate	20 g
Fiber	1 g
Protein	12 g
Calcium	342 mg
Magnesium	0 mg
Potassium	163 mg

Eggplant and Zucchini Lasagna

Try this unique version of a family favorite. The smooth flavors of the eggplant and zucchini make a lip-smacking combination.

Makes 6 servings

Tip

If you need to avoid dairy foods, you can replace the ricotta cheese and mozzarella cheese with 3 cups (750 mL) shredded GF mozzarella-style rice cheese and omit the Romano cheese.

- **Preheat oven to 350°F (180°C)**
- **13- by 9-inch (33 by 23 cm) glass baking dish**

9	GF lasagna noodles	9
1	jar (23 oz/650 mL) GF tomato pasta sauce (preferably with spinach)	1
1½ cups	shredded part-skim mozzarella cheese	375 mL
1	Japanese eggplant, thinly sliced	1
1½ cups	light ricotta cheese	375 mL
1	zucchini, thinly sliced	1
¼ cup	grated Romano cheese	60 mL
	Salt and freshly ground black pepper	

1. In a large pot of boiling water, cook lasagna according to package instructions until tender but firm (al dente). Drain.
2. Spread a thin layer of pasta sauce in baking dish. Top with 3 lasagna noodles, making sure they don't overlap. Cover with one-quarter of the sauce. Sprinkle with one-third of the mozzarella. Arrange eggplant on top. Cover with one-third of the remaining sauce, then half the ricotta. Add 3 more noodles and top with layers of tomato sauce and half the remaining mozzarella. Arrange zucchini on top. Cover with the remaining sauce, then the remaining ricotta. Top with the remaining noodles.

Nutrients per serving	
Calories	362
Fat	13 g
Sodium	613 mg
Carbohydrate	37 g
Fiber	5 g
Protein	21 g
Calcium	479 mg
Magnesium	48 mg
Potassium	516 mg

Tip

Use kosher salt if you can — it tastes better than iodized table salt and (ideally) contains no additives.

3. Pour ½ cup (125 mL) water into the pasta sauce jar and swish to catch any remaining sauce; pour over lasagna. Sprinkle with the remaining mozzarella and Romano cheese.
4. Cover with foil and bake in preheated oven for 45 to 50 minutes or until sauce is bubbling and cheese is melted. Remove foil and bake for 15 minutes. Broil for 5 minutes or until top is browned. Let stand for 10 minutes before serving. Season to taste with salt and pepper.

Health Tip

- Top with some fresh herbs before serving to raise the alkalizing effect of this recipe.

Celery Root and Mushroom Lasagna

If you're tired of the same old thing, try this delightfully different lasagna, which combines celery root and mushrooms with more traditional tomatoes and cheese. To complete the unusual but appetizing flavors, add a sprinkle of toasted walnuts.

Makes 6 to 8 servings

Tip

Make this using whole wheat lasagna noodles or oven-ready noodles, if you prefer. If using oven-ready noodles, do not toss with olive oil and use only 1 tbsp (15 mL) oil when softening the vegetables.

Nutrients per serving (1 of 8)	
Calories	329
Fat	15 g
Sodium	986 mg
Carbohydrate	31 g
Fiber	4 g
Protein	20 g
Calcium	436 mg
Magnesium	60 mg
Potassium	985 mg

- **Large (minimum 5-quart) oval slow cooker, stoneware greased**

9	brown rice lasagna noodles (see tip, at left)	9
2 tbsp	olive oil, divided	30 mL
4 cups	shredded, peeled celery root (about 1 medium)	1 L
2 tbsp	freshly squeezed lemon juice	30 mL
1	large sweet onion (such as Spanish or Vidalia), finely chopped	1
1 lb	cremini mushrooms, stems removed, caps sliced	500 g
4	cloves garlic, minced	4
1 tbsp	fresh thyme leaves (or 1 tsp/5 mL dried thyme, crumbled)	15 mL
1 tbsp	fresh rosemary leaves, finely chopped (or 1 tsp/5 mL dried rosemary, crumbled)	15 mL
4 cups	tomato sauce, divided	1 L
2 cups	ricotta cheese	500 mL
2 cups	shredded part-skim mozzarella cheese	500 mL
½ cup	toasted chopped walnuts (optional)	125 mL

1. Cook lasagna noodles in a pot of boiling salted water, until slightly undercooked, or according to package instructions, undercooking by 2 minutes. Drain, toss with 1 tbsp (15 mL) oil and set aside.
2. In a bowl, toss celery root with lemon juice. Set aside.
3. In a skillet, heat the remaining oil over medium heat for 30 seconds. Add onion and mushrooms and cook, stirring, for 2 minutes. Add garlic, thyme and rosemary and cook, stirring, for 1 minute. Add celery root and 2 cups (500 mL) tomato sauce and bring to a boil. Remove from heat.

Tip

This dish can be partially prepared before it is cooked. Complete steps 1 through 4. Cover and refrigerate overnight. In the morning, continue with step 5.

4. Spread 1 cup (250 mL) tomato sauce over bottom of prepared slow cooker stoneware. Cover with 3 noodles. Spread with half of the ricotta, half of the mushroom mixture and one-third of the mozzarella. Repeat. Cover with final layer of noodles. Pour the remaining tomato sauce over top. Sprinkle with the remaining mozzarella.

5. Cover and cook on Low for 6 hours or on High for 3 hours, until mushrooms are tender and mixture is hot and bubbly. Garnish with toasted walnuts, if desired.

Health Tip

- This healthy dish is a good choice as your acidifying food for the day, to keep your pH balanced.

Green Pad See Ew

In this leafy green vegetarian version of a signature Thai dish, slippery rice noodles are bathed in a simple soy-lime sauce, while tofu and egg provide additional protein. Make sure you have all the ingredients prepped and ready, or what should be a simple job will become confusing.

Makes 4 to 6 servings

Tip

To maintain more control over the saltiness of dishes, use reduced-sodium soy sauce. Depending on the type, 1 tbsp (15 mL) regular soy sauce can contain 1,000 mg or more of sodium. Reduced-sodium soy sauce contains about half that amount.

- **Wok**

¼ cup	reduced-sodium soy sauce (GF, if needed)	60 mL
1 tbsp	freshly squeezed lime juice	15 mL
1 tbsp	granulated sugar	15 mL
2	large eggs (optional)	2
	Kosher salt or coarse sea salt	
8 oz	½-inch (1 cm) wide dried rice noodles	250 g
¼ cup	vegetable oil	60 mL
12 oz	medium tofu, drained and cut into ½-inch (1 cm) cubes	375 g
6	cloves garlic, slivered	6
1 lb	Chinese broccoli, stems, leaves and florets separated and cut (see tip, opposite)	500 g
2 tbsp	ready-to-use vegetable broth (GF, if needed) or water	30 mL
2 tbsp	slivered fresh basil leaves	30 mL

1. In a small measuring cup, combine soy sauce, lime juice and sugar.
2. In a small bowl, lightly whisk eggs (if using) with salt.
3. In a large pan of boiling salted water over medium heat, cook noodles for 5 to 8 minutes, until tender but firm. Drain.
4. Meanwhile, heat wok over high heat for 1 minute. Add oil and swirl to coat bottom of pan. Add eggs (if using) and fry undisturbed for about 1 minute, until very puffy. Flip over and then, using a slotted spoon, transfer to a large plate, leaving oil in wok. Using a spoon, break egg into large chunks.

Nutrients per serving (1 of 6)	
Calories	348
Fat	15 g
Sodium	424 mg
Carbohydrate	45 g
Fiber	3 g
Protein	12 g
Calcium	540 mg
Magnesium	39 mg
Potassium	175 mg

Tip

To prepare Chinese broccoli for this recipe, trim, separating stems from leaves and florets. Using a vegetable peeler, peel the thickest stems and cut in half lengthwise. Cut stems crosswise into ½-inch (1 cm) pieces. Coarsely chop leaves and florets.

5. In wok over high heat, add tofu (be careful, as it will spatter) and cook, shaking pan often, for 3 to 5 minutes, until golden. Using a slotted spoon, transfer tofu to a plate, leaving oil in wok.
6. Add garlic to wok and stir-fry for 20 seconds. Add Chinese broccoli, salt lightly to taste, and stir-fry for about 1 minute, until leaves are slightly wilted. Add broth, cover and cook for 3 to 4 minutes, until stems are tender-crisp. Add noodles and soy sauce mixture and, using tongs, toss gently to combine. Add eggs and toss briefly. Remove from heat. Season to taste with salt. Transfer to a serving platter or individual bowls. Top with tofu and sprinkle with basil. Serve immediately.

Health Tip

- Fresh herbs add to the already high alkalizing effect of this recipe.

Soy-Braised Tofu

It's amazing how tofu soaks up the mouthwatering Asian flavors in this recipe. Use it as a centerpiece to a meal of vegetarian dishes that might include stir-fried bok choy or wilted greens garnished with toasted sesame seeds.

Makes 4 servings

Tips

To drain tofu, place a layer of paper towels on a plate. Set tofu in the middle. Cover with another layer of paper towel and a heavy plate. Set aside for 30 minutes. Peel off paper and cut into cubes.

Refrigerate any leftovers for use in other dishes, such as stir-fried mixed vegetables, or salads, such as an Asian-inspired coleslaw. You can also transform this flavorful tofu into a wrap. Place on lettuce leaves, garnish with shredded carrots and fold.

Nutrients per serving	
Calories	144
Fat	9 g
Sodium	610 mg
Carbohydrate	9 g
Fiber	1 g
Protein	10 g
Calcium	180 mg
Magnesium	68 mg
Potassium	290 mg

- **Large (minimum 6-quart) slow cooker**

1 lb	firm tofu, drained and cut into 1-inch (2.5 cm) cubes (see tip, at left)	500 g
1/4 cup	reduced-sodium soy sauce	60 mL
1 tbsp	puréed gingerroot	15 mL
1 tbsp	pure maple syrup	15 mL
1 tbsp	toasted sesame oil	15 mL
1 tbsp	freshly squeezed lemon juice	15 mL
1 tsp	minced garlic	5 mL
1/2 tsp	cracked black peppercorns	2 mL

1. In slow cooker stoneware, combine soy sauce, gingerroot, maple syrup, toasted sesame oil, lemon juice, garlic and peppercorns. Add tofu and toss gently until coated on all sides. Cover and refrigerate for 1 hour.
2. Toss well. Cover and cook on Low for 5 hours or on High for 2 1/2 hours, until tofu is hot and has absorbed the flavor.

Health Tip

- Although extra-firm tofu is a slightly acidifying food, other forms of tofu are alkalizing and will help to balance your pH.

Quick Quinoa Stir-Fry with Vegetables and Tofu

Quinoa is a mild, slightly sweet grain with hints of corn, nuts and grass. Here, it's studded with assorted vegetables and sesame seeds, creating a substantial stir-fry worthy of its billing as a main course.

Makes 4 servings

Tips

To prepare 4 cups (1 L) cooked quinoa, combine 1⅓ cups (325 mL) quinoa and 2⅔ cups (650 mL) water in a medium saucepan. Bring to a boil over medium-high heat. Reduce heat to low, cover and simmer for 12 to 15 minutes or until water is just barely absorbed. Cover and let stand for 5 to 6 minutes. Fluff with a fork and let cool completely, then transfer to an airtight container and refrigerate until chilled.

To toast sesame seeds, place up to 3 tbsp (45 mL) seeds in a medium skillet set over medium heat. Cook, shaking the skillet, for 3 to 5 minutes or until seeds are golden brown and fragrant. Let cool completely before use.

Nutrients per serving	
Calories	313
Fat	9 g
Sodium	361 mg
Carbohydrate	46 g
Fiber	7 g
Protein	16 g
Calcium	175 mg
Magnesium	161 mg
Potassium	649 mg

2 tsp	vegetable oil, divided	10 mL
8 oz	extra-firm tofu, drained, cut into 1-inch (2.5 cm) cubes and patted dry	250 g
12 oz	frozen stir-fry vegetables, thawed and patted dry	375 g
3	cloves garlic, minced	3
1 tbsp	minced gingerroot	15 mL
4 cups	cooked quinoa (see tip, at left), chilled	1 L
⅓ cup	thinly sliced green onions	75 mL
¼ cup	teriyaki sauce	60 mL
1 tbsp	toasted sesame seeds (see tip, at left)	15 mL

1. In a large skillet, heat half the oil over medium-high heat. Add tofu and cook, stirring, for 3 to 4 minutes or until golden. Using a slotted spoon, transfer tofu to a plate.
2. In the same skillet, heat the remaining oil over medium-high heat. Add stir-fry vegetables and cook, stirring, for 2 minutes. Add garlic and ginger; cook, stirring, for 30 seconds. Return tofu to the pan and add quinoa, green onions and teriyaki sauce; cook, stirring, for 2 to 3 minutes or until well coated and warmed through. Serve sprinkled with sesame seeds.

Health Tips

- If you have a gastrointestinal issue that is affected by sesame seeds, omit them when preparing this recipe.
- This dish is high in the minerals that act as buffers to reduce acid in our tissues.

Tofu Quinoa Scramble

Health food gets fancy, turning tofu, quinoa and vegetables into a truly delectable meal.

Makes 4 servings

Tip

To prepare 1 cup (250 mL) cooked quinoa, combine ⅓ cup (75 mL) quinoa and ⅔ cup (150 mL) water in a medium saucepan. Bring to a boil over medium-high heat. Reduce heat to low, cover and simmer for 12 to 15 minutes or until water is just barely absorbed. Cover and let stand for 5 to 6 minutes. Fluff with a fork and let cool completely.

1 tbsp	extra virgin olive oil	15 mL
1	large red bell pepper, chopped	1
1 cup	chopped mushrooms	250 mL
16 oz	extra-firm or firm tofu, drained and coarsely mashed with a fork	500 g
1 cup	cooked quinoa (see tip, at left), cooled	250 mL
¼ cup	chopped green onions	60 mL
1 tbsp	reduced-sodium tamari or soy sauce (GF, if needed)	15 mL
Pinch	freshly ground black pepper	Pinch

1. In a small skillet, heat oil over medium-high heat. Add red pepper and mushrooms; cook, stirring, for 4 to 5 minutes or until softened.
2. Add tofu, quinoa, green onions and tamari; cook, stirring, for 5 to 6 minutes or until tofu is golden brown. Season with pepper.

Nutrients per serving	
Calories	217
Fat	10 g
Sodium	157 mg
Carbohydrate	16 g
Fiber	4 g
Protein	14 g
Calcium	103 mg
Magnesium	33 mg
Potassium	238 mg

Side Dishes

Yummy Asparagus

The title says it all — both kids and adults will be back for more.

Makes 4 servings

Tip

For the best taste and freshness, choose asparagus with a bright green stalk and tightly closed, purple-tinged stalks. To prepare asparagus, break off the tough root end.

Nutrients per serving	
Calories	47
Fat	3 g
Sodium	21 mg
Carbohydrate	3 g
Fiber	2 g
Protein	2 g
Calcium	34 mg
Magnesium	11 mg
Potassium	157 mg

1 tbsp	butter	15 mL
1	bunch asparagus, ends trimmed	1
1	clove garlic, minced	1
1 tbsp	freshly grated Parmesan cheese	15 mL

1. In a medium saucepan, melt butter over medium heat. Sauté asparagus and garlic, shaking pan constantly, until just tender, about 5 minutes.
2. Sprinkle with cheese and let it melt before serving.

This recipe courtesy of dietitian Roberta Lowcay.

Roasted Beets with Warm Dill Sauce

Pickled beets were a staple in most old-time prairie pantries. Here's a take on fresh beets, one that's reminiscent of that old-fashioned flavor.

Makes 6 servings

Nutrients per serving	
Calories	87
Fat	0 g
Sodium	128 mg
Carbohydrate	20 g
Fiber	5 g
Protein	3 g
Calcium	26 mg
Magnesium	38 mg
Potassium	534 mg

- **Preheat oven to 350°F (180°C)**

12	small beets, scrubbed	12
1⁄3 cup	white wine vinegar	75 mL
2 tbsp	granulated sugar	30 mL
1 tbsp	chopped fresh dill	15 mL

1. Wrap beets individually in foil. Bake for 1 hour or until tender. Cool beets slightly, then slip off skins and slice.
2. In a small saucepan, combine vinegar and sugar; cook over medium-high heat for 1 minute or until sugar is dissolved. Toss with warm beets. Sprinkle with fresh dill and serve immediately.

Sesame-Glazed Baby Bok Choy

Baby bok choy are delicious cooked whole and glazed to complement dishes of Asian flavors.

Makes 4 servings

Tip

Bok choy is a mild member of the cabbage family that comes in bunches of soft white stems and green leaves. It is most familiar used in stir-fries. The large bunches are usually cut in half or chopped. Be sure to wash boy choy carefully, paying attention to root ends.

Nutrients per serving	
Calories	64
Fat	5 g
Sodium	271 mg
Carbohydrate	5 g
Fiber	0 g
Protein	1 g
Calcium	36 mg
Magnesium	9 mg
Potassium	99 mg

- **Bamboo steamer (optional)**

1 tbsp	vegetable oil	15 mL
1	clove garlic, finely chopped	1
1 tsp	finely chopped gingerroot	5 mL
1 tbsp	packed brown sugar	15 mL
1 tbsp	soy sauce (GF, if needed)	15 mL
1 tsp	grated lime zest	5 mL
2 tbsp	freshly squeezed lime juice	30 mL
1 tsp	sesame oil	5 mL
6 to 8	small bok choy (see tip, at left)	6 to 8
	Kosher or sea salt	
1 tsp	black sesame seeds (optional)	5 mL

1. In a small saucepan, heat oil over medium heat. Add garlic and ginger and sauté until fragrant but not browned, 1 to 2 minutes. Stir in brown sugar, soy sauce, and lime zest and simmer, stirring, while sugar melts. Remove from heat and add lime juice and sesame oil. Set aside.
2. Slice bok choy in half lengthwise if large. Steam in a bamboo steamer over simmering water, or place in a shallow skillet in ½ inch (1 cm) lightly salted water and cook, covered, until tender, 3 to 4 minutes. Drain.
3. Toss steamed bok choy with soy glaze. Add salt or a dash of sesame oil to taste. Serve hot, garnished with black sesame seeds, if desired.

Health Tips

- Use a reduced-sodium soy sauce to reduce the sodium in this recipe.
- If you have a GI condition that is aggravated by seeds, omit the optional sesame seeds.

Chinese Broccoli with Nori Mayonnaise

This Pan-Asian dish stars Chinese broccoli stems, served at room temperature with a yummy dip. Reserve the leaves for other dishes.

Makes 2 servings

Tips

To promote even cooking, cut thick stems of Chinese broccoli in half lengthwise.

Look for toasted nori and pickled ginger in well-stocked supermarkets. To chop nori, fold it along the serrations, then use kitchen scissors to cut it into tiny pieces.

8 oz	Chinese broccoli stems, trimmed and peeled	250 g
½ cup	mayonnaise or vegan alternative	125 mL
1	sheet toasted nori, chopped	1
1 tbsp	finely chopped pickled ginger, drained (or ½ tsp/2 mL puréed gingerroot)	15 mL
1 tsp	rice vinegar	5 mL
¼ tsp	freshly squeezed lemon juice	1 mL
¼ tsp	kosher salt or coarse sea salt	1 mL

1. In a covered steamer basket above 1 inch (2.5 cm) of boiling water, steam stems over medium-low heat for about 10 minutes, until tender-crisp. Immediately rinse with cold water to stop the cooking, drain and set aside to cool to room temperature. Pat dry.
2. Meanwhile, in a medium measuring cup, combine mayonnaise, nori, ginger, rice vinegar, lemon juice and salt.
3. Serve stems with nori mayonnaise alongside for dipping.

Health Tip

- This recipe is both high in fiber and highly alkalizing.

Nutrients per serving	
Calories	246
Fat	20 g
Sodium	959 mg
Carbohydrate	27 g
Fiber	3 g
Protein	4 g
Calcium	58 mg
Magnesium	24 mg
Potassium	395 mg

Sautéed Red Chard with Lemon and Pine Nuts

This colorful and easy addition to the dinner table makes eating your greens a pleasure, not a chore. Serve it over brown rice or whole grains.

Makes 2 servings

Tips

To prepare the chard for this recipe, trim, separating stems and thick center ribs from the leaves. Using a sharp knife, cut stems and ribs into ½-inch (1 cm) pieces. Chop the leaves coarsely. Set aside in separate piles.

Bottled reconstituted lemon and lime juices usually contain additives. To avoid them, use freshly squeezed juice. Squeeze a whole lemon or lime and store the leftover juice in a small container in the fridge or freeze it in 1 tbsp (15 mL) portions in an ice-cube tray.

Nutrients per serving	
Calories	204
Fat	20 g
Sodium	592 mg
Carbohydrate	6 g
Fiber	2 g
Protein	4 g
Calcium	187 mg
Magnesium	55 mg
Potassium	498 mg

2 tbsp	extra virgin olive oil	30 mL
2 tbsp	pine nuts	30 mL
1	small bunch red chard (12 oz/375 g), trimmed, leaves chopped and stems cut into ½-inch (1 cm) pieces (see tip, at left)	1
2	large cloves garlic, chopped	2
½ tsp	kosher salt or coarse sea salt	2 mL
⅛ tsp	freshly ground black pepper	0.5 mL
2 tsp	freshly squeezed lemon juice	10 mL
½ cup	shredded smoked Gouda cheese (optional)	125 mL

1. In a large skillet over medium heat, heat oil until shimmery. Fry pine nuts, stirring often, for about 2 minutes, until golden. Using a slotted spoon, transfer nuts to a small bowl.
2. Add chard stems to same skillet and cook over medium heat, stirring often, for about 5 minutes, until softened. Stir in garlic for 20 seconds. Add chard leaves, salt and pepper and cook, stirring often, for about 5 minutes, until leaves are wilted and tender and stems are tender-crisp. Stir in lemon juice and remove from heat. Stir in pine nuts.
3. Transfer to a microwave-safe serving bowl or individual plates. Sprinkle with cheese (if using). Heat in microwave on High for 1 minute or until cheese is molten.

Health Tip

- If your percentage of acidifying foods is already high for the day, omit the optional smoked Gouda cheese in this recipe.

Old-School Collard Greens

A dish of long-simmered collards is a culinary classic from the American South. Serve over grits for a Southern dining experience, or simply over brown rice.

Makes 2 servings

Tips

To prepare the collards for this recipe, use a sharp knife to trim leaves from stems, discarding stems and thick center ribs. Coarsely chop leaves.

Braise collards for 30 to 60 minutes or longer, depending on how soft and satiny you like them.

2 tbsp	extra virgin olive oil	30 mL
1	onion, finely chopped	1
2	large cloves garlic, chopped	2
1	bunch collard greens (10 to 12 oz/300 to 375 g), trimmed and coarsely chopped	1
1 cup	ready-to-use vegetable broth (GF, if needed)	250 mL
1 cup	water	250 mL
1/2 tsp	kosher salt or coarse sea salt	2 mL
1/4 tsp	granulated sugar	1 mL
1/8 tsp	freshly ground black pepper	0.5 mL
1 tbsp	white wine vinegar	15 mL
1 to 2 tbsp	unsalted butter or non-dairy alternative	15 to 30 mL
Dash	hot pepper sauce (optional)	Dash

1. In a large saucepan over medium heat, heat oil until shimmery. Add onion and cook, stirring often, for about 5 minutes, until softened and turning golden. Stir in garlic for 20 seconds. Stir in collards for 1 minute, until combined and slightly wilted. Stir in broth, water, salt, sugar and pepper. Cover, reduce heat to low and simmer for about 45 minutes, until very tender (see tip, at left).
2. Stir in vinegar and butter. Season to taste with salt. Serve with a slotted spoon and drizzle with cooking liquid to taste. If desired, add a dash of hot sauce to taste.

Health Tip

- Skip the optional hot pepper sauce if you have a GI condition that is worsened by spicy foods.

Nutrients per serving	
Calories	249
Fat	20 g
Sodium	587 mg
Carbohydrate	16 g
Fiber	7 g
Protein	4 g
Calcium	240 mg
Magnesium	21 mg
Potassium	336 mg

Balsamic Roasted Fiddleheads

This recipe provides an easy two-step roasting technique for fiddleheads.

Makes 2 servings

- **Preheat oven to 400°F (200°C)**
- **Rimmed baking sheet**

8 oz	fiddleheads, trimmed	250 g
1 tbsp	extra virgin olive oil	15 mL
1/2 tsp	kosher salt or coarse sea salt	2 mL
	Freshly ground black pepper	
1/4 cup	freshly grated Parmesan cheese (optional)	60 mL
2 tsp	balsamic vinegar	10 mL

1. In a saucepan of boiling salted water over medium heat, blanch fiddleheads, covered, for about 5 minutes, until tender-crisp and lighter green. Drain, then immediately rinse with cold water to stop the cooking. Drain and pat dry.
2. Transfer fiddleheads to baking sheet and, using a spatula, toss with oil, salt and pepper to taste. Arrange in a single layer and sprinkle cheese (if using) overtop.
3. Roast in preheated oven for about 10 minutes, until fiddleheads are tender but firm and cheese is browned. Drizzle with vinegar and toss with spatula, scraping browned bits from bottom of pan. Serve immediately.

Nutrients per serving	
Calories	103
Fat	7 g
Sodium	483 mg
Carbohydrate	7 g
Fiber	0 g
Protein	5 g
Calcium	38 mg
Magnesium	39 mg
Potassium	426 mg

Mushroom Ragoût

This elegant mix of mushrooms in a richly flavored sauce is a favorite for vegetarians when accompanied by grilled polenta or tucked into an omelet. It's also a delicious side with roast beef or turkey.

Makes 4 to 6 servings

Tips

A soft-bristle pastry brush is a handy tool for gently brushing dirt from mushrooms.

You can rinse off the shiitake stems and save them for when you're making vegetable stock.

8 oz	cremini mushrooms	250 g
8 oz	king oyster mushrooms	250 g
8 oz	shiitake mushrooms	250 g
1/2 cup	olive oil, divided	125 mL
	Salt and freshly ground black pepper	
1/2 cup	minced shallots	125 mL
2	cloves garlic, minced	2
2 1/2 cups	ready-to-use vegetable broth (GF, if needed)	625 mL
2 tsp	chopped fresh thyme	10 mL
1 tsp	balsamic vinegar	5 mL
2 tbsp	butter	30 mL
1/4 cup	coarsely chopped fresh flat-leaf (Italian) parsley	60 mL

1. Trim off cremini stems and thinly slice caps. Set aside.
2. Trim off bottom of king oyster stems and separate top from bottom. Thinly slice the mushroom tops. Cut the stem in half and slice into half-moons. Set aside.
3. Remove shiitake stems and discard. Thinly slice mushroom caps. Set aside.
4. In a large skillet, heat 2 tbsp (30 mL) oil over medium-high heat and swirl to completely coat pan. Add cremini mushrooms in a single layer. Let them sit for 1 minute, then stir. Let them sit for another minute. Season lightly with salt and pepper and stir until mushrooms brown, 2 to 3 minutes. Transfer mushrooms to a large bowl. Repeat the same cooking method with king oyster and shiitake mushrooms. Set aside.

Nutrients per serving (1 of 6)	
Calories	253
Fat	22 g
Sodium	101 mg
Carbohydrate	13 g
Fiber	4 g
Protein	3 g
Calcium	21 mg
Magnesium	25 mg
Potassium	452 mg

Tip

Use kosher salt if you can — it tastes better than iodized table salt and (ideally) contains no additives.

5. In the same skillet, heat the remaining oil over medium heat. Add shallots and garlic and sauté for 1 minute. Return cooked mushrooms to the pan with the cooking juices collected in the bowl. Add broth, thyme, 1 tsp (5 mL) salt and ½ tsp (2 mL) pepper.
6. Reduce heat to medium-low and simmer mushroom mixture until liquid is reduced and slightly thickened, 5 to 6 minutes.
7. Add balsamic vinegar and stir in butter to lightly thicken and add sheen to the sauce. Toss with parsley and taste for seasoning.

Health Tips

- Fresh herbs increase the alkalizing effect of this recipe.
- Substitute your own vegetable stock for the ready-to-use broth to reduce the sodium in this recipe.

Roasted Garlic Sweet Pepper Strips

These pepper strips will add a dash of color and flavor to any meal.

Makes 4 servings

Tips

Add a sprinkle of fresh herbs, such as parsley or basil, to oil mixture.

This is a delicious and colorful way to serve bell peppers.

These peppers can be prepared ahead of time and served cold.

Nutrients per serving	
Calories	103
Fat	7 g
Sodium	24 mg
Carbohydrate	8 g
Fiber	2 g
Protein	2 g
Calcium	28 mg
Magnesium	16 mg
Potassium	282 mg

- **Preheat oven to 400°F (200°C)**

4	large bell peppers (combination of green, red and yellow)	4
2 tbsp	olive oil	30 mL
1½ tsp	crushed garlic	7 mL
1 tbsp	freshly grated Parmesan cheese	15 mL

1. On baking sheet, bake whole peppers for 15 to 20 minutes, turning occasionally, until blistered and blackened. Place in paper bag; seal and let stand for 10 minutes.
2. Peel off charred skin from peppers; cut off tops and bottoms. Remove seeds and ribs; cut into 1-inch (2.5 cm) wide strips and place on serving platter.
3. Mix oil with garlic; brush over peppers. Sprinkle with cheese.

Moroccan Vegetable Tagine

Saffron, lemon and parsley add scrumptious scents to this colorful and healthy blend of vegetables. This recipe makes a good side dish. Or ladle it over couscous for an extra 5.9 g of protein per serving. Partnering the vegetables instead with brown rice adds just 2.7 g protein per serving, but it increases the alkalizing effect of the dish.

Makes 8 servings

Tips

Nothing can really substitute for the flavor of saffron, but the pretty yellow-orange color it creates can be mimicked with ½ tsp (2 mL) ground turmeric.

There are about 2⅓ cups (575 mL) of diced tomatoes in a 19-oz (540 mL) can and about 2 cups (500 mL) of drained chickpeas in a 19-oz can.

Nutrients per serving	
Calories	199
Fat	3 g
Sodium	434 mg
Carbohydrate	39 g
Fiber	7 g
Protein	6 g
Calcium	76 mg
Magnesium	39 mg
Potassium	554 mg

1 tbsp	olive oil	15 mL
2	onions, chopped	2
2	cloves garlic, finely chopped	2
2	Yukon gold potatoes, peeled and cubed	2
2	large carrots, cut into short sticks	2
½	large sweet potato, peeled and cut into short sticks	½
1 tbsp	grated gingerroot	15 mL
1 tsp	ground cumin	5 mL
1 tsp	ground cinnamon	5 mL
1	can (19 oz/540 mL) diced tomatoes, with juice	1
1	can (19 oz/540 mL) chickpeas, drained and rinsed	1
4 cups	ready-to-use vegetable broth	1 L
Pinch	saffron strands (optional)	Pinch
¼ cup	chopped fresh parsley	60 mL
	Juice of 1 lemon	
	Salt and freshly ground black pepper	
2 tbsp	hot pepper sauce (optional)	30 mL

1. In a large saucepan, heat oil over medium-high heat. Add onions, garlic, potatoes, carrots, sweet potato, ginger, cumin and cinnamon; cook, stirring often, for 10 minutes.
2. Stir in tomatoes; cook for 2 minutes. Stir in chickpeas, broth and saffron (if using); bring to a boil. Reduce heat, cover and simmer for 30 minutes, until vegetables are just tender. Stir in parsley and lemon juice. Season to taste with salt and pepper. Stir in hot sauce (if using).

This recipe courtesy of dietitian Donna Bottrell.

Health Tip

- Replace the ready-made vegetable stock with a homemade version to reduce the sodium in this recipe.

Vegetable Biryani

Here's a tasty and nutritious side dish that is very easy to make.

Makes 4 servings

Tip

For the best flavor, toast cumin and coriander seeds and grind them yourself. To toast seeds: Place in a dry skillet over medium heat and cook, stirring, until fragrant, about 3 minutes. Immediately transfer to a spice grinder or mortar and grind finely.

Nutrients per serving	
Calories	455
Fat	13 g
Sodium	778 mg
Carbohydrate	78 g
Fiber	10 g
Protein	8 g
Calcium	110 mg
Magnesium	117 mg
Potassium	873 mg

- **Medium to large (3½- to 5-quart) slow cooker**
- **Lightly greased slow cooker stoneware**

3 tbsp	vegetable oil, divided	45 mL
1 tsp	cumin seeds	5 mL
½ tsp	ground turmeric	2 mL
2 cups	cubed peeled potatoes (½-inch/ 1 cm cubes)	500 mL
1	red or sweet onion, thinly sliced on the vertical	1
2	carrots, diced	2
2 cups	diced fennel bulb	500 mL
1½ cups	long-grain brown rice, rinsed and drained	375 mL
2 tsp	ground cumin	10 mL
1 tsp	ground coriander	5 mL
1 tsp	salt	5 mL
1 tsp	cracked black peppercorns	5 mL
2	green cardamom pods, crushed	2
4 cups	ready-to-use vegetable broth (GF, if needed)	1 L

1. In a skillet, heat 2 tbsp (30 mL) oil over medium-high heat. Add cumin seeds and cook until they sizzle, about 10 seconds. Stir in turmeric. Add potatoes and cook, stirring, until they begin to brown, about 3 minutes. Add red onion and cook, stirring, for 1 minute. Add carrots and fennel and cook, stirring, until well coated with mixture. Transfer to a bowl and set aside.
2. Add the remaining oil, rice, ground cumin and coriander, salt, peppercorns and cardamom pods to pan and cook, stirring, until well coated. Add broth and bring to a boil. Boil for 2 minutes.

Tip

Before removing the core of a fennel bulb, chop off the top shoots (which resemble celery) and discard. If desired, save the feathery green fronds to use as a garnish. If the outer sections of the bulb seem old and dry, peel them with a vegetable peeler before using.

3. Using a slotted spoon, layer half the rice mixture over bottom of prepared stoneware. Spread vegetables over it. Add the remaining rice mixture, plus all of the liquid. Place a clean tea towel, folded in half (so you will have two layers), over top of stoneware to absorb moisture. Cover and cook on Low for 6 hours or on High for 3 hours, until rice is tender and liquid has been absorbed. Serve hot.

Health Tips

- Use homemade stock instead of the ready-made version to increase the health benefits of this recipe.
- Use sea salt instead of iodized salt; the trace minerals will increase the alkalizing impact.
- If you are experiencing flare-ups from a GI condition, brown or wild rice, both insoluble fiber foods, may worsen symptoms. Keep track of foods and symptoms in your health, life and diet diary to help identify troublesome foods.

Steamed Asian Vegetable Medley

This versatile, delicately flavored dish encourages families to enjoy a variety of vegetables. Choose a selection from each of the color groups, ensuring good color and flavor contrast.

Tip

Allow ¾ cup (175 mL) assorted vegetables per person and let each family member make a choice for the dish.

Nutrients per serving (based on a ¾-cup (175 mL) assortment of snow peas, carrots, red bell peppers and water chestnuts without any flavoring)

Calories	46
Fat	0 g
Sodium	21 mg
Carbohydrate	10 g
Fiber	2 g
Protein	1 g
Calcium	17 mg
Magnesium	14 mg
Potassium	293 mg

Green: Sugar snap peas, snow peas, finely chopped bok choy, chopped spinach

Yellow/orange: Baby corn, julienned yellow or orange bell peppers, yellow squash slices, carrot slices

Red: Julienned red bell peppers, cherry tomatoes, radishes

White: Bean sprouts, water chestnuts, turnip strips

Sesame oil

Soy sauce (GF, if needed)

Toasted sesame seeds (optional)

1. In a medium saucepan, bring 1 cup (250 mL) water to a boil. Place steamer basket over boiling water and fill with vegetables. Drizzle with a small amount of sesame oil and soy sauce. Cover and steam until vegetables are tender-crisp.
2. Transfer to a serving dish and sprinkle with toasted sesame seeds, if desired.

This recipe courtesy of Eileen Campbell.

Health Tips

- Choose reduced-sodium soy sauce to lower the sodium in this recipe.
- If you have a GI condition that is aggravated by seeds, omit the optional sesame seeds in this recipe.

Roasted Root Vegetables with Wild Mint

This mouthwatering blend of root vegetables is sure to please any palate.

Makes 6 servings

- **Preheat oven to 400°F (200°C)**
- **Roasting pan or rimmed baking sheet**

6	new potatoes, cut into chunks	6
3	carrots, cut into chunks	3
2	parsnips, cut into chunks	2
1	red onion, quartered	1
2 tbsp	olive oil	30 mL
2 tbsp	chopped fresh mint (preferably wild)	30 mL
1 tsp	freshly squeezed lemon juice	5 mL
	Salt and freshly ground black pepper	

1. In a large bowl, toss together potatoes, carrots, parsnips, onion and olive oil. Spread vegetables out in single layer in roasting pan or on baking sheet.
2. Roast about 1 hour, turning occasionally, until tender and caramelized. Stir in fresh mint and lemon juice. Season to taste with salt and pepper.

Health Tip

- Fresh herbs raise the alkalizing effect of this dish.

Nutrients per serving	
Calories	162
Fat	5 g
Sodium	22 mg
Carbohydrate	31 g
Fiber	4 g
Protein	5 g
Calcium	36 mg
Magnesium	7 mg
Potassium	142 mg

Baked Summer Vegetable Layers

Typical Italian flavors are blended in this tasty side dish.

Makes 4 servings

- **Preheat oven to 425°F (220°C)**
- **8-inch (20 cm) shallow baking dish, greased**

4	potatoes, peeled and thinly sliced, divided	4
1	onion, thinly sliced	1
1	small zucchini, thinly sliced	1
	Chopped fresh oregano or basil leaves (optional)	
	Salt and freshly ground black pepper	
2	tomatoes, sliced	2

1. In prepared baking dish, arrange half the potatoes in an even layer. Spread onion and then zucchini on top. If desired, sprinkle evenly with oregano or basil. Sprinkle lightly with salt and pepper.
2. Repeat with the remaining potatoes and top with tomato slices. If desired, sprinkle evenly with herbs again. Add ¼ cup (60 mL) water.
3. Cover and bake in preheated oven for 20 minutes. Uncover and bake for 20 minutes more or until potatoes are tender.

Nutrients per serving	
Calories	174
Fat	0 g
Sodium	41 mg
Carbohydrate	39 g
Fiber	6 g
Protein	5 g
Calcium	36 mg
Magnesium	60 mg
Potassium	1129 mg

Baked Winter Vegetable Layers

Root vegetables are particularly appropriate for this recipe, since they all require approximately the same cooking time. For a change, use parsnips, red onions and thinly sliced carrots.

Makes 4 servings

- **Preheat oven to 375°F (190°C)**
- **9-inch (23 cm) deep pie plate, greased**

1 tbsp	butter or margarine	15 mL
6	green onions, sliced	6
2	large potatoes, sliced	2
1	large beet, peeled and sliced	1
	Salt and freshly ground black pepper	

1. In a nonstick skillet, melt butter over medium heat. Add onions and cook, stirring, for 5 minutes or until tender.

2. In pie plate, layer potato, half of cooked onions, beet and more onions in pie plate. Sprinkle each layer lightly with salt and pepper. Add a small amount of water.

3. Cover and bake in preheated oven for about 1 hour or until vegetables are tender.

Health Tip

- Use clarified butter or ghee instead of butter or margarine to raise the health factor another notch.

Nutrients per serving	
Calories	49
Fat	3 g
Sodium	20 mg
Carbohydrate	5 g
Fiber	1 g
Protein	1 g
Calcium	11 mg
Magnesium	13 mg
Potassium	203 mg

Baked Parsnip Fries

Parsnips have a surprising sweetness that contrasts wonderfully to the bite of parsley. For extra-crisp fries, add the salt and pepper after cooking.

Makes 4 servings

- **Preheat oven to 400°F (200°C)**
- **Large rimmed baking sheet, lined with foil and sprayed with nonstick cooking spray**

1 lb	parsnips, cut into 3-inch (7.5 cm) long by 1⁄4-inch (0.5 cm) thick sticks	500 g
1⁄4 tsp	fine sea salt	1 mL
1⁄8 tsp	freshly ground black pepper	0.5 mL
1 tbsp	extra virgin olive oil	15 mL
1 tbsp	chopped fresh flat-leaf (Italian) parsley	15 mL

1. In a large bowl, combine parsnips, salt, pepper and oil, tossing to coat. Spread in a single layer on prepared baking sheet.
2. Bake in preheated oven for 15 minutes. Gently turn parsnips over and bake for 12 to 17 minutes or until crisp. Serve immediately, sprinkled with parsley.

Nutrients per serving	
Calories	115
Fat	4 g
Sodium	187 mg
Carbohydrate	21 g
Fiber	6 g
Protein	1 g
Calcium	42 mg
Magnesium	33 mg
Potassium	431 mg

Sweet Potato, Apple and Raisin Casserole

The combination of ginger and cinnamon adds punch to the flavors of this high-fiber dish.

Makes 6 servings

Tips

The darker the skin of the sweet potato, the moister it is.

Chopped dates or apricots can replace the raisins.

Prepare casserole without apples up to the day before. Add apples, toss and bake just prior to serving.

Nutrients per serving	
Calories	187
Fat	6 g
Sodium	82 mg
Carbohydrate	34 g
Fiber	3 g
Protein	2 g
Calcium	33 mg
Magnesium	28 mg
Potassium	342 mg

- **Preheat oven to 350°F (180°C)**
- **Baking dish, sprayed with nonstick vegetable spray**

1 lb	sweet potatoes, peeled and cubed	500 g
3/4 tsp	ground ginger	3 mL
1/4 cup	liquid honey or pure maple syrup	60 mL
3/4 tsp	ground cinnamon	3 mL
2 tbsp	margarine, melted	30 mL
1/4 cup	raisins	60 mL
2 tbsp	chopped walnuts	30 mL
3/4 cup	cubed peeled sweet apples	175 mL

1. Steam or microwave sweet potatoes just until slightly underdone. Place in baking dish.
2. In small bowl, combine ginger, honey, cinnamon, margarine, raisins, walnuts and apples; mix well. Pour over sweet potatoes and bake, uncovered, for 20 minutes or until tender.

Health Tip

- To reduce the acid load of this dish, swap the high acidifying walnuts for pecans.

Scalloped Potatoes with a New Twist

An old-fashioned comfort food, updated for today.

Makes 6 servings

Tips

Use the slicing blade of a food processor to slice potatoes thinly.

The dark green leaves of celery are most flavorful.

If the GF chicken stock powder is unsalted, season the potatoes with salt to taste.

Nutrients per serving	
Calories	190
Fat	6 g
Sodium	81 mg
Carbohydrate	32 g
Fiber	5 g
Protein	3 g
Calcium	28 mg
Magnesium	43 mg
Potassium	777 mg

- **Preheat oven to 350°F (180°C)**
- **Food processor**
- **10-cup (2.5 L) casserole dish**

1	onion, finely chopped	1
½ cup	celery leaves	125 mL
3 tbsp	butter or margarine	45 mL
2 tbsp	potato starch	30 mL
2 tbsp	GF chicken stock powder	30 mL
3 to 4 cups	water	750 mL to 1 L
¼ tsp	freshly ground black pepper	1 mL
2 lbs	potatoes, thinly sliced	1 kg

1. In food processor, process onion, celery leaves, butter, potato starch, chicken stock powder, 3 cups (750 mL) water and ground pepper until combined. Set aside.
2. Spread potatoes evenly in casserole dish. Pour sauce over top. If necessary, add extra water so potatoes are almost covered. The amount depends on the size and shape of the casserole.
3. Bake, uncovered, in preheated oven for 75 to 90 minutes or until potatoes are fork-tender.

Variation

For a potluck dish, double or triple the recipe and use a 20- to 30-cup (5 to 7.5 L) casserole and increase the baking time by 15 to 30 minutes or until fork-tender.

Cauliflower "Mashed Potatoes"

This delicious, dairy-free alternative to mashed potatoes is certain to please.

Makes 4 servings

Tips

Remove the tougher stems from the cauliflower; they will not blend as well as the florets.

Chopping the ingredients in a food processor before blending creates a smooth purée with very little liquid, ensuring a creamy result.

Nutrients per serving	
Calories	326
Fat	27 g
Sodium	732 mg
Carbohydrate	17 g
Fiber	4 g
Protein	10 g
Calcium	33 mg
Magnesium	101 mg
Potassium	558 mg

- **Food processor**
- **Blender**

1 cup	raw cashews	250 mL
3 tbsp	nutritional yeast	45 mL
1 tsp	fine sea salt	5 mL
3 cups	chopped cauliflower (see tip, at left)	750 mL
3 tbsp	extra virgin olive oil	45 mL
1 tbsp	freshly squeezed lemon juice	15 mL

1. In food processor, process cashews, nutritional yeast and salt until flour-like in consistency. Add cauliflower, olive oil and lemon juice. Process at high speed until finely chopped, stopping motor to scrape down sides of work bowl as necessary.

2. Transfer mixture to blender and blend on high speed until smooth and creamy. Transfer to a bowl. Serve immediately or cover and refrigerate for up to 4 days.

Variations

For an even creamier dish, soak 2 cups (500 mL) raw cashews in 4 cups (1 L) warm water for 15 minutes. Drain, then add to ingredients in step 2, along with an additional 1 cup (250 mL) chopped cauliflower florets and ½ cup (125 mL) filtered water.

Herbed Cauliflower "Mashed Potatoes": In step 2, add 1 tbsp (15 mL) chopped fresh chives, 1 tsp (5 mL) chopped fresh rosemary and ½ tsp (2 mL) chopped fresh thyme leaves.

Health Tip

- Nutritional yeast are not live yeast, and this food is nutrient-rich. If you are sensitive to yeast because of an allergy or a history of gastrointestinal yeast overgrowth, omit this ingredient.

Horseradish Mashed Potatoes

Horseradish makes these mashed potatoes especially suited for beef or pork. Serve them at once or cover and refrigerate for up to 2 days and then reheat (see tip, at left). They also freeze well.

Makes 4 servings

Tips

Reheat refrigerated potatoes in a covered baking dish in a 300°F (150°C) oven for 30 minutes or until hot.

The Prince Edward Island Potato Board does not recommend using an electric mixer because it makes the potatoes "gluey." It is their number one telephone complaint.

4	Yukon Gold or other good mashing potatoes, peeled and cut into chunks	4
½ cup	sour cream	125 mL
2 tbsp	prepared horseradish	30 mL
1	green onion, thinly sliced	1
	Salt and freshly ground black pepper	

1. In a medium saucepan, cook potatoes in boiling water for 20 minutes or until just tender. Drain and return to saucepan. Then mash potatoes.
2. Add sour cream and horseradish. Beat with a potato masher until potatoes are smooth and fluffy (see tip, at left). Stir in onions and salt and pepper to taste.

Health Tip

- Horseradish contains compounds called glucosinolates, which the body converts to compounds that support detoxification.

Nutrients per serving	
Calories	194
Fat	4 g
Sodium	80 mg
Carbohydrate	37 g
Fiber	5 g
Protein	5 g
Calcium	68 mg
Magnesium	50 mg
Potassium	955 mg

Fragrant Coconut Rice

The robustness of a spicy curry would nicely complement the creamy sweetness of this rice.

Makes 4 servings

Tip

Coconut milk should be suitable for people who are allergic to gluten. However, some brands contain guar gum, which, although it does not contain gluten, is not recommended for people with celiac disease. Also it may be processed in a facility where gluten is present. Check the label.

1½ cups	coconut milk (see tip, at left)	375 mL
1 cup	water	250 mL
1	2-inch (5 cm) cinnamon stick	1
1 cup	brown basmati or long-grain brown rice, rinsed and drained	250 mL

1. In a saucepan over medium-high heat, bring coconut milk, water and cinnamon stick to a rapid boil.
2. Stir in rice and return to a boil. Reduce heat to low. Cover and simmer until rice is tender and liquid is absorbed, about 50 minutes. Discard cinnamon stick.

Health Tip

- If you are experiencing flare-ups from a GI condition, brown or wild rice, both insoluble fiber foods, may worsen symptoms. Keep track of foods and symptoms in your health, life and diet diary to help identify troublesome foods.

Nutrients per serving	
Calories	339
Fat	19 g
Sodium	13 mg
Carbohydrate	39 g
Fiber	4 g
Protein	5 g
Calcium	51 mg
Magnesium	35 mg
Potassium	243 mg

Basic Brown Rice Pilaf

Even whole-grain skeptics will love this simple yet flavorful brown rice dish.

Makes 6 servings

2 tsp	extra virgin olive oil	10 mL
1 cup	finely chopped celery	250 mL
1/2 cup	finely chopped onion	125 mL
1 cup	long-grain brown rice	250 mL
1/8 tsp	freshly ground black pepper	0.5 mL
2 cups	ready-to-use reduced-sodium chicken or vegetable broth (GF, if needed)	500 mL

1. In a large saucepan, heat oil over medium-high heat. Add celery and onion; cook, stirring, for 3 minutes. Add rice and cook, stirring, for 2 minutes.
2. Stir in pepper and broth. Bring to a boil. Reduce heat to low, cover and simmer for 40 to 45 minutes or until broth is absorbed. Let stand, covered, for 5 minutes, then fluff with a fork.

Health Tip

- If you are experiencing flare-ups from a GI condition, brown or wild rice, both insoluble fiber foods, may worsen symptoms. Keep track of foods and symptoms in your health, life and diet diary to help identify troublesome foods.

Nutrients per serving	
Calories	140
Fat	3 g
Sodium	63 mg
Carbohydrate	27 g
Fiber	2 g
Protein	3 g
Calcium	24 mg
Magnesium	48 mg
Potassium	201 mg

Red Beans and Red Rice

Here's a fresh twist on the classic Southern dish of red beans and rice. Bulked up with muscular red rice, it is very hearty — with the addition of salad, it's a meal in itself.

Makes 8 servings

Tips

Wehani rice is widely available in well-stocked supermarkets or natural foods stores. Bhutanese, Thai or Camargue red rice can be substituted, although the cooking times vary.

If you're using chicken broth to cook the rice, you may not need the added salt.

When using any canned product, such as beans, check the label to make sure ingredients containing gluten have not been added.

You can cook your own beans or use 1 can (14 to 19 oz/398 to 540 mL) no-salt-added red kidney or small red beans, drained and rinsed.

Nutrients per serving	
Calories	219
Fat	3 g
Sodium	191 mg
Carbohydrate	40 g
Fiber	6 g
Protein	9 g
Calcium	49 mg
Magnesium	33 mg
Potassium	428 mg

1 tbsp	olive oil	15 mL
1	onion, finely chopped	1
1	green bell pepper, finely chopped	1
4	stalks celery, diced	4
4	cloves garlic, minced	4
1 tsp	dried thyme	5 mL
1/2 tsp	salt (see tip, at left)	2 mL
1/2 tsp	cracked black peppercorns	2 mL
1/4 tsp	cayenne pepper	1 mL
1 cup	Wehani red rice (see tip, at left), rinsed and drained	250 mL
2 cups	water or ready-to-use reduced-sodium chicken broth (GF, if needed)	500 mL
2 cups	rinsed drained cooked or canned red beans	500 mL
2 cups	cooked green peas	500 mL

1. In a Dutch oven, heat oil over medium heat for 30 seconds. Add onion, bell pepper, celery and garlic and cook, stirring, until pepper is softened, about 5 minutes. Add thyme, salt, peppercorns and cayenne and cook, stirring, for 1 minute.
2. Add rice and toss to coat. Add water and bring to a boil. Reduce heat to low. Cover and simmer until rice is tender and most of the water is absorbed, about 1 hour. Stir in beans and peas and cook, covered, until heated through, about 10 minutes.

Variations

Red Rice, Sausage and Beans: To turn this into a heartier dish, perfect for a pot luck or buffet, add 4 oz (125 g) diced gluten-free kielbasa along with the peas.

Substitute brown rice or a mixture of brown rice and wild rice for the red rice.

Speedy Weeknight Lo Mein

Turn the kitchen into your new favorite fast-food joint with these outstanding and easy noodles.

Makes 4 servings

Tip

Make sure to use fine sea salt in the water you use to cook the noodles. Conventional table salt contains chemicals and additives, whereas sea salt contains an abundance of naturally occurring trace minerals.

Variation

To make the lo mein heartier, add 1 to 1½ cups (250 to 375 mL) cooked shrimp or diced cooked chicken when adding the pasta to the vegetables.

8 oz	quinoa spaghetti pasta or multigrain spaghetti pasta	250 g
1 tsp	ground ginger	5 mL
2 tbsp	reduced-sodium tamari or soy sauce (GF, if needed)	30 mL
2 tbsp	mirin or sherry	30 mL
1 tsp	toasted sesame oil	5 mL
2 tsp	vegetable oil	10 mL
10 oz	frozen stir-fry vegetables, thawed and patted dry	300 g
½ cup	thinly sliced green onions	125 mL

1. In a large pot of boiling salted water (see tip, at left), cook pasta according to package directions until al dente. Drain, reserving ¼ cup (60 mL) pasta water.
2. In a small cup, combine ginger, tamari, mirin and sesame oil.
3. In a large skillet, heat vegetable oil over medium-high heat. Add stir-fry vegetables and cook, stirring, for 3 minutes. Stir in pasta, ginger mixture and green onions; cook, tossing gently, for about 2 minutes or until heated through. If necessary, stir in enough of the reserved pasta water to moisten.

Health Tip

- Mirin is a type of Japanese rice wine. If you are sensitive to alcohol or allergic to fermented foods, omit it from the recipe.

Nutrients per serving	
Calories	303
Fat	5 g
Sodium	390 mg
Carbohydrate	55 g
Fiber	5 g
Protein	11 g
Calcium	41 mg
Magnesium	54 mg
Potassium	336 mg

Desserts and Beverages

Almond Flax Seed Energy Cookies

Almonds not only make these cookies delicious, but also deliver a significant nutritional boost.

Makes 12 cookies

Tips

Look for roasted almonds lightly seasoned with sea salt. If using unsalted roasted almonds (or toasted almonds), add 1⁄8 tsp (0.5 mL) fine sea salt to the recipe.

Store cooled cookies in an airtight container at room temperature for up to 5 days. Or wrap them in plastic wrap, then foil, completely enclosing them, and freeze for up to 6 months. Let thaw at room temperature for 2 to 3 hours before serving.

Nutrients per cookie	
Calories	182
Fat	11 g
Sodium	30 mg
Carbohydrate	19 g
Fiber	4 g
Protein	5 g
Calcium	71 mg
Magnesium	71 mg
Potassium	236 mg

- **Preheat oven to 325°F (160°C)**
- **12-cup muffin pan, sprayed with nonstick cooking spray**

2⁄3 cup	ground flax seeds (flaxseed meal)	150 mL
1⁄2 cup	unsweetened natural almond or peanut butter	125 mL
1⁄3 cup	liquid honey or brown rice syrup	75 mL
1⁄3 cup	plain almond milk	75 mL
2⁄3 cup	raisins	150 mL
2⁄3 cup	lightly salted roasted almonds, chopped	150 mL

1. In a large bowl, whisk together ground flax seeds, almond butter, honey and milk until well combined. Stir in raisins and almonds until just combined.
2. Roll dough into 12 balls of equal size. Press each ball into a prepared muffin cup.
3. Bake in preheated oven for 25 to 30 minutes or until edges are golden brown and tops appear somewhat dry. Let cool in pan on a wire rack for 5 minutes, then transfer to the rack to cool.

Crispy Brown Rice Treats

It's always a good idea to have a few no-nonsense recipes in your repertoire. Crispy rice treats are just that, and this variation on the classic offers both good health and great taste.

Makes 16 bars

Tips

For the dried fruit, try raisins, cranberries, cherries or chopped apricots. For the nut or seed butter, try almond butter, peanut butter or sunflower butter.

Store the rice treats in an airtight container at room temperature for up to 3 days.

- **9-inch (23 cm) square metal baking pan, sprayed with nonstick cooking spray**

4 cups	crisp brown rice cereal	1 L
1/2 cup	finely chopped dried fruit	125 mL
1/2 cup	unsweetened natural nut or seed butter	125 mL
1/3 cup	brown rice syrup or liquid honey	75 mL
2 tsp	vanilla extract (GF, if needed)	10 mL

1. In a large bowl, combine rice cereal and dried fruit.
2. In a small saucepan over medium-low heat, heat nut butter and brown rice syrup for 2 to 3 minutes or until warm and blended. Remove from heat and stir in vanilla.
3. Add the nut butter mixture to the cereal mixture, stirring until combined. Spread in prepared baking pan. Cover and refrigerate for 1 hour or until set. Cut into 16 bars.

Nutrients per bar	
Calories	121
Fat	5 g
Sodium	36 mg
Carbohydrate	18 g
Fiber	2 g
Protein	2 g
Calcium	37 mg
Magnesium	29 mg
Potassium	101 mg

Pear Almond Torte

This thin torte is prepared completely in the food processor. Serve warm from the oven or cold straight from the fridge.

Makes 6 to 8 servings

Tips

To quickly peel pears, use a vegetable peeler.

The torte can be made up to 2 days ahead. Cover with plastic wrap and refrigerate.

A ripe pear will yield slightly when you apply gentle thumb pressure near the base of the stem. Ripen pears in a paper bag on the counter. Check daily — ripening may take 1 to 6 days.

Nutrients per serving (1 of 8)	
Calories	353
Fat	19 g
Sodium	98 mg
Carbohydrate	45 g
Fiber	4 g
Protein	5 g
Calcium	100 mg
Magnesium	49 mg
Potassium	263 mg

- **Food processor**
- **9-inch (23 cm) springform pan, lightly greased and dusted with rice flour**

Topping

2 tsp	granulated sugar	10 mL
1 tsp	ground cinnamon	5 mL
1/2 tsp	ground nutmeg	2 mL
2	pears, peeled, cored and cut into eighths	2
1/3 cup	slivered almonds	75 mL

Base

1/2 cup	almond flour	125 mL
1/2 cup	brown rice flour	125 mL
1 tsp	xanthan gum	5 mL
2 tsp	GF baking powder	10 mL
1/4 tsp	salt	1 mL
1/2 cup	butter, softened	125 mL
1 cup	granulated sugar	250 mL
1 tsp	almond extract (GF, if needed)	5 mL
2	large eggs	2

1. *Topping:* In a medium bowl, stir together sugar, cinnamon and nutmeg; add pears and toss until evenly coated; set aside.
2. *Base:* In a small bowl, combine almond flour, rice flour, xanthan gum, baking powder and salt until mixed; set aside.
3. In food processor, combine butter, sugar and almond extract; pulse until smooth and creamy. Scrape down sides. Add eggs, one at a time, pulsing just until mixed. Add flour mixture; pulse until mixed. Scrape batter into prepared pan. Spread to edges and smooth top with a moist rubber spatula.

Variation

In season, substitute apples, plums, peaches or apricots for the pears. Use enough fruit to cover the base generously and finish a whole piece of fruit.

4. Arrange the coated pear wedges in a circle over the batter and sprinkle with almonds. Let stand for 30 minutes. Meanwhile, preheat oven to 325°F (160°C).
5. Bake in preheated oven for 50 to 55 minutes or until top is a rich golden color and a cake tester inserted in the center comes out clean. Transfer to a rack. Run a knife around the inside edge of pan. Let stand 10 minutes, then remove ring. Serve warm or let cool completely on base on rack.

Health Tip

- Pears are higher in fructose than most fruits, so this treat may increase the risk of diarrhea for some people.

Chocolate Zucchini Cake

Rich, moist and decadently chocolaty, this cake is an excellent way to eat your vegetables. It's delicious to the last crumb.

Makes 9 servings

Tip

Store the cooled cake, loosely wrapped in foil or waxed paper, in the refrigerator for up to 1 week. Alternatively, wrap it in plastic wrap, then foil, completely enclosing cake, and freeze for up to 6 months. Let thaw at room temperature for 4 to 6 hours before serving.

- **Preheat oven to 350°F (180°C)**
- **8-inch (20 cm) square metal baking pan, sprayed with nonstick cooking spray**

1 1⁄4 cups	quinoa flour	300 mL
3⁄4 cup	natural cane sugar or granulated sugar	175 mL
1⁄3 cup	unsweetened cocoa powder (not Dutch process)	75 mL
3⁄4 tsp	baking soda	3 mL
1⁄2 tsp	fine sea salt	2 mL
1	large egg, at room temperature, lightly beaten	1
1⁄3 cup	unsweetened applesauce	75 mL
1⁄4 cup	buttermilk	60 mL
1⁄4 cup	vegetable oil	60 mL
1 tsp	vanilla extract (GF, if needed)	5 mL
1 cup	shredded zucchini	250 mL
1⁄2 cup	miniature semisweet chocolate chips (GF, if needed)	125 mL

1. In a medium bowl, whisk together quinoa flour, sugar, cocoa powder, baking soda and salt.
2. Add egg, applesauce, buttermilk, oil and vanilla to flour mixture. Using an electric mixer on medium-low speed, beat for 1 minute, until blended. Scrape sides and bottom of bowl with a spatula. Beat on medium speed for 1 minute. Gently stir in zucchini.
3. Spread batter evenly in prepared pan.
4. Bake in preheated oven for 15 minutes. Sprinkle with chocolate chips. Bake for 7 to 11 minutes or until a toothpick inserted in the center comes out with a few moist crumbs attached. Let cool completely in pan on a wire rack.

Nutrients per serving	
Calories	263
Fat	11 g
Sodium	281 mg
Carbohydrate	37 g
Fiber	4 g
Protein	4 g
Calcium	29 mg
Magnesium	15 mg
Potassium	98 mg

Raspberry Custard Cake

As this delicious, old-fashioned dessert cooks, the batter separates into a light soufflé-like layer on top, with a rich, creamy custard on the bottom. Serve hot or warm, accompanied by a light cookie, with whipped cream on the side, if desired.

Makes 6 servings

Variation

Blueberry Custard Cake: Substitute blueberries for the raspberries.

- **Large (minimum 5-quart) oval slow cooker**
- **6-cup (1.5 L) baking or soufflé dish, lightly greased**

1 cup	granulated sugar, divided	250 mL
2 tbsp	butter, softened	30 mL
4	large eggs, separated	4
	Grated zest and juice of 1 lemon	
Pinch	salt	Pinch
1/4 cup	all-purpose flour	60 mL
1 cup	milk	250 mL
1 1/2 cups	raspberries, thawed if frozen	375 mL
	Confectioners' (icing) sugar	

1. In a bowl, beat 3/4 cup (175 mL) sugar with butter until light and fluffy. Beat in egg yolks until incorporated. Stir in lemon zest and juice. Add salt, then flour and mix until blended. Gradually add milk, beating to make a smooth batter.
2. In a separate bowl, with clean beaters, beat egg whites until soft peaks form. Add the remaining sugar and beat until stiff peaks form. Fold into lemon mixture, then fold in raspberries.
3. Pour mixture into prepared dish. Cover tightly with foil and secure with a string. Place dish in slow cooker stoneware and add boiling water to reach 1 inch (2.5 cm) up the sides. Cover and cook on High for about 3 hours or until the cake springs back when touched lightly in the center. Dust lightly with confectioners' sugar and serve.

Health Tip

- If this recipe puts your percentage of acidifying foods over 20% for the day, increase the amount of alkalizing foods in your diet for the next 24 hours. Testing the pH of your urine and saliva first thing in the morning and checking that value against other days from your Health Life & Diet Diary will help you stay on track.

Nutrients per serving	
Calories	264
Fat	8 g
Sodium	67 mg
Carbohydrate	44 g
Fiber	2 g
Protein	7 g
Calcium	92 mg
Magnesium	17 mg
Potassium	161 mg

Five-Minute Cheesecake Cups with Raspberries

This quick, lower-fat cheesecake recipe will put a smile on everyone's face!

Makes 2 servings

- **Food processor**
- **Two ¾-cup (175 mL) ramekins or dessert glasses**

1 cup	nonfat cottage cheese	250 mL
1 tbsp	agave nectar or liquid honey	15 mL
½ tsp	vanilla extract (GF, if needed)	2 mL
⅔ cup	raspberries	150 mL
2 tbsp	finely chopped lightly salted roasted pistachios	30 mL

1. In food processor, combine cottage cheese, agave nectar and vanilla; purée until smooth.
2. Divide mixture between ramekins. Top with raspberries and pistachios.

Health Tip

- If you suspect that seeds may worsen the symptoms of your GI condition, omit the pistachios. This dessert tastes great without them too!

Nutrients per serving	
Calories	181
Fat	5 g
Sodium	321 mg
Carbohydrate	18 g
Fiber	4 g
Protein	16 g
Calcium	79 mg
Magnesium	15 mg
Potassium	161 mg

Maple Pumpkin Micro-Pies

These maple-pumpkin mini sweets — crispy, creamy and wonderfully spiced — are easy enough for a weeknight dessert and good enough for company.

Makes 16 servings

Tips

These are best eaten soon after baking.

An equal amount of ground cinnamon may be used in place of the pumpkin pie spice.

Nutrients per serving	
Calories	56
Fat	0 g
Sodium	47 mg
Carbohydrate	13 g
Fiber	1 g
Protein	1 g
Calcium	14 mg
Magnesium	6 mg
Potassium	49 mg

- **Preheat oven to 400°F (200°C)**
- **Baking sheet, lined with parchment paper**

1 cup	pumpkin purée (not pie filling)	250 mL
1/4 cup	pure maple syrup, liquid honey or brown rice syrup	60 mL
1 tsp	pumpkin pie spice	5 mL
16	wonton wrappers	16
	Nonstick cooking spray	
1 tbsp	turbinado (raw) sugar	15 mL

1. In a medium bowl, whisk together pumpkin purée, maple syrup and pumpkin pie spice.
2. Place one wonton wrapper on a work surface. Spoon 1 tbsp (15 mL) filling into center of wrapper. Using a pastry brush or a fingertip, moisten the edges of the wrapper with water. Fold in half to form a triangle, pressing the edges to seal. Repeat with the remaining wontons and filling.
3. Arrange filled wontons on prepared baking sheet. Lightly spray both sides of wontons with cooking spray and sprinkle tops with turbinado sugar.
4. Bake in preheated oven for 14 minutes. Carefully turn wontons over and bake for 4 to 5 minutes or until golden. Let cool on pan on a wire rack.

Trendy Pastry

Though not quite as tender as pastry made with shortening or butter, this pastry, made with vegetable oil, is just as easy to work with.

Makes enough pastry for 1 double-crust or 2 single-crust 9-inch (23 cm) pies

Tips

If the pastry cracks while you're handling it, don't worry: just use the excess to patch.

This pastry can also be made into tart shells to fill with custard and fresh fruit or to make mini-quiches or hors d'oeuvre tartlets.

Nutrients per single-crust pastry	
Calories	272
Fat	11 g
Sodium	301 mg
Carbohydrate	42 g
Fiber	2 g
Protein	4 g
Calcium	58 mg
Magnesium	2 mg
Potassium	137 mg

1½ cups	sorghum flour	375 mL
1 cup	cornstarch	250 mL
½ cup	tapioca starch	125 mL
1 tbsp	granulated sugar	15 mL
2 tsp	GF baking powder	10 mL
1 tsp	salt	5 mL
1	large egg	1
½ cup	ice water	125 mL
⅓ cup	vegetable oil	75 mL
2 tbsp	cider vinegar	30 mL

Food Processor Method

1. In a food processor, combine sorghum flour, cornstarch, tapioca starch, sugar, baking powder and salt; pulse until combined. Set aside.
2. In a small bowl, whisk together egg, ice water, oil and vinegar.
3. With food processor running, add egg mixture through feed tube in a slow, steady stream. Process until dough just holds together. Do not let it form a ball.

Traditional Method

1. In a large bowl, sift sorghum flour, cornstarch, tapioca starch, sugar, baking powder and salt. Set aside.
2. In a small bowl, whisk together egg, ice water, oil and vinegar.
3. Stirring with a fork, sprinkle egg mixture, a little at a time, over the flour mixture to make a soft dough.

For Both Methods

4. Divide dough in half. Gently gather each piece into a ball and flatten into a disc. Place the pastry disc between two sheets of parchment paper. Using quick, firm strokes of the rolling pin, roll out the dough into a circle about 1 inch (2.5 cm) larger than the diameter of an inverted pie plate. Carefully remove the top sheet of parchment paper and invert the pastry over the pie plate, easing it in. Carefully peel off the remaining sheet of parchment paper.

Tips

You can freeze the pastry for up to 3 months. Thaw in refrigerator. Bring to room temperature before rolling out.

While rolling out the first half of the dough, cover the remaining half to prevent it from drying out.

5. To prepare another single-crust pie, repeat step 4 with the remaining dough. To prepare the top crust for a double-crust pie, roll out the remaining dough as directed above, then set aside.

For a Single-Crust Pie

Trim excess pastry to edge of pie plate, patch any cracks with trimmings, and press edges with a fork. Or, for a more attractive finish, using a sharp knife, trim the pastry evenly, leaving a 1-inch (2.5 cm) overhang. Tuck pastry under to form a raised double rim. Flute or crimp the edges.

To Bake an Unfilled Pastry Shell

To prevent pastry from shrinking or puffing up, prick bottom and sides with a fork. Bake in oven preheated to 425°F (220°C) for 18 to 20 minutes or until golden. Let cool completely before filling.

To Bake a Filled Pastry Shell

Do not prick the pastry. Spoon filling into unbaked pastry shell and bake according to individual recipe directions.

For a Double-Crust Pie

For instructions on finishing and baking, see recipe for Strawberry Rhubarb Pie, page 380.

Strawberry Rhubarb Pie

When fresh local rhubarb and strawberries are at their prime, it's the perfect time to make pie.

Makes 6 to 8 servings

Tip

For the best flavor and color, purchase fresh local berries while they're in season. Choose firm stalks of rhubarb that are fresh and crisp; slender stalks are more tender than thick ones.

Nutrients per serving (1 of 8)	
Calories	141
Fat	0 g
Sodium	3 mg
Carbohydrate	36 g
Fiber	2 g
Protein	1 g
Calcium	59 mg
Magnesium	13 mg
Potassium	241 mg

- **9-inch (23 cm) deep-dish pie plate**

4 cups	chopped fresh rhubarb (or frozen rhubarb, thawed)	1 L
2 cups	quartered fresh strawberries	500 mL
1 cup	granulated sugar	250 mL
⅓ cup	tapioca starch	75 mL
2 tsp	freshly squeezed lemon juice	10 mL
	Trendy Pastry (page 378)	

1. In a large bowl, toss together rhubarb, strawberries, sugar and tapioca starch. Add the lemon juice. Let stand for 15 minutes. Meanwhile, preheat oven to 425°F (220°C).
2. Roll out pastry for a double-crust pie and press the bottom pastry into pie plate as directed on page 378. Spoon filling into the unbaked pie shell and moisten the edge. Carefully remove the top sheet of parchment paper from the top pastry, invert and cover the filling. Carefully peel off the remaining sheet of parchment paper. Trim pastry, leaving a ¾-inch (2 cm) overhang. Fold overhang under bottom pastry rim, seal and flute edge.
3. Make numerous ½-inch (1 cm) slits near the center of the pie through the crust to the filling or cut out a 1-inch (2.5 cm) circle in the center of the crust.
4. Position the oven racks to divide the oven into thirds. Place a baking sheet on the bottom rack to catch the drips if pie boils over. Bake in preheated oven on the top rack for 20 minutes. Reduce heat to 350°F (180°C) and bake for 40 to 50 minutes or until crust is golden and filling is bubbly. Shield edges with foil if they are browning too quickly. Let cool completely on a rack.

Variation

To make a rhubarb pie, substitute rhubarb for the strawberries and increase the granulated sugar to 1¼ cups (300 mL).

The Ultimate Baked Apples

These luscious apples, simple to make yet delicious, are the definitive autumn dessert.

Makes 8 servings

Tip

When buying nuts, be sure to source them from a purveyor with high turnover. Because nuts are high in fat (but healthy fat), they tend to become rancid very quickly. This is especially true of walnuts. Taste before you buy, if possible. If they are not sweet, substitute an equal quantity of pecans.

- **Large (minimum 5-quart) oval slow cooker**

1/2 cup	chopped toasted walnuts	125 mL
1/2 cup	dried cranberries	125 mL
2 tbsp	packed brown sugar	30 mL
1 tsp	grated orange zest	5 mL
8	apples, cored	8
1 cup	cranberry juice	250 mL
	Vanilla-flavored yogurt or whipped cream or vegan alternative (optional)	

1. In a bowl, combine walnuts, cranberries, sugar and orange zest. To stuff the apples, hold your hand over the bottom of the apple and, using your fingers, tightly pack core space with filling. One at a time, place filled apples in slow cooker stoneware. Drizzle cranberry juice evenly over tops.
2. Cover and cook on Low for 8 hours or on High for 4 hours, until apples are tender.
3. Transfer apples to a serving dish and spoon cooking juices over them. Serve hot with a dollop of yogurt, if desired.

Nutrients per serving	
Calories	194
Fat	5 g
Sodium	4 mg
Carbohydrate	39 g
Fiber	5 g
Protein	2 g
Calcium	22 mg
Magnesium	27 mg
Potassium	268 mg

Cinnamon Applesauce

This applesauce couldn't be easier to make and it's a great source of fiber.

Makes about 3 cups (750 mL)

Tip

To remove the skin and core from an apple, cut a small amount from both the top and bottom of the apple. Use a vegetable peeler to remove the skin. Cut into four equal parts and, using a paring knife held on an angle, remove the core.

- **Food processor**

4 cups	chopped peeled apples	1 L
1 tsp	freshly squeezed lemon juice	5 mL
2 tsp	ground cinnamon	10 mL

1. In food processor, combine apples, lemon juice and cinnamon; process until smooth, stopping the machine once or twice to scrape down the sides of the work bowl.
2. Transfer to a bowl. Serve immediately or cover and refrigerate for up to 4 days.

Variation

Substitute pears for the apples and add a pinch of freshly grated nutmeg.

Nutrients per ½ cup (125 mL)	
Calories	46
Fat	0 g
Sodium	1 mg
Carbohydrate	12 g
Fiber	2 g
Protein	0 g
Calcium	14 mg
Magnesium	5 mg
Potassium	94 mg

Pumpkin Rice Pudding

The combination of flavors and the chewy but crunchy texture of this luscious pudding make it hard to resist.

Makes 8 servings

Tips

Cook 1 cup (250 mL) raw rice to get the 2 cups (500 mL) of cooked rice required for this recipe.

If you don't have evaporated cane juice sugar, use dark brown sugar instead.

If you prefer, use 1½ tsp (7 mL) pumpkin pie spice instead of the cinnamon, nutmeg and cloves.

Nutrients per serving	
Calories	255
Fat	3 g
Sodium	61 mg
Carbohydrate	52 g
Fiber	4 g
Protein	7 g
Calcium	123 mg
Magnesium	66 mg
Potassium	341 mg

- **Small (3½-quart) slow cooker, stoneware greased**

2 cups	cooked brown rice (see tip, at left)	500 mL
1½ cups	pumpkin purée (not pie filling)	375 mL
1 cup	dried cranberries or dried cherries	250 mL
1 cup	evaporated skim milk	250 mL
½ cup	packed evaporated cane juice sugar or muscovado sugar (see tip, at left)	125 mL
2	large eggs	2
1 tsp	ground cinnamon (see tip, at left)	5 mL
½ tsp	grated nutmeg	2 mL
¼ tsp	ground cloves	1 mL
	Toasted chopped pecans (optional)	
	Vanilla-flavored yogurt or whipped cream (optional)	

1. In prepared slow cooker stoneware, combine rice, pumpkin purée and cranberries.
2. In a bowl, whisk together milk, sugar, eggs, cinnamon, nutmeg and cloves until smooth and blended. Stir into pumpkin mixture. Cover and cook on High for 3 hours, until pudding is set. Serve warm, garnished with toasted pecans and a dollop of yogurt, if desired.

Health Tip

- Pumpkin is an alkalizing food, as are the spices in this recipe. Enjoy this slow-cooked dessert with the knowledge that it provides minerals that buffer or reduce the acid levels in your body.

Nut Milk

Most people do not realize how simple it is to make non-dairy milk at home. This recipe contains three ingredients and takes no more than 5 minutes to make.

Makes about 4 cups (1 L)

Tips

Soaking the almonds will make the milk a bit creamier. If you have time, soak them for 30 minutes in 4 cups (1 L) warm water. When the soaking time has been completed, drain, discard the soaking liquid and rinse the almonds under cold running water until the water runs clear.

You can also strain the nut milk through cheesecloth or a nut-milk bag placed over a pitcher large enough to accommodate the liquid.

Nutrients per 1 cup (250 mL)	
Calories	206
Fat	18 g
Sodium	97 mg
Carbohydrate	8 g
Fiber	4 g
Protein	8 g
Calcium	102 mg
Magnesium	98 mg
Potassium	252 mg

- **Blender**
- **Fine-mesh sieve**

1 cup	whole raw almonds (see tip, at left)	250 mL
4 cups	filtered water	1 L
Pinch	fine sea salt	Pinch

1. In blender, combine almonds, water and salt. Blend on high speed for 45 seconds or until liquid becomes milky white and no visible pieces of almond remain.
2. Transfer to sieve and strain (see tip, at left). Serve immediately or cover and refrigerate for up to 3 days. Discard pulp or save for another use.

Variations

For slightly sweet nut milk, omit the salt and add a pinch of ground cinnamon and 1 or 2 pitted dates.

Almond Berry Milk: After processing the nut milk in step 1, add 1 cup (250 mL) of your favorite berry (such as blueberries or strawberries) and blend at high speed until smooth.

Cashew, Hazelnut or Coconut Milk: Substitute an equal quantity of raw cashews, raw hazelnuts or unsweetened dried shredded coconut for the almonds.

Fruity Milkshake

Pour this delicious shake into a stainless steel container and enjoy it on your way to work or as a pick-me-up snack. By all means, double or triple this recipe to make as much as you need.

Makes 3 servings

Tip

You can purchase ground flax seeds (which may be called flaxseed meal), grind whole seeds in the blender before adding the remainder of the ingredients, or grind them in a coffee or spice grinder. If you grind your own, ensure that your blender, coffee grinder or spice grinder is used for gluten-free foods only, to avoid the risk of cross-contamination.

- **Blender**

1/2	small banana	1/2
1 1/2 cups	strawberries	375 mL
1 cup	fortified GF non-dairy milk	250 mL
1/2 cup	GF soy yogurt or yogurt	125 mL
1 tbsp	ground flax seeds (flaxseed meal)	15 mL

1. In blender, combine banana, strawberries, milk, yogurt and flax seeds. Blend for 1 minute.

Variations

Try using a flavored yogurt.

If you prefer to use lower-sugar fruit, try kiwifruit, peaches, apricots, blueberries or blackberries.

Nutrients per serving	
Calories	113
Fat	3 g
Sodium	42 mg
Carbohydrate	19 g
Fiber	3 g
Protein	5 g
Calcium	172 mg
Magnesium	33 mg
Potassium	328 mg

Strawberry Cheesecake Smoothie

This smoothie is so sinfully sweet you won't believe it's good for you. The blend of rich cashews, aromatic vanilla and sweet strawberries is a match made in heaven.

Makes 1 serving

Tips

To soak the cashews, place in a bowl and cover with warm water. Cover and set aside for 10 minutes. Drain, discarding soaking water.

Coconut oil is solid at room temperature. It has a melting temperature of 76°F (24°C), so it is easy to liquefy. To melt it, place in a shallow glass bowl over a pot of simmering water.

Nutrients per serving	
Calories	735
Fat	66 g
Sodium	106 mg
Carbohydrate	29 g
Fiber	7 g
Protein	15 g
Calcium	136 mg
Magnesium	228 mg
Potassium	640 mg

- **Blender**

1 cup	Nut Milk (page 384) or hemp milk	250 mL
½ cup	hulled strawberries	125 mL
⅓ cup	raw cashews, soaked (see tip, at left)	75 mL
2 tbsp	melted coconut oil (see tip, at left)	30 mL
½ tsp	raw vanilla extract (GF, if needed)	2 mL

1. In blender, combine nut milk, strawberries, soaked cashews, coconut oil and vanilla. Blend until smooth. Serve immediately.

Variations

Mixed Berry Cheesecake Smoothie: Substitute ¼ cup (60 mL) blueberries, 3 to 4 raspberries and 2 to 3 blackberries for the strawberries.

If you prefer a sweeter smoothie, add 1 to 2 tbsp (15 to 30 mL) raw agave nectar.

Almond Banana Smoothie

Nutmeg adds a new twist to a family favorite.

Makes 1 to 2 servings

Tip

Although many of the recipes call for unflavored soy milk, some flavored soy milks work equally well in fruit smoothies. Feel free to substitute your favorite flavor.

- **Blender**

1 cup	soy milk	250 mL
3 tbsp	chopped almonds	45 mL
2	bananas, cut into chunks	2
Pinch	ground nutmeg	Pinch

1. In blender, combine soy milk, almonds, bananas and nutmeg. Secure lid and blend (from low to high if using a variable-speed blender) until smooth.

Health Tip

- Bananas are high in potassium and are known to bulk up loose stools, so they're a good choice when diarrhea symptoms are present.

Nutrients per serving (1 of 2)	
Calories	260
Fat	7 g
Sodium	58 mg
Carbohydrate	31 g
Fiber	4 g
Protein	6 g
Calcium	181 mg
Magnesium	73 mg
Potassium	581 mg

Apple Pear Lemonade

This is a simple way to make fresh lemonade sweetened only with fruit.

Makes about 2½ cups (625 mL)

Tips

Typically a medium-sized lemon will yield about 3 tbsp (45 mL) fresh lemon juice.

To yield the maximum juice from citrus fruits, let them sit at room temperature for 30 minutes before juicing. Use the palm of your hand to roll the fruit on the counter to release the juices before slicing and squeezing.

- **Juicer**

2	apples, quartered	2
2	pears, quartered	2
½ cup	freshly squeezed lemon juice (see tip, at left)	125 mL
¼ cup	filtered water	60 mL
Pinch	ground cinnamon	Pinch

1. In juicer, process apples and pears.
2. Transfer resulting juice to a container and whisk in lemon juice, water and cinnamon. Serve immediately or cover and refrigerate for up to 2 days.

Health Tip

- Stay well hydrated for improved health. Increased thirst, dry mouth, fatigue and light-headedness are some of the signs of dehydration.

Nutrients per ½ cup (125 mL)	
Calories	85
Fat	0 g
Sodium	2 mg
Carbohydrate	23 g
Fiber	4 g
Protein	1 g
Calcium	12 mg
Magnesium	10 mg
Potassium	188 mg

Grapey Pear Juice

Most people never think to juice whole grapes, but they yield a delicious drink.

Makes about 1½ cups (375 mL)

Tip

Grapes are likely to contain high amounts of pesticides and herbicides. When purchasing, buy organic grapes if possible.

Nutrients per ½ cup (125 mL)	
Calories	110
Fat	0 g
Sodium	2 mg
Carbohydrate	29 g
Fiber	4 g
Protein	1 g
Calcium	19 mg
Magnesium	11 mg
Potassium	258 mg

- **Juicer**

2 cups	red grapes, divided (see tip, at left)	500 mL
2	pears, quartered, divided	2

1. In juicer, process ¼ cup (60 mL) grapes and 1 pear quarter. Repeat until all the grapes and pears have been juiced. Whisk and serve immediately.

Variation

Grapey Apple Juice: Substitute an equal quantity of white grapes for the red grapes, and apples for the pears.

Cherries Jubilee

This delicious smoothie serves as a healthy start to your day or a great snack anytime.

Makes 3 servings

Nutrients per serving	
Calories	155
Fat	3 g
Sodium	40 mg
Carbohydrate	32 g
Fiber	4 g
Protein	4 g
Calcium	120 mg
Magnesium	49 mg
Potassium	506 mg

- **Blender**

1 cup	soy or rice milk	250 mL
1 cup	pitted cherries	250 mL
2	pineapple wedges, cut into chunks	2
2	frozen banana chunks	2
1 tbsp	flax seeds	15 mL
⅛ tsp	almond extract (GF, if needed)	0.5 mL

1. In blender, combine soy milk, cherries, pineapple, banana, flax seeds and almond extract. Secure lid and blend (from low to high if using a variable-speed blender) until smooth.

Orange Aid

This refreshing beverage is great during any season. The citrus fruits are alkalizing and will help balance your pH.

Makes 3 servings

Nutrients per serving	
Calories	101
Fat	1 g
Sodium	6 mg
Carbohydrate	25 g
Fiber	3 g
Protein	2 g
Calcium	28 mg
Magnesium	16 mg
Potassium	464 mg

- **Blender**

3/4 cup	freshly squeezed orange juice	175 mL
2 tsp	freshly squeezed lemon juice	10 mL
2	nectarines, halved	2
1	orange, sectioned and seeded	1
1	cantaloupe wedge, cubed	1

1. In blender, combine orange juice, lemon juice, nectarines, orange and cantaloupe. Secure lid and blend (from low to high if using a variable-speed blender) until smooth.

Ginger Sun Tea

Ginger adds that special touch to a summertime cooler.

Makes about 6 cups (1.5 L)

Tips

You can substitute 3 teabags for the loose green tea.

If you don't have fresh stevia, you can use 1 tsp (5 mL) dried.

Nutrients per 1/2 cup (125 mL)	
Calories	9
Fat	0 g
Sodium	0 mg
Carbohydrate	2 g
Fiber	0 g
Protein	0 g
Calcium	3 mg
Magnesium	1 mg
Potassium	15 mg

- **8-cup (2 L) clear glass container**

1	2-inch (5 cm) piece gingerroot (unpeeled), thinly sliced	1
4 tbsp	green tea leaves	60 mL
1 tbsp	bruised fresh stevia leaves	15 mL
6 cups	warm water	1.5 L
2 tbsp	ginger syrup	30 mL
	Lemon slices	

1. In container, combine ginger, tea leaves, stevia leaves and water. Cover with a lid or clear plastic wrap. Let stand in direct sun, preferably outside, for 3 hours.
2. Strain through a fine sieve into a serving pitcher. Stir in syrup and chill. To serve, fill glasses with ice. Pour in tea and garnish with lemon slice.

Contributing Authors

Alexandra Anca with Theresa Santandrea-Cull
Complete Gluten-Free Diet & Nutrition Guide
Recipes from this book are found on pages 178, 192, 248, 260, 334 and 385.

Andrew Chase
The Asian Bistro Cookbook
Recipes from this book are found on pages 204, 231, 238, 306, 314 and 316.

Cinda Chavich
The Wild West Cookbook
Recipes from this book are found on pages 272, 274, 304, 305, 320, 344 (bottom) and 357.

Pat Crocker
The Healing Herbs Cookbook
Recipes from this book are found on pages 210, 253, 254, 257, 327, 329 and 390 (bottom).

Pat Crocker
The Smoothies Bible, Second Edition
Recipes from this book are found on pages 387, 389 (bottom) and 390 (top).

Dietitians of Canada
Simply Great Food
Recipes from this book are found on pages 172, 173, 228 (bottom), 264, 273, 275, 279, 282, 297, 344 (top), 353 and 356.

Judith Finlayson
The Complete Gluten-Free Whole Grains Cookbook
Recipes from this book are found on pages 171, 185, 208, 288, 330, 365 and 367.

Judith Finlayson
The Healthy Slow Cooker, Second Edition
Recipes from this book are found on pages 170, 188, 236, 246, 276, 280, 284, 286, 336, 340 and 383.

Judith Finlayson
The Vegetarian Slow Cooker
Recipes from this book are found on pages 169, 197, 198 (bottom), 214, 234, 237, 240, 324, 326, 328, 354, 375 and 381.

George Geary
500 Best Sauces, Salad Dressings, Marinades & More
Recipes from this book are found on pages 225 (bottom), 226, 227, 228 (top), 261, 266 and 267.

Margaret Howard
The 250 Best 4-Ingredient Recipes
Recipes from this book are found on pages 219, 221, 270 (top), 281, 292, 295, 312, 358, 359 and 364.

Jan Main
200 Best Lactose-Free Recipes
Recipes from this book are found on pages 179, 251, 256 and 262.

Douglas McNish
Eat Raw, Eat Well
Recipes from this book are found on pages 168, 189, 202, 217, 222, 242 and 382.

Douglas McNish
Raw, Quick & Delicious
Recipes from this book are found on pages 167, 180, 216, 218, 223, 363, 384, 386, 388 and 389 (top).

The Organic Gourmet
Recipes from this book are found on pages 232, 265, 313 and 321.

Jane Rodmell
All the Best Recipes
Recipes from this book are found on pages 198 (top), 206, 220, 230, 258, 278, 283, 293, 298, 302, 310, 345 and 350.

Susan Sampson
The Complete Leafy Greens Cookbook
Recipes from this book are found on pages 244, 250, 252, 255, 268, 269, 322, 338, 346, 347, 348 and 349.

Camilla V. Saulsbury
5 Easy Steps to Healthy Cooking
Recipes from this book are found on pages 196, 199, 203, 215, 308, 341, 360, 366, 368, 370, 371, 376 and 377.

Camilla V. Saulsbury
500 Best Quinoa Recipes
Recipes from this book are found on pages 181, 194, 209, 317, 318, 342 and 374.

Donna Washburn and Heather Butt
The Best Gluten-Free Family Cookbook
Recipes from this book are found on pages 166, 174, 182, 195, 200, 212, 290, 296, 333 and 372.

Donna Washburn and Heather Butt
Easy Everyday Gluten-Free Cooking
Recipes from this book are found on pages 176, 184, 186, 190, 294, 301, 332, 362, 378 and 380.

Katherine E. Younker, Editor
America's Complete Diabetes Cookbook
Recipes from this book are found on pages 270 (bottom), 352 and 361.

Resources

Call your local public health office for associations and support organizations near you.

Agency for Healthcare Research and Quality, U.S. Department of Health & Human Services: www.ahrq.gov

British Dietetic Association: www.bda.uk.com

British Society of Gastroenterology: www.bsg.org.uk

Canadian Celiac Association: www.celiac.ca

Canadian Digestive Health Foundation: www.cdhf.ca

Centers for Disease Control and Prevention: www.cdc.gov/chronicdisease

Continence Foundation of Australia: www.continence.org.au/pages/bristol-stool-chart.html

Crohn's and Colitis Foundation of Canada: www.ccfc.ca

Crohn's and Colitis UK: www.crohnsandcolitis.org.uk

Dietitians of Canada: www.dietitians.ca

Dietitians Association of Australia: http://daa.asn.au

Dr. Jeff Health Center: http://drjeffhealthcenter.com

EatRight Ontario, Resources, Irritable Bowel Syndrome: www.eatrightontario.ca/en/Articles/Digestion-Digestive-health/Irritable-Bowel-Syndrome.aspx#.U6mKdyhJl9k

European Crohn's and Colitis Organisation: www.ecco-ibd.eu

European Federation of Crohn's and Ulcerative Colitis Associations: www.efcca.org

Food as Medicine Institute, National College of Natural Medicine: http://foodasmedicineinstitute.com

Gastroenterological Society of Australia, GI Health and Nutrition Centre: www.gesa.org.au/consumer.asp?cid=1&id=1

Health Canada, Eating Well with Canada's Food Guide: www.hc-sc.gc.ca/fn-an/food-guide-aliment/index-eng.php

Health Canada, It's Your Health: www.hc-sc.gc.ca/hl-vs/iyh-vsv/index-eng.php

HealthLink BC, Healthy Eating Guidelines for People with Irritable Bowel Syndrome: www.healthlinkbc.ca/healthyeating/irritable-bowel-syndrome.html

IBS Network: www.theibsnetwork.org

International Confederation of Dietetic Associations: www.internationaldietetics.org

International Foundation for Functional Gastrointestinal Disorders: www.iffgd.org

Irritable Bowel Syndrome Self Help and Support Group: www.ibsgroup.org/ibsassociation.org

Johns Hopkins Medicine: www.hopkinsmedicine.org

Mayo Clinic: www.mayoclinic.org

National Institute for Health and Care Excellence, Gastrointestinal Conditions Overview: http://pathways.nice.org.uk/pathways/gastrointestinal-conditions

USDA, Choose My Plate: www.choosemyplate.gov

References and Background Reading

Books

El-Hashemy S, Downorowicz E, Rouchotas P, et al. *Family Medicine & Integrative Primary Care: Standards & Guidelines*. Toronto: CCNM Press, 2011. Gastroenterology, gastroesophageal reflux disease; p. 133–35.

Smith, F. *An Introduction to Principles & Practices of Naturopathic Medicine*. Toronto: CCNM Press, 2008.

Journal Articles

Adams JB, Johansen LJ, Powell LD, et al. Gastrointestinal flora and gastrointestinal status in children with autism — Comparisons to typical children and correlation with autism severity. *BMC Gastroenterology*, 2011 Mar 16; 11: 22.

Adeva MM, Souto G. Diet-induced metabolic acidosis. *Clin Nutr*, 2011 Aug; 30(4): 416–21.

Adibi SA, Ruiz C, Glaser P, Fogel MR. Effect of intraluminal pH on absorption rates of leucine, water, and electrolytes in human jejunum. *Gastroenterology*, 1972 Oct; 63(4): 611–18.

Alfaro V, Ródenas J, Palaclos L, et al. Blood acid-base changes during acute experimental inflammation in rats. *Can J Physiol Pharmacol*, 1996 Mar; 74(3): 313–19.

Almomani EY, Kaur S, Alexander RT, Cordat E. Intercalated cells: More than pH regulation. *Diseases*, 2014 Apr 8; 2(2): 71–92.

Altman KW, Haines GK 3rd, Hammer G, Radosevich JA. The H+/K+ –ATPase (proton) pump is expressed in human laryngeal submucosal glands. *Laryngoscope*, 2003 Nov; 113(11): 1927–30.

Beckmann M, Lloyd AJ, Haldar S, et al. Dietary exposure biomarker-lead discovery based on metabolomics analysis of urine samples. *Proc Nutr Soc*, 2013 Aug; 72(3): 352–61.

Bonjour JP. Nutritional disturbance in acid-base balance and osteoporosis: A hypothesis that disregards the essential homeostatic role of the kidney. *Br J Nutr*, 2013 Oct; 110(7): 1168–77.

Bücker R, Azevedo-Vethacke M, Groll C, et al. Helicobacter pylori colonization critically depends on postprandial gastric conditions. *Sci Rep*, 2012; 2: 994.

Colombel JF, Sandborn WJ, Reinisch W, et al; SONIC Study Group. Infliximab, azathioprine, or combination therapy for Crohn's disease. *N Engl J Med*, 2010 Apr 15; 362(15): 1383–95.

Costea I, Mack DR, Lemaitre RN, et al. Interactions between the dietary poly-unsaturated fatty acid ratio and genetic factors determine susceptibility to pediatric Crohn's disease. *Gastroenterology*, 2014 Apr; 146(4): 929–31.

de Nadai TR, de Nadai MN, Albuquerque AA, et al. Metabolic acidosis treatment as part of a strategy to curb inflammation. *Int J Inflam*, 2013 June 6 (epub): 601424.

Engberink MF, Bakker SJ, Brink EJ, et al. Dietary acid load and risk of hypertension: The Rotterdam Study. *Am J Clin Nutr*, 2012 Jun; 95(6): 1438–44.

Evans DF, Pye G, Bramley R, et al. Measurement of gastrointestinal pH profiles in normal ambulant human subjects. *Gut*, 1988 Aug; 29(8): 1035–41.

Farraye FA, Odze RD, Eaden J, et al; AGA Institute Medical Position Panel on Diagnosis and Management of Colorectal Neoplasia in Inflammatory Bowel Disease. AGA medical position statement on the diagnosis and management of colorectal neoplasia in inflammatory bowel disease. *Gastroenterology*, 2010 Feb; 138(2): 738–45.

Fenton TR, Tough SC, Lyon AW, et al. Causal assessment of dietary acid load and bone disease: A systematic review & meta-analysis applying Hill's epidemiologic criteria for causality. *Nutr J*, 2011 Apr 30; 10: 41.

Flint HJ. The impact of nutrition on the human microbiome. *Nutr Rev*, 2012 Aug; 70 Suppl 1: S10–13.

Gennari FJ, Weise WJ. Acid-base disturbances in gastrointestinal disease. *Clin J Am Soc Nephrol*, 2008 Nov; 3(6): 1861–68.

Heinzmann SS, Merrifield CA, Rezzi S, et al. Stability and robustness of human metabolic phenotypes in response to sequential food challenges. *J Proteome Res*, 2012 Feb 3; 11(2): 643–55.

Horowitz S. Acid-base balance, health, and diet. *Altern and Complement Ther*, 2009 Dec; 15(6): 292–96.

Hussain Z, Quigley EM. Systematic review: Complementary and alternative medicine in the irritable bowel syndrome. *Aliment Pharmacol Ther*, 2006 Feb 15; 23(4): 465–71.

Johansson ME, Ambort D, Pelaseyed T, et al. Composition and functional role of the mucus layers in the intestine. *Cell Mol Life Sci*, 2011 Nov; 68(22): 3635–41.

Kanbara A, Hakoda M, Seyama I. Urine alkalization facilitates uric acid excretion. *Nutr J*, 2010 Oct; 9: 45.

Khan KJ, Dubinsky MC, Ford AC, et al. Efficacy of immunosuppressive therapy for inflammatory bowel disease: A systematic review and meta-analysis. *Am J Gastroenterol*, 2011 Apr; 106(4): 630–42.

Kim K, Mall C, Taylor SL, et al. Mealtime, temporal, and daily variability of the human urinary and plasma metabolomes in a tightly controlled environment. *PLoS One*, 2014 Jan 24; 9(1): e86223.

Koufman JA. Low-acid diet for recalcitrant laryngopharyngeal reflux: Therapeutic benefits and their implications. *Ann Otol Rhinol Laryngol*, 2011 May; 120(5): 281–87.

Lampe JW, Navarro SL, Hullar MA, Shojaie A. Inter-individual differences in response to dietary intervention: Integrating omics platforms towards personalised dietary recommendations. *Proc Nutr Soc*, 2013 May; 72(2): 207–18.

Lands WE. Dietary fat and health: The evidence and the politics of prevention — Careful use of dietary fats can improve life and prevent disease. *Ann NY Acad Sci*, 2005 Dec; 1055: 179–92.

MacArtain P, Gill CI, Brooks M, et al. Nutritional value of edible seaweeds. *Nutr Rev*, 2007 Dec; 65(12 Pt 1): 535–43.

Manderscheid RW, Ryff CD, Freeman EJ, et al. Evolving definitions of mental illness and wellness. *Prev Chronic Dis*, 2010 Jan; 7(1): A19.

Mascarenhas C, Nunoo R, Asgeirsson T, et al. Outcomes of ileocolic resection and right hemicolectomies for Crohn's patients in comparison with non-Crohn's patients and the impact of perioperative immunosuppressive therapy with biologics and steroids on inpatient complications. *Am J Surg*, 2012 Mar; 203(3): 375–78.

McKenzie YA, Alder A, Anderson W, et al; Gastroenterology Specialist Group of the British Dietetic Association. British Dietetic Association evidence-based practice guidelines for the dietary management of irritable bowel syndrome in adults. *J Hum Nutr Diet*, 2012 Jun; 25(3): 260–74.

Minich DM, Bland JS. Acid-alkaline balance: Role in chronic disease and detoxification. *Altern Ther Health Med*, 2007 Jul–Aug; 13(4): 62–65.

Mithal A, Bonjour JP, Boonen S, et al; IOF CSA Nutrition Working Group. Impact of nutrition on muscle mass, strength, and performance in older adults. *Osteoporosis Int*, 2013 May; 24(5): 1555–66.

Morris CG, Low J. Metabolic acidosis in the critically ill: Part 1 — Classification and pathophysiology. *Anaesthesia*, 2008 Mar; 63(3): 294–301.

Mullin GE. Popular diets prescribed by alternative practitioners — Part 1. *Nutr Clin Pract*, 2010 Apr; 25(2); 212–14.

Nicoll R, McLaren Howard J. The acid-ash hypothesis revisited: A reassessment of the impact of dietary acidity on bone. *J Bone Miner Metab*, 2014 Feb 21: 1–7.

Olendzki BC, Silverstein TD, Persuitte GM, et al. An anti-inflammatory diet as treatment for inflammatory bowel disease: A case series report. *Nutr J*, 2014 Jan 16; 13: 5.

Pampel FC, Krueger PM, Denney JT. Socioeconomic disparities in health behaviors. *Annu Rev Sociol*, 2010 Aug; 36: 349–70.

Parks SK, Chiche J, Pouyssegur J. pH Control Mechanisms of Tumor Survival and Growth. *J Cell Physiol*, 2011 Feb; 226(2): 299–308.

Philpott H, Gibson P, Thien F. Irritable bowel syndrome — An inflammatory disease involving mast cells. *Asia Pac Allergy*, 2011 Apr; 1(1): 36–42.

Pongratz G, Straub RH. Role of peripheral nerve fibres in acute and chronic inflammation in arthritis. *Nat Rev Rheumatol*, 2013 Feb; 9(2), 117–26.

Poupin N, Calvez J, Lassale C, et al. Impact of the diet on net endogenous acid production and acid-base balance. *Clin Nutr*, 2012 Jun; 31(3): 313–21.

Rosborg I, Nihlgård B, Gerhardsson L. Inorganic constituents of well water in one acid and one alkaline area of South Sweden. *Water, Air, and Soil Pollution*, 2003 Jan; 142(1–4): 261–77.

Rosner MH. Metabolic acidosis in patients with gastrointestinal disorders: Metabolic and clinical consequences. *Pract Gastroenterol*, Nutrition Issues in Gastroenterology, Series #73, 2009 Apr: 42–52.

Roth LW, Polotsky AJ. Can we live longer by eating less? A review of caloric restriction and longevity. *Maturitas*, 2012 Apr; 71(4), 315–19.

Rulis AM, Levitt JA. FDA's food ingredient approval process: Safety assurance based on scientific assessment. *Regul Toxicol Pharm*, 2009 Feb; 53(1): 20–31.

Schöllgen I, Huxhold O, Schüz B, Tesch-Römer C. Resources for health: Differential effects of optimistic self-beliefs and social support according to socioeconomic status. *Health Psychol*, 2011 May; 30(3): 326–35.

Schwalfenberg GK. The alkaline diet: Is there evidence that an alkaline pH diet benefits health? *J Environ Public Health*, 2011 Oct 12 (epub): 727630.

Shaheen NJ. Highlights from the New ACG Guidelines for the Diagnosis and Management of GERD. *Gastroenterol Hepatol (NY)*, 2013 Jun; 9(6): 377–79.

Simopoulos AP. Omega-3 fatty acids in inflammation and autoimmune diseases, *J Am Coll Nutr*, 2002 Dec; 21(6): 495–505.

Slattery ML, Lundgreen A, Welbourn B, et al. Oxidative balance and colon and rectal cancer: Interaction of lifestyle factors and genes. *Mutat Res*, 2012 Jun 1; 734(1–2): 30–40.

Stefanini GF, Saggioro A, Alvisi V, et al. Oral cromolyn sodium in comparison with elimination diet in the irritable bowel syndrome, diarrheic type. Multicenter study of 428 patients. *Scand J Gastroenterol*, 1995 Jun; 30(6): 535–41.

Tanabe M, Takahashi T, Shimoyama K, et al. Effects of rehydration and food consumption on salivary flow, pH and buffering capacity in young adult volunteers during ergometer exercise. *J Int Soc Sports Nutr*, 2013 Oct 28; 10(1): 49.

Vormann J, Remer T. Dietary, metabolic, physiologic, and disease-related aspects of acid-base balance: Foreword to the contributions of the second International Acid-Base Symposium. *J Nutr*, 2008 Feb; 138(2): 413S–14S.

Waterman M, Xu W, Stempak JM, et al. Distinct and overlapping genetic loci in Crohn's disease and ulcerative colitis: Correlations with pathogenesis. *Inflamm Bowel Dis*, 2011 Sep; 17(9): 1936–42.

Weigert J, Obermeier F, Neumeier M, et al. Circulating levels of chemerin and adiponectin are higher in ulcerative colitis and chemerin is elevated in Crohn's disease. *Inflamm Bowel Dis* 2010 Apr; 16(4): 630–37.

Welch AA, Mulligan A, Bingham SA, Khaw KT. Urine pH is an indicator of dietary acid-base load, fruit and vegetables and meat intakes: Results from the European Prospective Investigation into Cancer and Nutrition (EPIC)-Norfolk population study. *Br J Nutr*, 2008 Jun; 99(6): 1335–43.

Wolpert PW, Shaughnessy D, Houchin DN, et al. Tissue pH: A new clinical tool. *Arch Surg*, 1970 Aug; 101(2): 308–13.

Wongdee K, Teerapornpuntakit J, Riengrojpitak S, et al. Gene expression profile of duodenal epithelial cells in response to chronic metabolic acidosis. *Mol Cell Biochem*, 2009 Jan; 321(1–2): 173–88.

Web Articles

Bruno G. Acid-alkaline balance and health: An examination of the data. *Vitamin Retailer Magazine*, 2013 Apr 1; 4. Available at: http://vitaminretailer.com/?p=1390. Accessed January 2014.

Centers for Disease Control and Prevention. Nutrition for everyone. Available at: http://www.cdc.gov/nutrition/everyone/basics/index.html. Accessed January 2014.

Encyclopaedia Britannica's Guide to the Nobel Prizes. Immune system. Available at: https://www.britannica.com/nobelprize/article-215537. Accessed January 2014.

Health Canada. Sugar substitutes. Available at: http://www.hc-sc.gc.ca/fn-an/securit/addit/sweeten-edulcor/index-eng.php. Accessed January 2013.

Health Canada. Trans fat. Available at: http://www.hc-sc.gc.ca/fn-an/nutrition/gras-trans-fats/index-eng.php. Accessed January 2013.

Kitts J, Beaton B, Cook C, et al; Health Council of Canada. Self-management support for Canadians with chronic health conditions: A focus for primary health care. Available at: http://healthcouncilcanada.ca/rpt_det.php?id=372. Accessed January 2014.

National Institutes of Health, Office of Dietary Supplements. Omega-3 fatty acids and health. Available at: http://ods.od.nih.gov/factsheets/Omega3FattyAcidsandHealth-HealthProfessional. Accessed January 2013.

OpenStax College. 105 negative feedback loops. *Anatomy & Physiology*. OpenStax-CNX Web site. April 5, 2013. Available at: http://cnx.org/content/col11496/1.6/. Accessed June 2014.

OpenStax College. 216 pH scale-01. *Anatomy & Physiology*. OpenStax-CNX Web site. May 16, 2013. Available at: http://cnx.org/content/col11496/1.6/. Accessed June 2014.

OpenStax College. *Anatomy & Physiology*. OpenStax-CNX Web site. June 19, 2013. Available at: http://cnx.org/content/col11496/1.6/. Accessed June 2014.

OpenStax College. *Atoms, Isotopes, Ions, and Molecules: The Building Blocks*. OpenStax-CNX Web site. February 20, 2014. Available at: http://cnx.org/content/m44390/1.9/. Accessed June 2014.

USDA National Nutrient Database for Standard Reference, Release 18 (SR18). Low acid diet. Available at: http://health-diet.us/lowaciddiet. Accessed December 2013.

U.S. Department of Health and Human Services, National Digestive Diseases Information Clearinghouse (NDDIC). The digestive system and how it works. Available at: http://digestive.niddk.nih.gov/ddiseases/pubs/yrdd. Accessed January 2013.

U.S. Food and Drug Administration. Ingredients, additives, GRAS & packaging guidance documents & regulatory information. Available at: http://www.fda.gov/food/guidanceregulation/guidancedocumentsregulatoryinformation/ingredientsadditivesgraspackaging/default.htm. Accessed January 2013.

Library and Archives Canada Cataloguing in Publication

Smith, Fraser, 1968-, author
The pH balance health & diet guide for GERD, IBS & IBD : practical solutions, diet management + 175 recipes / Dr. Fraser Smith, BA, ND, Susan Hannah, BA, BScH, Dr. Daniel Richardson, BS, MSc, PhD.

Includes index.
ISBN 978-0-7788-0492-5 (pbk.)

1. Nutrition. 2. Health. 3. Acid-base equilibrium. 4. Acid-base imbalances—Diet therapy. 5. Gastrointestinal system—Diseases—Diet therapy. I. Hannah, Susan, 1956-, author II. Richardson, Daniel, 1942-, author III. Title. IV. Title: pH balance health and diet guide for GERD, IBS and IBD.

RA784.S62 2014 613.2 C2014-904365-1

Index

C

D

H

I

N

O

P

Q

R

S

T

U

V

W

X

Y

Z